MAYO CLINIC

Book of
Alternative
Medicine
&
Home
Remedies

TWO ESSENTIAL HOME HEALTH BOOKS IN ONE

MAYO CLINIC

Book of Alternative Medicine

SECOND EDITION

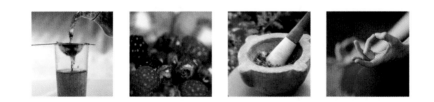

Introduction

The best way to manage an illness is to prevent it from happening in the first place. As the cost of health care continues to rise and worries about flu pandemics and other disease outbreaks become more prevalent, greater responsibility is being — and will continue to be — placed on each of us to stay healthy and avoid illness.

It's in this environment — one in which Americans are seeking greater control of their health — that we've seen explosive growth in the field of alternative medicine. People are looking for more "natural" or "holistic" ways to maintain good health — not only their physical health, but also their mental and spiritual health. At the same time, an increasing number of treatments once considered "on the fringe" are slowly being incorporated into conventional medicine.

We decided to write this book because we recognize the need for reliable and easy-to-understand information when it comes to alternative medicine. The purpose of *Mayo Clinic Book of Alternative Medicine* isn't only to inform you about various products and practices, but to guide you as to which appear to be of benefit and may help treat or prevent disease and which are of no benefit and could even be dangerous. The intent of this book is to help promote self-care — steps you can take on your own to achieve and maintain health and wellness. However it's important that you include your doctor's advice in the decisions you make.

A note about the title of the book: As nontraditional products and practices gain greater acceptance as potential forms of healing, the terms used to describe them are evolving as well. Today, the term *integrative medicine* is often used to describe this evolving form of health care in which alternative therapies proved effective in scientific studies are being integrated with conventional care. But we're also aware that the latest changes in the medical field take time to filter down to the general public. *Alternative medicine* is still the term most commonly used to describe practices that aren't typically part of conventional medical care, or that are slowly being blended into conventional care.

That's why we decided to title this publication *Mayo Clinic Book of Alternative Medicine.* We feel it best describes to the reader what this book is about — nontraditional therapies to promote health and wellness. Inside, you'll find the latest information on how you might put some of these practices to work for you. By combining the best of complementary and conventional health care practices to meet your individual needs, you'll be practicing integrative medicine.

As you read through the pages ahead, here are a few important points to keep in mind. Some therapies don't fit neatly into a specific category. Reflexology, for instance, could go in either the hands-on therapies chapter or the chapter on energy therapies — it has components of both. Aromatherapy is another example. Some view it as a form of energy medicine, while others see it as a mind-body technique. We placed the therapies in the chapters we felt they fit best, but we recognize that many of them cross boundaries.

It's also important to understand that what's considered alternative today may be conventional tomorrow. In addition, using a particular therapy to treat one condition may be an accepted medical practice, but using it to treat another condition may not. A case in point is chiropractic care. There are numerous studies to back up the effectiveness of chiropractic therapy for treatment of low back pain. However, use of chiropractic techniques to treat high blood pressure would still be considered an alternative practice by many because there's not sufficient evidence that it's effective.

In the end, the names and classifications of the various therapies are going to become increasingly less important. What is important, is finding the best evidence-based products and practices that work with conventional medicine to improve your health — mind, body and spirit.

Brent A. Bauer

Brent Bauer, M.D.
Medical Editor

Table of Contents

Part 1

Today's New Medicine

Making wellness the focus of care

People who take an active role in their health care experience better health and improved healing. It's a common-sense concept gaining scientific roots.

As studies continue to reveal the important role the mind plays in healing and in fighting disease, a transformation is slowly taking place in hospitals and clinics across the country. Doctors, in partnership with their patients, are turning to practices once considered "alternative" as they attempt to treat the whole person — mind and spirit, as well as body.

In Part 1, we take a look at how alternative medicine is making inroads into conventional care, blending the best of nontraditional therapies with the best of high-tech medicine. We also discuss the important role you play in maintaining good health with the choices you make each day.

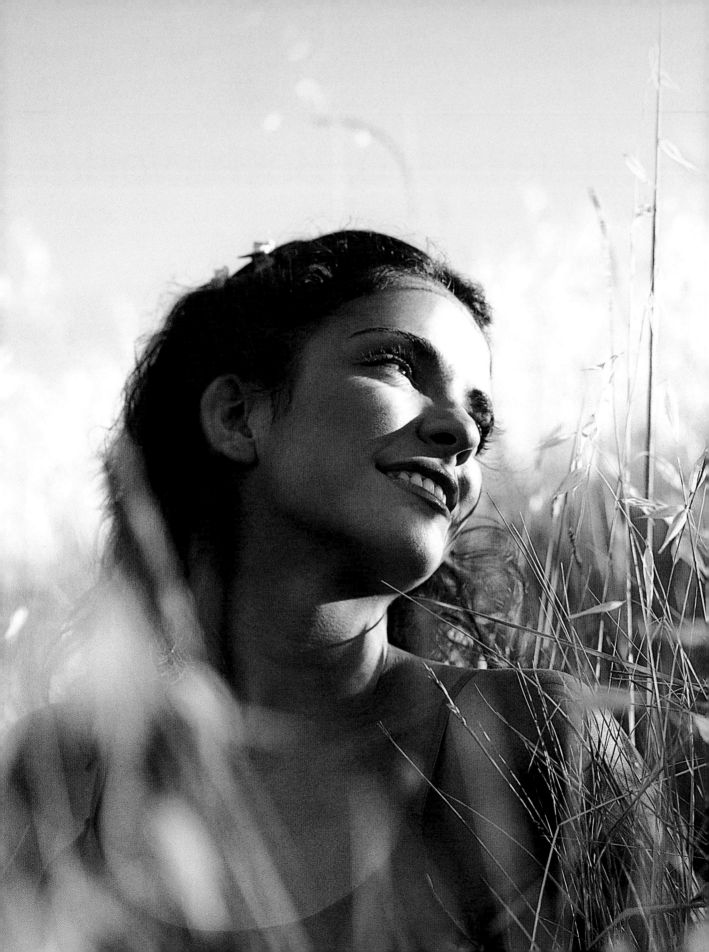

Chapter 1
The Best of Both Worlds

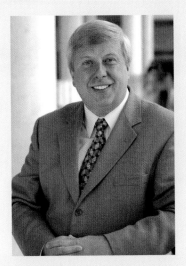

Brent Bauer, M.D.
Director, Complementary
and Integrative Medicine
Program

❝ *Thanks to increased research during the past two decades, doctors are now better able to understand the role these 'alternative' therapies can play in helping treat and prevent disease.* ❞

Kairos is a Greek word meaning "the critical time," and it's often thought of as the point in time when crisis and opportunity are equally balanced. Health care in the United States appears to be at a kairos moment — a combination of an aging population and wonderful, yet expensive, medical technology has resulted in skyrocketing costs. At the same time, many people feel that medicine, in spite of its amazing advances, has become too technical and "cold."

In response to some of these changes, an opportunity has risen that may hold the promise of a new paradigm for better health. Called "unconventional" or "alternative" medicine in the early '90s, then "complementary and alternative medicine" (CAM) until recently, new therapies and treatments are emerging to meet the needs of our physical, mental and spiritual health. Many of these therapies — such as massage therapy, herbal supplements and meditation — have been with us for a thousand years or more. What's "new" is the growing recognition that these practices may hold special value in meeting our health needs. Thanks to increased research during the past two decades, doctors are now better able to understand the role these alternative therapies can play in helping treat and prevent disease. This blending of the best of both worlds — conventional medicine and alternative medicine — is known as integrative medicine.

In this chapter and in future chapters, we share some of the exciting research taking place at Mayo Clinic in the realm of integrative medicine. We also share some of the experience that our staff has had in working with thousands of individuals who have incorporated novel treatments into their health regimens. Unfortunately, there are pitfalls in this new realm — overhyped products on the Internet that promise to cure every ill; unexpected side effects from common herbs such as St. John's wort; and individuals who have died because they made the mistake of believing that everything that's "natural" is safe.

Keep in mind, at this point in time, there's more that we don't know about integrative medicine than we do know. On the other hand, integrative medicine offers some wonderful opportunities to improve your health. Imagine having a "tool" that you can use the next time you're stuck in traffic and you feel your stress level rising, or a simple technique that may allow you to treat your high blood pressure with less medication. These are just a couple of the many ways this book can help you develop new strategies for improving your health.

In the end, we are all unique creations — what works for one person may not work for another. But that's part of the beauty of being able to select from a growing array of treatments and therapies. If meditation doesn't appeal to you or meet your needs, music therapy might. The important thing is not the specific therapy or treatment, but making your health a top priority.

From alternative to integrative

Alternative medicine is actually an older and somewhat outdated term in today's medicine. So why, then, did we title this book "Book of Alternative Medicine?" Because *alternative medicine* is the term the general public most equates with health care practices that aren't — or typically haven't been — part of mainstream medicine.

Products and therapies that are slowly becoming more accepted as standard practice — such as fish oil supplements, acupuncture and meditation — are still often referred to as *alternative,* but really they're not. Today, fish oil tablets are prescribed to help lower high triglycerides, acupuncture to control the pain of fibromyalgia, and meditation to manage stress and anxiety.

The migration of these once questionable treatments into academic centers and community hospitals and clinics is known as *integrative medicine.* The concept behind integrative medicine is quite simple: The integration of alternative treatments, supported by research, with conventional medicine.

Does this mean all alternative therapies are OK to use? No. Some carry significant risks and others simply don't work. It does indicate, though, that certain therapies have merit and can aid in health and healing.

Integrative medicine

Integrative medicine describes an evolution taking place in many health care institutions: to treat the whole person — mind, body and spirit — not just the disease. This is done by combining the best of today's high-tech medicine with the best of non-traditional practices — products and therapies that have some high-quality evidence to support their use.

To date, 44 academic medical centers are now part of an organization called the Consortium of Academic Health Centers for Integrative Medicine. Its mission is to advance the principles and practices of integrative medicine.

Why the interest in doing so? Research continues to unveil the complex biology of how mind and body are intertwined, and how treating the mind and spirit can help to heal the body. It's also clear that interest in alternative practices isn't a fad. As more individuals turn to unconventional treatments, doctors need to be aware of their safety and effectiveness.

Guiding principles

Most integrative products and practices are based around a few common principles:

- **Prevention.** One of the main philosophies of integrative medicine is to take preventive steps to promote good health.
- **Natural healing.** Your body has the ability to heal itself. The purpose of treatment is to encourage the natural healing processes.
- **Active learning.** Integrative practitioners see themselves as facilitators — teachers who offer guidance. You're the one who actually produces the healing.
- **'Holistic' care.** The focus is on treating the whole person — addressing physical, emotional, social and spiritual needs.

What is integrative medicine?

"Integrative medicine is the practice of medicine that reaffirms the importance of the relationship between practitioner and patient, focuses on the whole person, is informed by evidence, and makes use of all appropriate therapeutic approaches, health care professionals and disciplines to achieve optimal health and healing."

Source: Consortium of Academic Health Centers for Integrative Medicine, updated May 2009

The changing focus of medicine

The philosophy of integrative medicine mirrors what is happening on the national health care scene. Many people believe that in order to fix the American health care system the focus of medicine has to change from a system concentrated on healing the sick to one focused on promoting wellness.

Realizing that a healthy employee is less expensive to insure than a sick one, employers are also taking greater steps to promote employee wellness — some even offering rewards to employees who quit smoking, lose weight, reduce their blood pressure or improve their blood cholesterol.

At the same time, doctor and patient relationships are changing. There was a time — not that long ago — when the patient met with the doctor, listened to what the doctor said, and, with little questioning, did what the doctor ordered.

Today, the doctor and patient relationship is more of a partnership. Doctor and patient work together as a team to determine the best course of action to take. Because patients are more educated and ask more questions, doctors need to be open to different ways of thinking and to treatments that may not always follow traditional practice.

Your role

So how do you fit into this changing system? First of all, instead of just treating you when you're sick, you may find

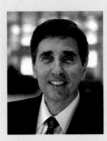

Some thoughts from Dr. Cortese

Would you like to be hospitalized tomorrow, even if it's at the best hospital in the world? Do you want to be sick tomorrow?

If you answered no to these questions, you're not alone. Thousands of people across the nation have told me they feel the same way.

But if no one *wants* to be hospitalized and no one *wants* to be sick, then it's time to establish a health care system that not only treats sickness, but also focuses on keeping people healthy.

As health care consumers, we need to be the No.1 priority in health care. By practicing prevention, we can make this happen — and help create a successful health care system.

Denis Cortese, M.D., emeritus CEO, Mayo Clinic

your doctor spending more time on tests, strategies and advice to keep you healthy.

However, as much as your doctor may help you, your health is your responsibility. You may see your doctor only once or twice a year. What are you doing the other 363 or 364 days out of the year to stay well?

Are you eating well — following a healthy diet? Are you getting enough exercise each day? Are you making efforts to relax and reduce stress? Are you taking steps to boost your immune system to help fight off disease?

Staying healthy doesn't have to be difficult — you may even find it fun! The pages that follow offer insight into steps you can take to stay healthy and prevent illness. These practices, products and therapies are intended to care for your whole self — mind, body and spirit.

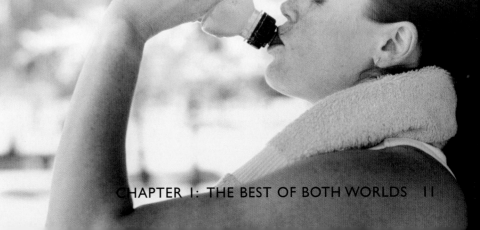

Integrative medicine at Mayo Clinic

Mayo Clinic's Complementary and Integrative Medicine Program was developed almost a decade ago to address interest by patients in products and practices not typically part of conventional medical care — treatments such as massage therapy, meditation and acupuncture. Specialty-trained doctors and other health professionals within the consultation service work with patients, and their doctors, to provide information on nontraditional therapies and to encourage healing and wellness through a variety of channels.

The treatments promoted through the Complementary and Integrative Medicine Program aren't substitutes for conventional medical care. They're used in concert with standard medical treatment to help alleviate a wide range of symptoms and conditions and to help promote a sense of well-being.

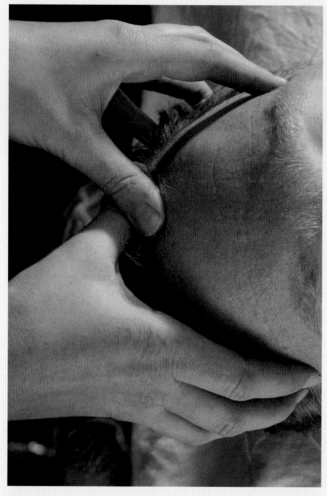

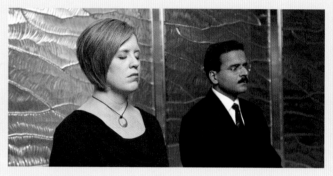

Meditation is an effective technique for managing stress and anxiety. At Mayo Clinic, individuals are taught how to meditate and then are given tools to help them perfect the technique on their own. A Mayo physician has even developed a meditation application for the iPhone, which allows people to practice meditation when they're away from home and could use a little extra support (see page 107).

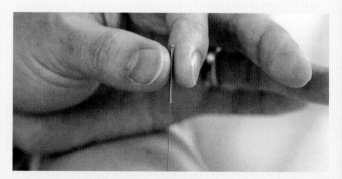

Massage is used in a variety of settings at Mayo Clinic. Individuals experiencing pain and other symptoms related to fibromyalgia, migraines, or back or neck problems may receive massage therapy. Massage is also used by patients and staff to reduce stress and anxiety. You may even receive a massage prior to or after surgery — to help reduce preoperative anxiety and postoperative pain and nausea.

At Mayo Clinic, licensed acupuncturists use acupuncture to treat a variety of conditions and symptoms. These include back, neck and shoulder pain, facial pain, symptoms associated with migraines and fibromyalgia, and infertility. A Mayo Clinic study found that a single acupuncture session also can reduce nausea following surgery.

Turning ideas into treatments

An important part of the mission of Mayo Clinic's Complementary and Integrative Medicine Program is to learn more about unconventional products and practices to determine if they can play a role in health and healing. The program is involved in several studies. Here are a few examples:

Massage therapy

Does your anxiety level and state of mind after cardiovascular surgery affect your recovery? The answer appears to be yes. Mayo researchers are involved in several studies to determine the beneficial role of massage in patient care. Two studies found that massage following surgery can lessen post-operative pain, anxiety and tension. These results were so positive that massage is now offered as part of routine postoperative care for individuals undergoing cardiac surgery at Mayo Clinic.

Other studies are evaluating the effects of massage in helping to reduce stress among clinic and hospital staff.

'Ambience' therapy

Researchers are studying whether playing music in hospital rooms — specifically, music mixed with sounds of nature — can reduce side effects and speed recovery after cardiovascular surgery. The music, known as "ambience" therapy, was produced by Chip Davis from the group Mannheim Steamroller.

Results suggest ambience therapy can reduce pain and anxiety by helping patients to relax.

Yoga

An important component of yoga is its methodic breathing, what's referred to as "paced respirations." This form of breathing is used to help alleviate stress and anxiety. Can it also help relieve hot flashes?

Participants in the study are breast cancer survivors who have limited treatment options for hot flashes because hormone therapy generally isn't advised for this group. If effective, the treatment should also work in women who don't have cancer.

Meditation

Researchers at Mayo Clinic have developed a short but effective meditation training strategy that has been taught to approximately 1,000 people. Several studies are under way evaluating the stress-reducing effects of this strategy in various study populations, ranging from Mayo physicians to community volunteers.

Ginseng

A common problem for individuals undergoing treatment for cancer is fatigue that typically accompanies chemotherapy or radiation therapy. Mayo researchers in the Complementary and Integrative Medicine Program in collaboration with the researchers from the Cancer Center evaluated the effects of the herb ginseng to determine if it can help offset cancer-related fatigue. The first study was positive. Researchers are now embarking on a second study to learn more about this possible treatment.

Ginkgo

Another potential side effect of cancer treatment is what some people refer to as "chemo brain" — a slowing of mental functioning that sometimes develops months after chemotherapy treatment. This phenomenon is thought to be related to oxidative stress on cells from the drug therapy.

To combat chemo brain, some people take antioxidant supplements, such as ginkgo. The question is, Do the supplements interfere with the effectiveness of cancer treatment? Mayo researchers hope to find out.

Mangosteen

Mayo Clinic researchers are evaluating whether this fruit contains novel anti-inflammatory compounds. Currently researchers are conducting a large trial in collaboration with the cardiology department to evaluate possible anti-inflammatory effects in people undergoing cardioversion therapy for atrial fibrillation.

Plant compounds

Mayo researchers are studying a 400-year-old catalogue of plants (botanicals) used by ancient healers of the South Pacific. The catalogue was written by German-Dutch naturalist Georg Eberhard Rumphius. Researchers are hoping to resurrect lost healing knowledge from ancient texts. The Dutch text has led to further exploration of a series of compounds that may hold promise as future therapies.

Popular treatments

The National Center for Complementary and Alternative Medicine and the National Center for Health Statistics are continuing their efforts to learn more about why people use alternative therapies and which are the most popular. The two organizations recently conducted a survey on use of alternative medicine. The results are based on interviews with 23,400 American adults.

People who use alternative medicine

In the United States, approximately 38 percent of adults — about 4 in 10 adults — use some form of alternative medicine. That's an increase from 2002, when approximately 36 percent of the adult population indicated use of alternative therapies.

The study also found that alternative products and practices are used by people of all backgrounds. However, use is greater among women, among those with higher levels of education and higher incomes, and among adults ages 50 to 59.

Approximately 50 percent of American Indians and Alaskans use alternative therapies. Use is lowest among Hispanics — about 24 percent.

For the first time, the study also gathered data on use of alternative medicine among American children. It found nearly 12 percent — about 1 in 9 children — have used alternative therapies.

Therapies used most often

The most commonly used form of alternative therapy is nonvitamin, nonmineral natural products — products such as fish oil, ginseng and garlic supplements. These therapies are discussed in further detail in Chapter 3, titled "Herbs and Other Dietary Supplements."

Other therapies that ranked at the top of the list included deep breathing, meditation, chiropractic and osteopathic care, and massage therapy.

Therapies that showed significant increases in use between 2002, when the survey was first done, and the latest survey in 2007, were deep breathing, meditation, massage and yoga.

Use by age

Age	Percentage who use it
1. 50-59	44.1%
2. 60-69	41.0%
3. 40-49	40.1%
4. 30-39	39.6%
5. 18-29	36.3%
6. 70-84	32.1%
7. 85+	24.2%
8. 12-17	16.4%
9. 5-11	10.7%
10. 0-4	7.6%

Source: National Center for Health Statistics, 2007

Most common therapies

Type of therapy	Percentage who use it
1. Natural products	17.7%
2. Deep breathing	12.7%
3. Meditation	9.4%
4. Chiropractic and osteopathic	8.6%
5. Massage	8.3%
6. Yoga	6.1%
7. Diet-based therapies	3.6%
8. Progressive relaxation	2.9%
9. Guided imagery	2.2%
10. Homeopathic treatment	1.8%

Natural products used most often

About 1 in 5 people surveyed use herbs and other dietary supplements (natural products) to enhance their health and promote wellness. The product most commonly used is fish oil tablets, which contain omega-3 fatty acids.

Other natural products topping the list include glucosamine, echinacea, flaxseed oil and ginseng.

The chart below lists the most popular natural products. The percentage represents the rate of use among adults who use dietary supplements.

Health conditions prompting use

People use alternative treatments for an array of diseases and conditions. American adults are most likely to use nontraditional practices to help treat pain including back pain or problems, neck pain or other neck problems, joint pain or stiffness, arthritis, or other musculoskeletal conditions.

Other reasons people turn to alternative medicine are to treat anxiety, prevent a head or chest cold, manage their cholesterol, control headaches, and improve insomnia.

Most common natural products*

Name of product	Percentage who use it
1. Fish oil/omega-3 fatty acids	37.4%
2. Glucosamine	19.9%
3. Echinacea	19.8%
4. Flaxseed oil/pills	15.9%
5. Ginseng	14.1%
6. Combination herb pills	13.0%
7. Ginkgo	11.3%
8. Chondroitin	11.2%
9. Garlic supplements	11.0%
10. Coenzyme Q10	8.7%

*Percentages among adults who used natural products in the last 30 days

Most common conditions

Condition	Percentage who cited it
1. Back pain	17.1%
2. Neck pain	5.9%
3. Joint pain	5.2%
4. Arthritis	3.5%
5. Anxiety	2.8%
6. Cholesterol	2.1%
7. Head or chest cold	2.0%
8. Other musculoskeletal	1.8%
9. Severe headache or migraine	1.6%
10. Insomnia	1.4%

Our top 10

Here's a brief rundown of what we consider to be the best integrative therapies at this point in time.

Research into complementary and alternative medicine is rapidly evolving. New studies are coming forward on an increasingly frequent basis and, many times, new studies conflict with older studies. To complicate matters even more, different forms can have different effects. This makes it difficult to state with authority which therapies are truly "the best." However, we've listed what we consider to be the top 10.

Therapy	What it's most commonly used for
Acupuncture	Nausea, fibromyalgia, and some forms of dental, postoperative and chronic pain (see page 120)
Guided imagery	Headache and some forms of pain (see page 100)
Hypnosis	Anxiety, pain and tension headache (see page 102)
Massage	Anxiety, back pain and fibromyalgia (see page 131)
Meditation	Anxiety, stress, fibromyalgia and high blood pressure (see page 103)
Music therapy	Relaxation, stress and depression (see page 109)
Spinal manipulation	Low back pain (see page 138)
Spirituality	Medical illness and chronic disease (see page 112)
Tai chi	Balance and strength and cardiovascular disease (see page 114)
Yoga	Anxiety, stress, depression, heart disease and high blood pressure (see page 115)

How to use this resource

Doctors and other staff in Mayo Clinic's Complementary and Integrative Medicine Program developed this publication to provide you straightforward information about various therapies being used and what's known about them.

With each treatment, we discuss the latest research, the safety and effectiveness of the product or practice, and any potential risks, should you decide to try it.

We also talk about the importance of good lifestyle habits to ensure you get the most out of the efforts you're making to improve your health.

Mayo Clinic Book of Alternative Medicine is a personal health guide that can help you achieve great health and fully enjoy life.

About the lights

A special feature of this book — which you'll find in upcoming pages — is our stoplight. Its purpose is to give you an at-a-glance overview as to how you should proceed with the therapy being discussed.

A shining red light means not to use the treatment or to use it very carefully and only under a doctor's close supervision. A therapy is given a red light when studies have found it to be unsafe or have found its risks far outweigh any benefits it may provide.

A shining yellow light means to use the therapy with caution. A treatment is given a yellow light when studies show it may be of benefit but that it also carries some risks. Therapies that have not been fully studied to determine their safety and effectiveness are also given a yellow light. In addition, a treatment may be given a yellow light if it's considered safe, but studies haven't found it to provide any benefit.

A shining green light means the therapy is generally safe for most people to use, and studies show it to be effective. (If you have a specific health condition, a therapy given a green light may not be appropriate for you.) Even when a green light is present, it's still important that you discuss the treatment with your doctor and use it appropriately.

How to be a smart consumer

As with any medical treatment, there can be risks. The same is true for integrative medicine. The risks depend on the specific therapy. Each therapy discussed in this book needs to be considered on its own. Just because one product is given a green light doesn't mean all similar products are green as well. If you're considering a specific therapy, think about safety and how you can minimize risks. And remember, just because a product is considered "natural" doesn't automatically mean that it's safe.

If you purchase a product for use, such as an herbal supplement, it's also important that you purchase the same supplement as used in a study in which the product was found effective. In other words, not all products labeled "Ginseng," for example, are the same. Some may contain much more of the herb than others.

In the last chapter of this book, we discuss specific steps that you can take to help ensure that your venture into integrative medicine is a safe, and beneficial, one.

Chapter 2

Good Health Begins With Good Choices

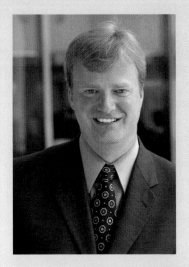

Paul Limburg, M.D., M.P.H.
Gastroenterology

" The fact is, if you spend most of your day lying on the couch and eating potato chips, taking a supplement to help you lose weight or practicing techniques to boost your immune system likely isn't going to do you much good. "

Congratulations! By reading this chapter, you've taken the first step in adopting a healthier lifestyle. And why is lifestyle important in a book about alternative medicine? The fact is, if you spend most of your day lying on the couch and eating potato chips, taking a supplement to help you lose weight or practicing techniques to boost your immune system likely isn't going to do you much good. To fend off disease and achieve better health, you need to take care of yourself.

Let's face it — most people, including doctors, find countless excuses for why they can't change their unhealthy behaviors. Change is difficult for everyone. However, adopting healthier habits doesn't have to be painful. And once you're able to learn new habits, the quality of your life can improve dramatically.

In the pages that follow, we focus on five key areas where good lifestyle choices have been shown to reduce the development of — or consequences related to — several common medical conditions, including cardiovascular disease, cancer and diabetes. These five areas are tobacco use, diet (including alcohol consumption), weight control, exercise and stress management. Clearly, trying to address all of these issues at once would be difficult. Therefore, we've included an easy-to-use checklist in the first few pages that can help you determine which of these factors are most relevant to your own personal health. We also provide recommendations for how to improve unhealthy habits.

As you begin, or continue, to think about making healthier lifestyle choices, keep in mind that the best results will come from long-term, rather than short-term, changes — a useful analogy might be to consider the process a marathon, not a sprint. What does this mean? First, start by finding an appropriate balance between positive lifestyle changes and family, job, social and other responsibilities. Don't let competing priorities get in the way of good health. Second, define milestones to help you monitor your progress. Reward yourself when you achieve your goals so that productive changes are reinforced. Just as importantly, challenge yourself when you fall short so that potential obstacles can be identified and avoided. Third, don't give up if your first attempt isn't successful. Learn from your effort, make necessary adjustments and try again, perhaps using an alternative approach. Last, involve people around you who might derive benefits from the healthy lifestyle habits you're trying to develop. Making changes can be easier if relatives, friends or colleagues are fully supportive.

In later chapters, we show you how complementary and alternative therapies can provide new opportunities to help you meet your wellness goals.

Assess your health

Over the next four pages we ask a few basic questions about your health to help you evaluate your lifestyle habits and determine your health risks.

If you breeze through the questions, you're probably already making good choices. If not, the questions should point to changes you can make for improvements.

The healthier you are, the greater the chances that other efforts you make to fight disease and stay healthy — including the use of complementary and alternative therapies — will be beneficial.

Do you use tobacco?

Do you smoke or use spit tobacco?

Yes _____ Tobacco use is a tough habit to break, but stopping could be the single most important health change you make. See pages 22-23 for tips on how to give up tobacco.

No _____ Go to the next question.

Basic tobacco quit plan

1. List five reasons for quitting.
2. Set a quit date.
3. Get rid of all tobacco on your quit date.
4. Get support from family, friends and co-workers.
5. Find alternatives to the habit, such as nicotine replacement products and lifestyle changes.

Tobacco facts

More than 440,000 Americans die of tobacco-related illnesses each year. If you smoke a pack of cigarettes a day and you quit, you'll save about $1,500 a year.

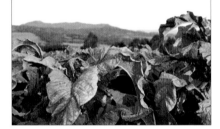

Do you get enough exercise?

How many minutes a week do you spend doing moderate or vigorous physical activities? Check the time that comes closest. (*Note*: For most people, moderate or vigorous activities include brisk walking, dancing, biking, swimming and running).

0 to 30 minutes _____
You need to be more physically active. If there are health reasons why you're not more active, ask your doctor about an exercise plan that's right for you.

30 to 90 minutes _____
You're off to a good start! Try to gradually increase the amount of time you exercise.

90 to 120 minutes _____
You're well on your way to being physically fit. If you're doing vigorous activity, you've reached a reasonable goal when you're doing 90 minutes or more a week.

120 minutes or more _____
You're an active person and probably at a good level of fitness. If weight loss is part of your plan, you may need at least 200 minutes a week of moderate physical activity.

Basic activity plan

1. Aim to do something nearly every day of the week.
2. Set a goal of a specific number of minutes or steps a week.
3. Keep a log to help remind you and track your progress.
4. Recruit a friend or family member to keep you company.
5. Build up slowly, but steadily.

If you're having difficulty or not feeling well while doing physical activities, see your doctor.

Fitness fact

More than 60 percent of American adults aren't physically active on a regular basis, and 25 percent aren't active at all. Even a modest walking program (see page 99) can improve your heart health, reduce stress and give you extra energy to do the things you enjoy.

How's your weight?

Determine your body mass index (BMI) and your waist circumference to see if you're in the healthy weight zone. To do this, you'll need a bathroom scale and a tape measure.

To determine your BMI use the handy BMI chart and write your BMI here. _____

Next, measure the narrowest part of your abdomen to determine your waist circumference and write the number here.

_____

If your BMI is less than 18.5, talk with your doctor. You may be at risk of health conditions associated with a low body weight.

If your BMI is within the range of 19 to 24, you're at a healthy weight.

If your BMI is 25 or greater, consider losing some weight.

As for your waist circumference, a healthy goal is 40 inches or less if you're a man and 35 inches or less if you're a woman.

Basic weight-loss plan

1. Set a weight-loss goal of 1 to 2 pounds a week.
2. Eat five or more servings of fruits and vegetables daily.
3. Work with your health care provider to develop an exercise plan.
4. Gradually increase the time you spend on physical activity to at least 30 minutes a day.
5. Recruit a friend or family member for support.

Body mass index (BMI)

You can determine your body mass index (BMI) by finding your height and weight on this chart. A BMI of 18.5 to 24.9 is considered the healthiest. People with a BMI under 18.5 are considered underweight. People with a BMI between 25 and 29.9 are considered overweight. People with a BMI of 30 or greater are considered obese.

	Healthy		Overweight					Obese				
BMI	19	24	25	26	27	28	29	30	35	40	45	50
Height						Weight in pounds						
4'10"	91	115	119	124	129	134	138	143	167	191	215	239
4'11"	94	119	124	128	133	138	143	148	173	198	222	247
5'0"	97	123	128	133	138	143	148	153	179	204	230	255
5'1"	100	127	132	137	143	148	153	158	185	211	238	264
5'2"	104	131	136	142	147	153	158	164	191	218	246	273
5'3"	107	135	141	146	152	158	163	169	197	225	254	282
5'4"	110	140	145	151	157	163	169	174	204	232	262	291
5'5"	114	144	150	156	162	168	174	180	210	240	270	300
5'6"	118	148	155	161	167	173	179	186	216	247	278	309
5'7"	121	153	159	166	172	178	185	191	223	255	287	319
5'8"	125	158	164	171	177	184	190	197	230	262	295	328
5'9"	128	162	169	176	182	189	196	203	236	270	304	338
5'10"	132	167	174	181	188	195	202	209	243	278	313	348
5'11"	136	172	179	186	193	200	208	215	250	286	322	358
6'0"	140	177	184	191	199	206	213	221	258	294	331	368
6'1"	144	182	189	197	204	212	219	227	265	302	340	378
6'2"	148	186	194	202	210	218	225	233	272	311	350	389
6'3"	152	192	200	208	216	224	232	240	279	319	359	399
6'4"	156	197	205	213	221	230	238	246	287	328	369	410

Note: Asians with a BMI of 23 or higher may have an increased risk of health problems.
Source: National Institutes of Health, 1998

Weight fact

More than two-thirds of Americans are overweight. Being overweight increases your risk of diabetes, arthritis, heart disease, cancer and sleep disorders. Slow, steady weight loss is the best way to get to a healthy weight.

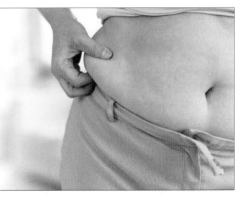

Is your diet healthy?

How many servings of:
Fruits do you eat each day?

_____

Vegetables do you eat each day?

_____

Total = _____

If your total is five or greater, you're doing great. Keep up the good work. If not, look for ways to add more fruits and vegetables to your diet.

Basic healthy-eating plan

1. Add one additional fruit or vegetable serving each week until you're getting five or more servings most days.
2. Look for ways to reduce fat in your diet and increase whole grains.
3. Eat three healthy meals — including breakfast — every day.
4. Try at least one new healthy recipe each week.

Nutrition fact

Eating the right foods can prevent disease. Fiber — found in fruits, vegetables and whole grains — may lower your risk of diabetes. Vitamins and other nutrients in fresh or frozen fruits and vegetables may reduce your risk of some cancers and cardiovascular disease. Replacing butter, lard and other solid fats with healthier fats such as olive, canola and peanut oils can help lower your risk of heart disease.

Alcohol and your health

Studies suggest that drinking moderate amounts of alcohol may increase levels of protective high-density lipoprotein (HDL, or "good") cholesterol and reduce the risk of cardiovascular disease. But it's important not to forget the risks of alcohol.

Even small amounts of alcohol can slow brain activity, affecting alertness, coordination and reaction time. Alcohol also can interfere with sleep and sexual function, induce headaches, and contribute to heartburn. Heavy drinking can increase risk of death from all causes.

Drinking alcohol can also increase blood triglycerides and blood pressure and interfere with the effectiveness of some blood pressure medications. And the American Cancer Society links alcohol use with increased risk of cancers of the breast, liver, mouth, throat and esophagus.

Until more is known about the effects of alcohol on overall health, if you don't drink don't start. If you do drink, use moderation. Moderation equates to one alcoholic drink a day for nonpregnant women and anyone age 65 or older. For men under age 65, moderation is no more than two drinks a day. Pregnant women shouldn't drink any alcohol.

One drink equals 5 ounces of wine, 12 ounces of beer or 1.5 ounces of 80-proof liquor.

How's your mood?

For at least the past two weeks, have you persistently felt anxious, down or depressed?

Yes _____ Talk to your doctor as soon as possible.

No _____ Go to the next question.

For at least the past two weeks, have you had little interest or pleasure in doing things?

Yes _____ Talk to your doctor as soon as possible.

No _____

Basic stress management plan

1. Exercise at least 30 minutes most days of the week to help relieve stress and anxiety.
2. Aim for an average of eight hours of sleep each night.
3. Stay connected with family and friends.
4. Consider starting a meditation program (see page 103).

Mood fact

Stress and a depressed mood can increase your risk of heart disease, and they can intensify physical symptoms, such as pain.

What are your biggest health threats?

Why is it important to know what threatens your health? It's not to scare you, but rather to help guide you in the choices you make regarding your health and safety. The news is full of stories about avian flu, terrorism, floods and hurricanes. These global issues are important, but they may not be the greatest threat to your health. What should you work hardest to avoid? Check out the biggest risks to your health and well-being.

Top 5 Leading Causes of Death in the United States

RANK	Most Common Causes of Death in All Ages	Causes of Death in Infants	Causes of Death in Children 1-14	Causes of Death in Young Adults 15-24	Causes of Death in Adults 25-44	Causes of Death in Adults 45-64	Causes of Death in Adults 65 and older
1	Heart Disease	Birth Defects	Accidents	Accidents	Accidents	Cancer	Heart Disease
2	Cancer	Premature Birth and Low Birth Weight	Cancer	Homicide	Cancer	Heart Disease	Cancer
3	Stroke	Sudden Infant Death Syndrome (SIDS)	Birth Defects	Suicide	Heart Disease	Accidents	Stroke
4	Lung Disease	Complications of Pregnancy	Homicide	Cancer	Suicide	Lung Disease	Lung Disease
5	Accidents	Accidents	Heart Disease	Heart Disease	Homicide	Diabetes	Alzheimer's Disease

Source: Centers for Disease Control and Prevention and National Center for Health Statistics, Deaths: Preliminary Data for 2007

Give up tobacco

A key strategy for living a longer, healthier life comes as no surprise — don't smoke. If you're a smoker, you're simply more likely to die prematurely. Smoking can take more than 10 years off your life.

But there's good news. Quitting now means health benefits start in just minutes, and your risk of heart disease is cut in half in as little as a year.

Strategies to help you quit

Success at quitting smoking is the result of planning and commitment, not luck. Develop a plan for how you'll cope with symptoms of nicotine withdrawal and how you'll survive urges to smoke.

Using more than one strategy to stop smoking might increase your chances of quitting successfully.

- **Medication.** Medication helps reduce cravings and eases withdrawal symptoms until the worst effects are over. You have many options — both prescription and over-the-counter products.
- **Cold turkey.** This is a sudden, decisive break from cigarettes. You stop smoking completely with little or no reduction beforehand. If you quit cold turkey, you're likely to experience symptoms of withdrawal, like nearly every-

one else who quits smoking. Some form of medication is usually recommended.

- **Taper down.** With this approach you gradually reduce the number of cigarettes you smoke until you don't smoke any at all. Medication is recommended with this approach as well.
- **Group support.** Whether it's an in-person support group, over the phone or online, seek the support of others who are trying to stop smoking.
- **Individual counseling.** This includes one-on-one contact with a trusted doctor, psychologist, nurse or counselor. This gives you a forum to discuss the barriers you have to quitting and, once you stop smoking, the urges you may have to light up again.
- **Telephone quit lines.** Counseling over the telephone has become an increasingly popular and accessible way for people to receive help for their smoking. Telephone counseling allows participants to receive an intensive intervention that's almost identical to face-to-face consultation.
- **Buddy system.** Ask a nonsmoking friend or family member to be available when you experience tough times or when you have a reason to celebrate.

Keep in mind that what works for some people won't work for others. Talk with your doctor about your options and what might work best for you.

No kidding

Tobacco is tobacco. One form isn't any less dangerous than another. Using other types of tobacco products or cigarette alternatives — light cigarettes, cigars, pipes, snuff and chewing tobacco — can endanger your health just as much as an regular cigarettes.

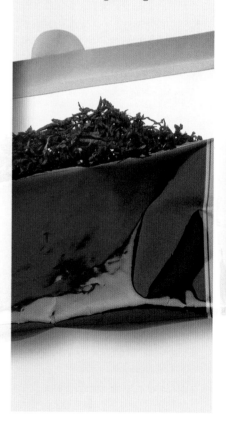

Medications to help you quit

Product	Pros	Cons	Cautions
Nicotine patch	Easy to use. Provides steady release of nicotine.	Can't quickly adjust amount to respond to craving. May cause skin irritation.	May not be appropriate if you have certain skin conditions.
Nicotine gum	Can chew it as often as needed. Keeps your mouth busy.	May cause gum or mouth soreness. May cause nausea or hiccups if chewed too fast.	As with all forms of nicotine replacement, don't use it while smoking.
Nicotine lozenges	Quickly satisfy cravings. Can use as needed.	May cause nausea, heartburn or hiccups.	Don't chew or swallow whole.
Nicotine inhaler	Keeps your hands and mouth busy. You control the dose.	May cause coughing and mouth or throat irritation.	May not be appropriate if you have lung disease, such as asthma.
Nicotine nasal spray	Reaches bloodstream quickly and works faster than other products.	May cause nasal, sinus and throat irritation, watery eyes and sneezing.	Not recommended for people with a nasal or sinus condition, allergies or asthma.
Bupropion (Zyban)	Easy-to-use pill. Doesn't contain nicotine.	Can cause insomnia and dry mouth.	Not appropriate for people with seizures or eating disorders, who already take medication containing bupropion, or who take an MAOI antidepressant.
Varenicline (Chantix)	Eases withdrawal symptoms. Blocks effects of nicotine if you resume smoking.	May cause stomach upset, headache and insomnia.	May not be appropriate for people with kidney disease.

Beyond the basics

Two alternative therapies people use to help them quit smoking are hypnosis (see page 102) and acupuncture (see page 120). While there isn't strong evidence that either is highly effective for smoking cessation, they're relatively safe. If you think they can help you quit, it might be worth it to give one or both a try.

7 benefits of exercise

Imagine that a new wonder formula has been created. It will prevent illness and disease, help you lose weight, fight stress and put you in a better mood. It can also slow the aging process and make you feel younger.

Now imagine that this formula doesn't cost a penny and you can take it several times a day or just once a day and still see results.

Sounds appealing, doesn't it? Well, this miracle formula is already available. It's called exercise. Regular, old-fashioned exercise is one of the most important things you can do to fight disease and enjoy life. The merits of exercise — ranging from preventing chronic diseases to boosting your confidence — are hard to ignore.

Here are seven ways exercise can have a positive impact on your health.

1. Strengthens your cardiovascular and respiratory systems

Exercise reduces the buildup of harmful deposits (plaques) in your arteries by increasing the concentration of high-density lipoprotein (HDL or "good") cholesterol in your blood.

Exercise also strengthens your heart so that it can pump blood more efficiently. And it reduces the risk of developing high blood pressure, even if you're already at increased risk of it.

Plus, exercise benefits your respiratory system by promoting rhythmic, deep breathing.

2. Keeps bones and muscles strong

Physical activity is likely the single most important factor in maintaining bone density. It

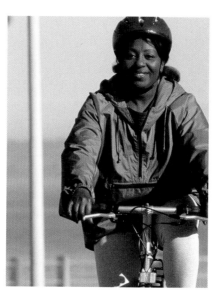

plays several roles in preventing and treating osteoporosis, perhaps most importantly by strengthening your bones.

3. Helps manage weight

Coupled with a healthy diet, exercise can help people lose weight, improving diseases and conditions associated with being overweight.

4. Prevents and manages diabetes

Regular exercise and a healthy diet reduce your risk of developing type 2 diabetes and can help control diabetes in individuals who already have it. Mild to moderate exercise helps the hormone insulin work better, lowering blood sugar levels.

5. Eases stress, depression and pain

Exercise fights stress, depression and pain by activating certain neurotransmitters — chemicals used by your nerve cells to communicate with one another.

These chemicals provide feelings of well-being that are associated with avoiding depression. They help you to relax and they provide "natural" pain relief.

6. Reduces your risk of certain cancers

Regular exercise may help lower the risk of cancers of the colon, breast, prostate, uterine lining (endometrium) and perhaps others.

Although it hasn't been proved, researchers think that exercise also helps combat colon cancer by causing digested food to move through the colon more quickly.

7. Helps you sleep better

Moderate exercise at least three hours before bedtime can help you relax and sleep better at night. A good night's sleep helps maintain your physical and mental health.

How fit are you?

Fitness isn't about how you look. It's about your health. Small increases in your fitness level can make a big difference in your overall well-being. Answer these questions.

Do you have enough energy to do the things you like to do?

① Rarely or never
② Sometimes
③ Always or most of the time

Do you have enough stamina and strength to carry out the daily tasks of your life?

① Rarely or never
② Sometimes
③ Always or most of the time

Can you walk a mile without feeling winded or fatigued?

① No
② Sometimes
③ Yes

Can you climb two flights of stairs without feeling winded or fatigued?

① No
② Sometimes
③ Yes

Can you do at least five push-ups before you need to stop for a rest?

① No
② Sometimes
③ Yes

Are you flexible enough to touch your toes while standing?

① No
② Sometimes
③ Yes

Can you carry on a conversation while doing light to moderate activities, such as brisk walking?

① No
② Sometimes
③ Yes

About how many days a week do you spend doing at least 30 minutes of moderately vigorous activity, such as walking briskly or raking leaves?

① Two days or less
② Three or four days
③ Five to seven days

About how many days a week do you spend doing at least 20 minutes of vigorous activity, such as jogging, participating in an aerobic dance class or playing singles tennis?

① None
② One to three
③ Four or more

About how many minutes do you walk during the day, including walking the dog, doing chores around the house, walking from your car to the office or store, or doing errands at work?

① Less than 30 minutes
② 30 to 60 minutes
③ More than 60 minutes

How did you score?

To the left of the answer you chose is a point value — 1, 2 or 3 points. Add up the points from your answers to determine your total score.

10 to 19 points. It's time to put getting into shape on your to-do list. Look for ways to get in 30 minutes or more of physical activity most days, even if it's just 10 minutes at a time.

20 to 25 points. You're on the right track, but your activity level could use a little boost. Look for ways to add more activity to your day or increase the intensity of your activities.

26 to 30 points. Way to go! You're well on your way to maintaining overall fitness. Keep up the good work.

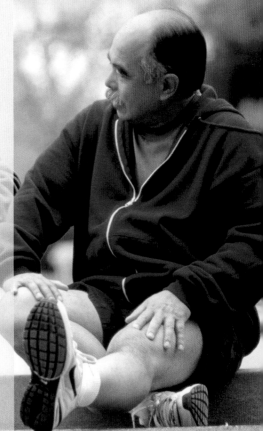

Living a more active life

Physical activity occurs from the moment you slip out of bed in the morning until you crawl back into bed at night. At its most basic level, physical activity simply means moving — every motion of your body burns calories.

Exercise is a more structured approach to physical activity intended to increase fitness.

Both are important. Studies indicate that daily physical activity can provide similar health benefits to structured exercise.

Adding activity to your day

Take advantage of any chance you have to be physically active. Here are a few ideas to help get you started. You can likely think of many other ways to make your day more active.

At home

- Exercise while watching television.
- Wash your car instead of going to the car wash.
- Use a push lawn mower instead of a riding one.
- Rake leaves and spend time in the garden.
- Use hand tools instead of power ones.
- Organize your closets or the garage.

At work

- Park at the far end of the parking lot and walk inside.
- Take the stairs and not the elevator, at least a few floors.
- Get up and visit with your co-workers instead of emailing them.
- Walk during your lunch hour.
- Periodically take an activity break. Get up, stretch your legs and move.

When out and about

- Park a little farther from your destination and walk.
- Bike or walk to the store.
- Avoid drive-throughs. Park the car and walk inside.
- Shop. You don't have to buy anything. Just walk the aisles and look at items.
- When golfing, walk the course instead of using a motorized cart.

When with your family

- Take a family walk after enjoying a meal.
- Participate in your kids' activities at the playground or park.
- Plan a family activity at least three times a week. This could be basketball in the driveway or a bike ride.
- Plan vacations that involve physical activities such as hiking, swimming, canoeing or skiing.

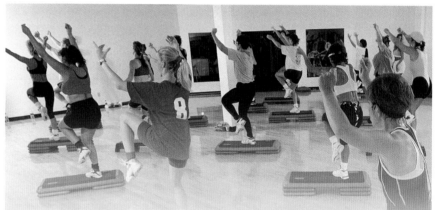

Cure for the common cold?

Researchers at the University of South Carolina in Columbia, S.C., investigated the relationship between different levels of physical activity and the risk of getting a cold (upper respiratory infection). The study included more than 500 healthy adults between the ages of 20 and 70.

The results found that participants who enjoyed a moderate amount of physical activity experienced 20 to 30 percent fewer colds than did individuals whose daily activities were limited and low in intensity.

One possible explanation is that moderate physical activity causes immune system cells to circulate more quickly, enhancing their ability to destroy viruses and bacteria.

Tired of always battling a cold? Get more physical activity each day and see what happens.

Aerobic exercise

One of the simplest and safest forms of exercise — and a great place to start if you're new to exercise — is aerobic activity.

Aerobic means with oxygen, as opposed to *anaerobic*, which means without oxygen. Aerobic activities, such as low to moderately intense walking or swimming, increase your breathing and heart rate as you continuously move your muscles at a regular pace.

Exercises carried out at an intense level placing heavy demands on your muscles and causing them to fatigue quickly are anaerobic. This includes fast running or intense weightlifting.

Both aerobic and anaerobic exercise play a role in achieving fitness. However, the greatest health benefits generally come from aerobic activities.

Beyond the basics

Tired of the same types of exercise? Check out these popular exercises and see what they have to offer:

- Pilates (see page 110)
- Tai chi (see page 114)
- Yoga (see page 115)

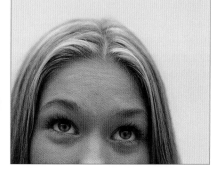

12-week walking program

Walking is an excellent exercise. It's simple, inexpensive, versatile and requires no equipment other than a good pair of walking shoes. If you're new to exercise, try this sample program, in which you slowly progress in the frequency and duration of your walking workout.

Week	Time (minutes)	Days a week	Total hours a week
1	20*	3	1
2	20	3	1
3-4	25	3	1.25
5-6	30	3-4	1.5-2
7-8	35	4-5**	2.5-3
9-10	40	4-5	3-3.5
11-12	40	5-6	3.5-4

*Older adults and people whose fitness is very limited may start out with just five to 10 minutes.

**If the days on which you can exercise are limited, you can continue to walk three or four days a week, instead of increasing the number of days, but gradually extend each walk to 45 or 60 minutes. On the other hand, if you have relatively little time on most days, you may benefit from more-frequent but shorter sessions.

This program can be adapted to many ability levels. A beginner might get a sufficient workout from a 10-minute walk around the neighborhood, and a more experienced walker can focus on increasing his or her speed, stride lengths or route, to make the workout more intense. Walking in a hilly area, for instance, may be a good choice for someone looking to boost endurance and build additional muscle tone in his or her legs. Note that walking with hand or ankle weights isn't recommended because adding these weights increases the stress and strain on your body.

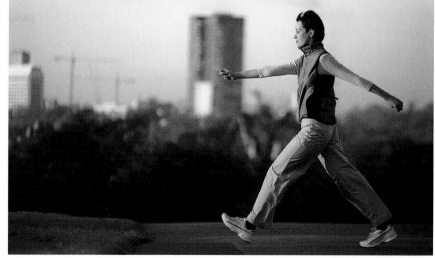

Eat for your health

If you're thinking that a healthy diet means eating bland and boring foods, think again.

It's true. You can eat your way to better health. What you put in your mouth every day has a direct effect on how you feel and how your body functions. A healthy diet — one that emphasizes vegetables, fruits and whole grains — may lower your risk of developing many diseases.

If you're thinking that a healthy diet means eating bland and boring foods, think again. It means enjoying great nutrition as well as great taste.

Eating better doesn't need to be complicated. The goal is to eat foods that not only taste good, but are good for you.

Vegetables and fruits

It's hardly news that vegetables and fruits are good for you. The real news is why. Every day more is being learned about how fresh produce supplies the body with a variety of substances to ward off illness.

People who typically eat generous helpings of vegetables and fruits run a lower risk of developing the leading killers of American adults: cardiovascular disease, high blood pressure, cancer and diabetes.

You're not a vegetable and fruit fan? You can be. You just have to know which ones to eat and how to prepare them. For example, instead of the familiar apples and oranges, try kiwi, Bing cherries or mangoes. To add more zest to your vegetables, sprinkle them with herbs.

Remember, much of what you eat is conditioned — that is, over time you've learned to like it. In the same respect, you can learn to enjoy new foods.

Carbohydrates

When it comes to carbohydrates, the key word to remember is *whole*, as in whole grains. The less refined a carbohydrate food is, the better it is for you. Whole grains abound with vitamins, minerals and other important nutrients.

This is why you want to choose whole-grain breads, pastas and cereals whenever you can, and select brown rice instead of white rice.

Contrary to what you may have heard or read, carbohydrates don't make you fat, excess calories do.

Protein and dairy

Despite what you may have learned as a child, it's not necessary to eat meat every day. Although rich in protein, many cuts of meat are high in saturated fat and cholesterol. When you do eat meat, try to eat only lean cuts.

A variety of other foods, including low-fat dairy products, seafood and legumes — dried beans, lentils and peas — furnish protein, too. Try to substitute these foods for meat on a regular basis.

These foods also provide other benefits. Low-fat dairy products are rich in calcium and vitamin D, and seafood supplies omega-3 fatty acids, which help protect against cardiovascular disease.

Fats

Not all fats are bad for you. Nuts, for instance, contain a type of oil that helps keep your heart and arteries free from harmful deposits. And people who replace much of the animal fat in their meals with liquid vegetable oils, such as olive or canola oil, can reduce their blood cholesterol level.

But while nuts and products such as vegetable oil may be beneficial, it's best to use them in moderation. That's because they also contain calories.

Sweets

Yes, it's true, the antioxidants in chocolate — especially dark chocolate — may provide some health benefits. But chocolate also contains plenty of added fat and calories.

When it comes to sweets, small is beautiful. You don't have to give up these foods entirely to eat well, but be smart about your selections and portion sizes.

Make sure you're getting enough antioxidants

Have you ever bitten into an apple, left it on the counter, and returned a few hours later to find it had turned brown? Or left your favorite pruning shears in the garden and discovered them later, covered in rust?

What, you might ask, does that have to do with your health? The answer is simple, although the process is complex: The same chemical reaction that caused the apple to discolor and the shears to rust (oxidation) occurs in your body.

The free radical effect

Your body continuously produces energy at the cellular level by building up and breaking down the substances that you eat and drink. Throughout this process, molecules that are missing an electron are created. These are called free radicals.

Because a free radical doesn't possess a full set of electrons, it's highly unstable and it "steals" an electron from any available substance to put itself in balance. When it does this, it alters the chemical structure of the cell from which it steals.

Free radicals help fight disease and break down toxins, but they're often produced in overabundance, resulting in an imbalance called oxidative stress.

Antioxidants to the rescue

To combat the effects of free radicals, your body produces antioxidants. Antioxidants readily give up one of their electrons but continue to stay in balance, sparing nearby cells from the damaging effects of free radicals.

At certain times, such as in the case of shock, infection or exposure to certain substances, naturally occurring antioxidants may not be able to neutralize the effects of all of the free radicals, and cellular damage may occur.

This damage is cumulative, and potentially can lead to degenerative diseases of the nervous system and eye, as well as cancer, diabetes and atherosclerosis.

Increasing your antioxidant intake

You can boost the antioxidants in your body and help fight disease by incorporating foods in your diet that are high in antioxidants — such as those that contain vitamins E, C and carotene, as well as the minerals selenium, copper, zinc and manganese.

Increasing antioxidant levels appears to enhance your health, although no direct link has been confirmed between antioxidant properties of certain foods and the prevention of disease.

Foods naturally highest in antioxidants tend to be those that are rich in color — red, purple, blue, orange and yellow. Dark chocolate, teas and several herbs also are packed with antioxidants.

In addition, how you prepare your foods affects antioxidant levels. For example, more of the antioxidants in tomatoes are available when tomatoes are cooked, whereas broccoli provides more antioxidants when it's raw. In many cases, unpeeled fruits are higher in antioxidants than are peeled forms.

How much is enough?

The Centers for Disease Control and Prevention (CDC) recommends that people eat at least five to seven servings a day of fruits and vegetables. In addition, the CDC recommends four to five servings of nuts, seeds or dry beans a week. All of these foods are good sources of antioxidants.

It's important, though, not to overdo it so that you're consuming a highly excessive amount. Excess consumption of antioxidants beyond your body's ability to use them could lead to increased production of free radicals.

In addition, it's probably best to get your antioxidants from food rather than supplements. Studies of beta carotene supplements indicate they don't protect against heart disease or cancer. To the contrary, they may increase disease risk. Two studies found an increased risk of lung cancer among smokers who took beta carotene supplements, and one found an increased risk of prostate cancer among men who took the supplements and drank alcohol.

10 disease-fighting foods

So then, just what foods should you eat to enjoy great health?

Here are our picks. These 10 foods can lay the groundwork for optimal health.

1. Whole grains

Whole grains are low in fat. And thanks to their fiber content, you eat less because you feel more satisfied. Eating whole grains can help lower your risk of cardiovascular disease, type 2 diabetes and some cancers.

Don't be fooled by the words *wheat bread* and *wheat flour*. Look for the word *whole*. Choose bread or cereal that has whole wheat, whole-wheat flour or another whole grain as the first ingredient on the label.

Look for breads with at least 3 grams of fiber in a serving, or cereals with at least 5 grams of fiber a serving — and preferably 8 or more.

2. Fish

Dietitians recommend that you aim for two servings of fish a week. Broiled, baked and grilled fish are better than fried.

If possible, go for fish such as salmon, tuna, trout, herring and sardines. They're rich in omega-3 fatty acids, which protect against heart disease by improving high-density lipoprotein (HDL, or "good") cholesterol and lowering triglycerides. Omega-3s also help lower blood pressure, may reduce the risk of an irregular heartbeat, and are thought to reduce inflammation that contributes to chronic illness.

However, it's important to pay attention to warnings regarding consumption levels of fish that may be affected by water contaminants, such as mercury and other toxins.

3. Walnuts and almonds

Nuts are high in calories but they're also nutrient dense. Almonds are loaded with calcium, iron, natural vitamin E and riboflavin. Walnuts are a good source of phosphorus, zinc, copper, iron, potassium and vitamin E, and the plant version of omega-3 fatty acids.

Nuts are naturally cholesterol-free. Studies suggest that they may even help reduce low-density lipoprotein (LDL, or "bad") cholesterol and reduce your risk of a heart attack.

Eat nuts in moderation. The serving size for nuts is 1 ounce. This equals about 14 walnut halves or about 22 almonds. One serving can take the place of the protein found in 1 ounce of meat.

4. Legumes

Legumes, which include a variety of dried beans, peas and lentils, are high in protein and make an excellent substitute for animal sources of protein.

Legumes have no cholesterol and very little fat. Unlike meat, legumes actually help reduce low-density lipoprotein (LDL, or "bad") cholesterol, and the minerals they contain may help control blood pressure.

Add legumes to chili, soups and casseroles in place of meat.

5. Soy

Claims that soy may reduce your cholesterol level and thereby lower your risk of cardiovascular disease are being re-examined after subsequent research found only minimal beneficial effects.

However, soy-based foods are still good for you because they contain less saturated fat than does meat, and they also provide fiber and protein.

It's best to eat soy in moderation, especially if you're at risk of or have had breast cancer. Soy contains phytochemicals that may produce weak estrogen activity. Studies are inconclusive as to whether soy may increase or decrease breast cancer risk.

6. Fat-free dairy products

Fortified skim milk is one of the best ways of getting needed calcium and vitamin D to help prevent osteoporosis.

There's also evidence that calcium can contribute to preventing high blood pressure, stroke, colon cancer and obesity. In addition, milk provides protein, minerals and B vitamins.

Fat-free cottage cheese, fat-free yogurt and fat-free cheeses have similar benefits.

7. Berries

Berries are rich in antioxidants and substances called flavonoids, which may help lower cancer and cardiovascular disease risk.

Blueberries are especially high in antioxidants, but blackberries, raspberries and strawberries aren't far behind.

If you're watching your weight, eat dried fruits sparingly because they're a concentrated source of calories.

8. Broccoli and cauliflower

Both broccoli and cauliflower are high in vitamin C. Broccoli also contains a good amount of vitamin A. These and other cruciferous vegetables — foods such as cabbage, Brussels sprouts, bok choy and kale — have naturally occurring phytochemicals that may help reduce the risk of colorectal cancer as well as other cancers.

Broccoli and cauliflower also contain fiber, have no cholesterol, and are naturally low in fat and calories.

9. Tomatoes

Tomatoes contain a number of nutrients, including vitamins C and B complex, as well as iron and potassium. They also contain the antioxidant lycopene.

Studies indicate that lycopene may lower the risk of heart attack, prostate cancer and possibly other types of cancer.

10. Green tea

Green tea is a major source of phytochemicals known as flavonoids, which may help lower the risk of some diseases.

It's particularly rich in a flavonoid called epigallocatechin gallate, which may inhibit the enzyme activity necessary for some forms of cancer growth.

Although green tea hasn't been shown in laboratory studies to prevent cancer or cardiovascular disease, some evidence suggests it may be of benefit.

Adding color to your meals

Red watermelon, purple grapes and orange sweet potatoes — all are examples of nature's wild color scheme. These bright fruits and vegetables are good for you, too. Different color classes of fruits and vegetables contain varying amounts of plant chemicals (phytochemicals) and other nutrients, offering many health benefits. Try to include these foods in your diet as much as possible.

Color family	Examples	Possible health benefits
Whites, tans, browns include the phytochemical allicin	Garlic, onions, scallions, leeks, bananas, pears, cauliflower	Lowers cholesterol and blood pressure; increases ability to fight infections
Blues, purples include the phytochemicals anthocyanin and phenolics	Blackberries, blueberries, purple grapes, raisins, eggplant, plums	Reduces risk of cancer and heart disease
Deep oranges, bright yellows include the nutrients bioflavonoid and carotenoid	Sweet potatoes, pumpkin, carrots, citrus fruits such as oranges, tangerines, grapefruit	Reduces risk of cancer, heart disease; maintains eyesight; strengthens immune system
Reds include the phytochemicals anthocyanin and lycopene	Tomatoes, watermelon, papaya, pink grapefruit, cherries, red apples, cranberries, red peppers	Reduces risk of heart disease and some cancers
Greens include the phytochemicals lutein and indole	Spinach, romaine lettuce, kale, collards, green peas, kiwi, broccoli, avocado	Protects against vision loss and cancer

Getting in a healthy groove

With everything that you have to do each day, making sure that you and your family eat healthy meals may seem like a difficult or time-consuming task.

When it comes to cooking, many people claim that they don't have the time. That's because healthy eating is often associated with complicated recipes, time-laden meal preparation and hours spent at the grocery store. However, you can prepare a healthy meal as quickly as you can an unhealthy one.

Here are some tips to help you eat well without a lot of fuss and hassle.

Plan by the week

It's more efficient to plan your meals for an entire week, especially if you shop for groceries on a weekly basis. This way, you'll know that you have all of the right ingredients on hand when it's time to prepare breakfast, lunch or dinner.

Look for shortcuts

Another way to help simplify meal preparation and save time is to purchase pre-cut vegetables and fruits, precooked meats, and packaged salads.

Frozen or canned vegetables may also come in handy for some dishes. Rinse the canned vegetables to help remove the sodium used in processing.

Shop from a list

Following a list helps keep you from impulse buying. Avoid shopping when you're hungry — you'll be tempted to grab anything that looks vaguely appetizing.

Read nutrition labels

When shopping, compare the nutrition labels of similar items to see if one is healthier than the others. You many find that one has less fat, fewer calories or more fiber.

Adapt to the seasons

Whenever you can, look for recently harvested produce — asparagus, peas and cherries in the spring; peaches, sweet corn and tomatoes in midsummer; and apples, pears and squash in the fall.

In the spring, summer and early fall months, you can find farmers markets in many areas. These markets offer local produce, which tends to be the freshest around.

Be adventurous

Discovering new foods and flavors is part of the joy of cooking and eating, so don't be afraid to explore unfamiliar cuisines. Keep in mind that the broadest range of health benefits comes from meals that feature a wide variety of foods.

Be flexible

Remember that every food you eat doesn't have to be an excellent source of nutrients. Nor is it out of the question to eat high-fat, high-calorie foods on occasion. The main thing is that you choose foods that promote good health more often than you choose those that don't.

Beyond the basics

It may seem easier to reach for a nutritional supplement than eat a healthy diet. However, supplements don't provide many of the benefits of whole foods. Fruits and vegetables, for example, contain naturally occurring food substances called phytochemicals, which may help protect you against cancer, heart disease, diabetes and high blood pressure.

If you depend on dietary supplements rather than eating a variety of whole foods, you miss the benefits of these substances. The best use of supplements is to "supplement" a good diet — not replace it.

For more information on what supplements might be appropriate for you, see Chapter 3.

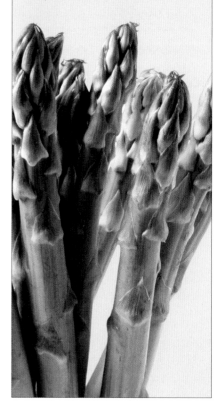

Your weight and your health

Your diet and your weight generally go hand in hand. A healthy diet can help you maintain a healthy weight.

The fact is, the more excess weight you carry, the greater your risk of developing certain health conditions. Among these conditions are:

- **High blood pressure.** Obese individuals are twice as likely to develop high blood pressure (hypertension) as are individuals who maintain a healthy weight.

- **Abnormal blood fats.** Being overweight is associated with low levels of high-density lipoprotein (HDL, or "good") cholesterol and high levels of triglycerides (another type of blood fat) in your bloodstream.

- **Type 2 diabetes.** More than 80 percent of adults with type 2 diabetes are overweight or obese.

- **Cardiovascular disease.** A weight gain of just 10 to 20 pounds can increase your risk of heart and blood vessel problems by 25 percent. A gain of 45 pounds or more increases the risk by more than 250 percent.

- **Other complications.** If you're overweight, your health is at increased risk of other conditions, including osteoarthritis, gallstones and sleep apnea. Many types of cancer also are associated with being overweight.

The right approach

If you really want to lose weight and keep the weight off, the best approach is to focus on healthy lifestyle changes and to follow an eating plan that's enjoyable, yet healthy and low in calories.

This approach will result in weight loss that you can live with — that is, that you can maintain over a long period of time. What you don't want is to gain the weight back.

True, achieving a healthy weight takes work — or more correctly, planning — but the rewards are great. Your efforts will result in a sustainable, enjoyable lifestyle that can improve your health and well-being. You'll feel better immediately and at the same time reduce your health risks.

Slow and steady wins the race

That there are so many diet plans to choose from these days attests to the fact that few of them work for most people or are effective for a long period of time. The term *diet* often implies something that's restrictive and negative and, therefore, temporary. Many diets will help people lose weight over a short period of time, but usually the weight is regained. People often find diets hard to sustain because they get tired of avoiding certain foods, loading up on others, or feeling deprived and hungry.

Weight loss is best — and most likely to be retained — when it's gradual and it results from a change in lifestyle habits. Think in terms of losing no more than 1 to 2 pounds a week. That's a goal that's realistic and achievable. A loss of just 5 to 10 percent of your body weight — no matter what you weigh — brings important health benefits and improves the quality of your life.

Here's a practical perspective on weight loss: 3,500 calories equals about 1 pound of body fat. To lose 1 pound in a week, you need to burn 3,500 calories more than you consume. That calculates to about 500 fewer calories a day. How do you do this? Eat fewer high-calorie foods, get more physical activity or, better yet, do both.

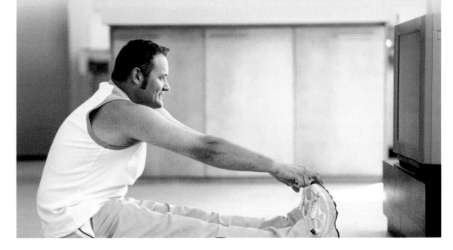

Find meaning in your life

Enjoying life is about taking part in activities and relationships that are meaningful to you — that motivate you to get up every morning.

Good health, remember, is more than your physical health, it also includes your mental health. Increasing evidence suggests that how you view life and the satisfaction you get from life have a major influence on your health.

If you're happy in what you're doing and you feel that your life has meaning and purpose, you're more likely to enjoy a healthy life. Without a sense of mission — a passion for something or someone — some people become vulnerable to depression or other illnesses.

Relationships

Strong social ties are one component of a purposeful life. Healthy relationships with family and friends appear to boost your physical health in a number of ways:

- **Bolster immunity.** Stress can suppress immunity. To the contrary, love and friendship reduce stress and strengthen immunity.
- **Improve mental health.** Having people to talk with provides a psychological buffer against stress, anxiety and depression.
- **Improve recovery.** Studies suggest that individuals who have a strong support system are likely to recover faster from a major health event than are those who don't.
- **Extend life.** More than a dozen studies link social support with a lower risk of early death.

Increasing evidence suggests that how you view life and the satisfaction that you get from life have a major influence on your health.

Activities

Another component of a purposeful life is spending your days doing what you enjoy.

A feeling of satisfaction comes in many different forms. For some individuals, their job provides meaning and enjoyment. Others find satisfaction in raising their children or caring for family members. For still others, real meaning in life may come from a hobby or civic duty.

Remember, satisfaction doesn't have to come in big packages. Something as simple as having coffee with friends may be what you look forward to and what gives you pleasure.

Spiritual ties

Similar to the benefits that come from strong relationships and meaningful activities, spiritual well-being is integral to health and happiness.

People often use the term *spirituality* interchangeably with *religion*. However, the terms aren't necessarily synonymous. Whereas religion refers to a system of beliefs and practices held by a group of believers, spirituality is more individualistic and self-determined.

Praying is one means of expressing your spirituality. Other activities people find to be spiritually soothing include spending time in nature or enjoying the pleasures of music, art or writing.

Spiritual beliefs and practices — whatever form they may take — help you connect to something greater than yourself. When you believe in some form of higher power, you strengthen your ability to cope with whatever life hands you.

Beyond the basics

Prayer is the most commonly used alternative practice. Can it actually improve your health? Studies suggest possibly so. For more on spirituality and prayer, see page 112.

What is your life purpose?

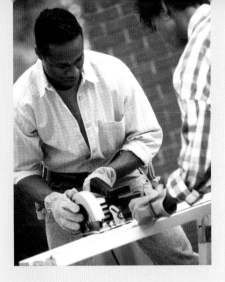

Meaningful activities support what you're trying to get out of life and help you feel connected to why you're here. They give you something to strive for, a reason to live and something to feel excited about each day.

Having a sense of purpose can keep you from waking up one morning, looking back on your life and saying, "What happened?"

A sense of purpose can mean different things to different people. For many of us, it includes a feeling that we matter — that others depend on us, are interested in us, and are concerned about what happens to us.

Spending time doing things that are meaningful to you and that you enjoy can help you feel better about yourself and improve your mood and your attitude toward life.

Researchers believe that engagement with life — purposeful activities and close relationships — is one of the main components of a high-quality life. Without a sense of mission — a passion for something or someone — some people become vulnerable to depression, which can lead to health problems.

So, then, how do you find your purpose?

Make a wish list

Allow yourself to dream about all of the things you'd like to do. Pay attention to your inner voice, asking yourself, "How can I use my talents?" and "What is really important to me?"

Write down those activities you see yourself doing, from part-time work to volunteering to hobbies. Try to include more than just solitary pursuits, such as reading, watching TV or walking.

Keep in mind that a list heavy on material things, for example, buying a new "toy" or redecorating your house, likely won't be satisfying for long.

Find a job you love

Going to work isn't work if you truly enjoy what you do each day. Many people who are successful at work — not just financially, but also emotionally — say they are following their passion, doing what they truly enjoy. If your job doesn't give you satisfaction, maybe you need to consider a different career.

Pursue interests and hobbies

What intellectual or physical pursuits do you find fascinating, fun or pleasurable? This might include researching your family history, attending concerts, playing golf or fixing up an old house.

The main thing is that your hobby brings you enjoyment. If it feels more like a duty, consider something else. Take part in interests and hobbies that make you feel energized, not drained.

Volunteer your time and talents

Many people say that one of the most fulfilling activities they do is community service and volunteer work. By volunteering your time and talents, you're also helping yourself. For decades, research has shown a link between quality of life and involvement with other people. Regular volunteering can improve your physical and psychological well-being and may even help you live longer. When you volunteer, you feel needed and valued, and you tend to feel better about yourself and the world around you. You're likely to be less isolated and less preoccupied with your own problems.

People who work to improve the world or to help others tend to maintain a sense of vitality that those who are more self-absorbed lack. Other benefits include making new friends and staying busy and productive.

Express your creativity

Expressing yourself in a creative way — writing, drawing, painting, sculpting, dancing, playing an instrument or making a film — enhances your enjoyment of life and gives it meaning.

Creativity isn't limited to a certain age range. Many people experience a burst of creativity in their later years. If you have the urge to create, go for it.

Learn to relax and stress less

Rest and relaxation are basic necessities. They're as fundamental to your health as physical activity and a nutritious diet.

If you're like many people, though, you don't get enough. And your body is paying for it.

Not enough rest and too little sleep can make it more difficult for you to concentrate, and you may become impatient with others, less interactive in your relationships and less productive at work.

Benefits of rest and relaxation

When it comes to your health, it's important to make sleep and relaxation a priority. Each day you may feel the need to complete a long list of tasks, and then with whatever time is left-over, sleep or relax.

Try this: Reverse the order. Set aside adequate time for sleep and relaxation and then see how many of the tasks on your list you can get done in the time you have remaining. You may be surprised.

There are many reasons why relaxation and a good night's sleep are important to your health. They:

- Slow your heart rate, meaning less work for your heart
- Reduce your blood pressure
- Increase blood flow to your major muscles
- Slow your breathing rate

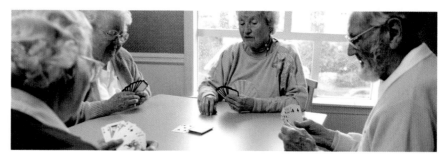

- Lessen muscle tension
- Reduce signs and symptoms of illness, such as headaches, nausea, diarrhea and pain
- Give you more energy
- Improve your concentration

Finding the right leisure activities

Leisure activities are important to good health because they can reduce stress and improve your outlook on life. Everyone needs an outlet — an opportunity to decompress.

Leisure activities — what you choose to do during your free time — vary from person to person. What someone else finds interesting and pleasurable you may find incredibly boring, or even stressful.

If you've been burying your nose in your work, you may not know what you like to do for leisure. One approach is to look at your self-care needs:

- **Are you getting enough physical activity and exercise?** Regular physical activity promotes both physical and mental health.

- **Do you challenge yourself mentally?** It's important to do things that are mentally stimulating.

- **Are you meeting your spiritual needs?** Depending on how you define spirituality, you might participate in organized religious activities or express yourself through music or art.

- **Are you using your creative abilities?** What gets your creative juices flowing? Maybe it's dancing, painting, cooking, or doing repair work on your house.

- **Do you have enough social contact with others.** Social interaction is important. If your answer is no, you might join a sports league or a book or dining club.

- **Is there novelty or adventure in your life?** Don't be afraid to experience new things. Consider traveling, hiking or learning a new skill or hobby.

- **Are you interested in service to others?** If you like helping others, look for opportunities to volunteer.

Recognizing stress

Modern-day life is full of time pressures and demands. In other words, it's stressful. But just because stress may be a regular component of your day, it doesn't have to get the best of you.

Too much stress

Many of the physical reactions that accompany stress can damage your long-term health. Stress can be a factor in a variety of illnesses, from headaches to heart disease. Stress may aggravate an existing health problem, or it may trigger an illness if you're already at risk.

- **Immune system.** The hormone cortisol produced during times of stress can suppress your immune system, increasing your susceptibility to infections, such as cold or flu.

- **Heart and blood vessel system.** During acute stress your heart beats more quickly, making you more susceptible to heart rhythm irregularities and chest pain (angina). If you're a Type A personality, acute stress may increase your heart attack risk. Increased blood clotting from persistent stress also can put you at risk of a heart attack, stroke or sudden death. High levels of cortisol can raise your blood lipids (cholesterol and triglycerides) and temporarily increase blood pressure.

- **Digestive system.** You may have a stomachache or diarrhea when stressed. This happens because stress hormones slow stomach acid release and stomach emptying. The same hormones also stimulate the colon, speeding passage of its contents.

- **Wound healing.** Studies show that stress decreases wound healing. One study found it took 60 percent longer for wounds to heal in people who were under stress.

- **Vaccine response.** Stress decreases the body's immune response to a vaccine.

- **Other illnesses.** Other studies suggest that stress may worsen symptoms of asthma, skin disorders, chronic pain, depression or anxiety. Stress has also been shown to increase risk of liver disease and decrease insulin sensitivity. A study involving children found that stress increases the frequency of illness in children.

Signs and symptoms of stress overload

Physical	Thoughts and feelings	Behaviors
Headache	Excessive worrying	Overeating or appetite loss
Chest pain	Anxiety	Increased arguing
Pounding heart	Anger	Angry outbursts
High blood pressure	Irritability	Increased alcohol and drug use
Shortness of breath	Depression	Increased smoking
Muscle aches	Sadness	Withdrawal or isolation
Clenched jaws	Restlessness	Crying spells
Grinding teeth	Mood swings	Neglecting responsibility
Tight, dry throat	Feeling insecure	Decreased productivity
Indigestion	Difficulty concentrating	Job dissatisfaction
Diarrhea or constipation	Confusion	Poor job performance
Stomach cramping	Forgetfulness	Increased use of sick time
Increased perspiration	Resentment	Burnout
Fatigue	Tendency to blame	Impatience
Insomnia	Negativity	Change in sleep patterns
Weight gain or loss	Guilt	Changes in relationships
Skin problems	Apathy	Nervous twitch or habit
Impaired sexual function	Feeling worthless	Decreased interest in sex

Problem solving: Think it through

To alleviate a stressful situation, brush up on your problem-solving skills by taking these steps:

1. **Identify. What's the cause of your stress?**

   - In concrete terms, what exactly is the problem?
   - Is the problem really that big? Would others think so?
   - Are you using this problem to avoid dealing with a much bigger one?
   - Is there any part of the problem over which you have control?

2. **Clarify. What would make the problem go away?**

   - What do you want to happen?
   - What do you want to prevent?
   - Are you attempting to solve the main problem that's causing you stress, or have you lost sight of the real stressor?

3. **Create. Think of all the possible ways in which you might solve your problem. Now isn't the time to judge whether one potential solution** is better than another. As you brainstorm, try to:

   - Recall past problems that you were able to solve. Could a similar solution work for this problem, too?
   - Ask friends, family and people you trust for advice.

4. **Choose. Of all your creative ideas, which make the most sense? Consider:**

   - What will likely happen if you choose this specific path?
   - How will using this solution make you — and others — feel in the end?
   - What are the possible positive and negative consequences?
   - Will you be able to carry it out?
   - Do you have the proper resources?
   - Do you realistically think it will solve the problem?

5. **Implement. Believe in yourself, be brave and try your solution out.**

   If you don't take action, you can't expect to reduce your stress.

6. **Reflect. In every outcome there is a lesson.**

   - Did your solution effectively solve the problem?
   - Is it solved well?
   - If not, what new plan might work?

Practicing problem-solving skills on stressors will help you better cope with stress as it comes at you.

Beyond the basics

In upcoming pages, you'll read about a number of techniques that can help you relax and reduce stress.

The best thing about mind and body therapies to relieve stress is that they're safe and often effective.

Therapies that can help you manage stress and that you'll want to learn more about include:

- Biofeedback (see page 98)
- Guided imagery (see page 100)
- Massage (see page 131)
- Meditation (see page 103)
- Muscle relaxation (see page 108)
- Music therapy (see page 109)
- Relaxed breathing (see page 111)
- Yoga (see page 115)

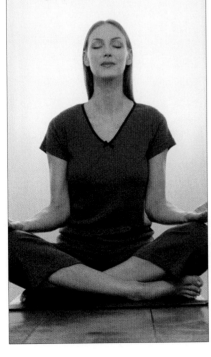

Tips for better sleep

If you have trouble sleeping, simple changes in your daily and bedtime routines may make sleep come easier. Here are a few suggestions:

- **Exercise and stay active.** Physical activity enhances deep and refreshing sleep. But avoid exercising too close to bedtime.
- **Don't eat too close to bedtime.** Having a full stomach increases your chances of experiencing heartburn while lying in bed.
- **Avoid or limit caffeine and alcohol.** Caffeine can prevent you from falling asleep. Alcohol can cause shallow sleeping and frequent awakenings.
- **Unwind.** If you lead a busy life, slow the pace of your activities in the evening. Do something relaxing before you go to bed.
- **Stick to a sleep schedule.** Go to bed and get up about the same time every day, including weekends.
- **Establish and follow a bedtime ritual.** In the evening, slow the pace of your activities before bedtime.
- **Create a comfortable sleep environment.** Keep your bedroom quiet, dark and comfortably cool.
- **Hide the alarm clock.** A visible readout of how long you've been unable to sleep may worry you needlessly and worsen the problem.
- **Don't 'try' to sleep.** If sleep doesn't come naturally, read a book, listen to music or watch television until you feel drowsy.
- **Avoid or limit naps to 30 minutes or less.** Naps can make it difficult to fall asleep at night.
- **Check your medications.** Ask your doctor if any of your medications — prescription, nonprescription and supplements you may be taking — can contribute to insomnia.

Are you getting enough sleep?

Many people think they're getting adequate sleep but really aren't. You may not be getting the right amount and quality of sleep if:
- You routinely ignore your alarm clock or catch a few extra minutes of sleep in the mornings.
- You wake up groggy and don't feel refreshed.
- You look forward to catching up on sleep on the weekends.
- You're irritable with co-workers, family and friends.
- You have difficulty concentrating or remembering.
- You have to fight to stay awake during long meetings or after a meal.
- You wake up repeatedly throughout the night.

Part 2

Guide to Alternative Therapies

Understanding the benefits and risks of popular treatments

Alternative medicine includes a diverse group of products, practices and therapies intended to treat and prevent illness.

As these treatments increasingly undergo scientific study, some are gradually incorporated into mainstream medicine, while others fall out of favor because they're considered ineffective or unsafe. For a number of alternative treatments, the jury is still out — either research results have been inconclusive or not enough research has been done to determine the effectiveness or safety of the therapy.

In Part 2, we take a look at various forms of alternative medicine and provide you with the latest information on what's known about the treatments — their benefits and their risks. We also offer information on how to incorporate specific treatments into your daily life.

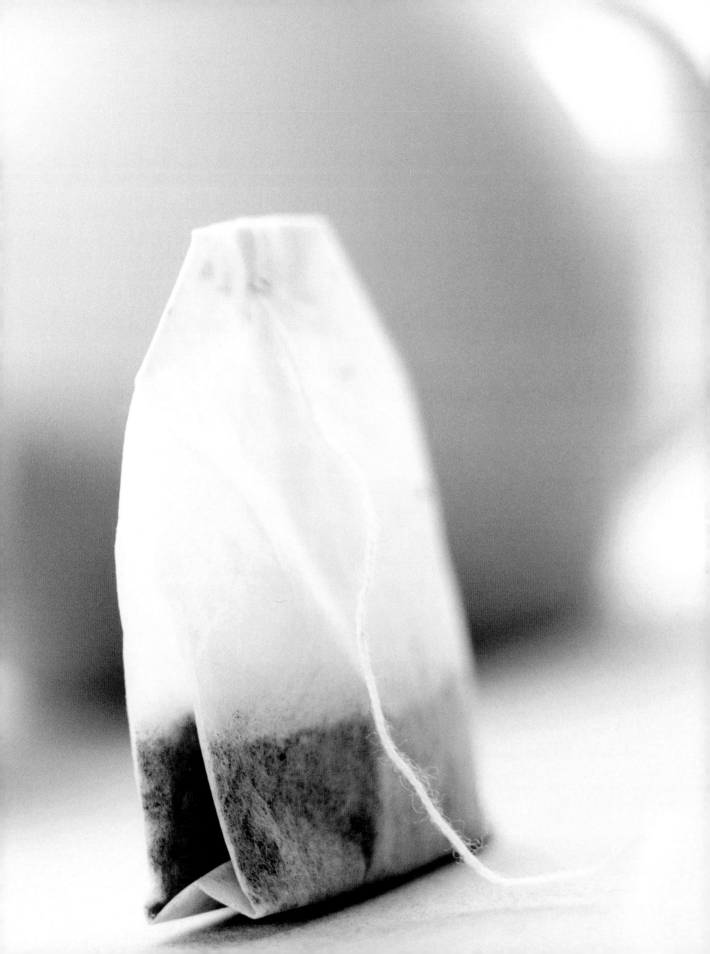

Chapter 3
Herbs and Other Dietary Supplements

A visit with Dr. Mark Lee

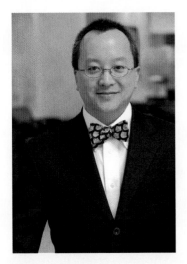

Mark Lee, M.D.
General Internal Medicine

There's growing evidence that certain supplements — when used in conjunction with modern medicine — can help you achieve and maintain good health. Supplements can be part of your overall wellness plan, provided you use them wisely.

The most common alternative therapy in use today is dietary supplements, which include herbs, vitamins and minerals. Since 1994, when the U.S. Congress passed the Dietary Supplement Health and Education Act, there's been a tremendous explosion of growth in the dietary supplement industry, with sales exceeding $20 billion annually, according to some estimates.

Most dietary supplements are derived from plants or herbs, though minerals, vitamins and even some hormones, such as DHEA and melatonin, are included in the category. People often take supplements because they believe that taking them is good for the prevention and treatment of many diseases, including arthritis, osteoporosis, infections and immune-related conditions. Supplements — especially herbal products — are also popular because of the perception that they're natural and, therefore, "good for you." But natural doesn't always translate into being safe. Any product that's strong enough to provide a potential benefit to the body can also be strong enough to cause harm. Tobacco, for example, is a "natural" product, and it's clearly not safe. Some natural products, such as nightshade or hemlock, can be extremely toxic when ingested and can even cause death.

Vitamins have generally proved to be safe. However, marketing campaigns and the antioxidant craze of the past decade have spurred the concept that "if a little is good for you, then a lot must be great." Megadose vitamin therapies are publicized as effective strategies to cure colds and infections, prevent Alzheimer's disease, and even prevent or cure cancer. Unfortunately, there's little scientific evidence to support these claims and their side effects have resulted in more of a problem rather than a panacea.

Despite these concerns, there's growing evidence that certain supplements — when used in conjunction with modern medicine — can help you achieve and maintain good health. Supplements can be part of your overall wellness plan, provided you use them wisely. When reading supplement labels, ask yourself these questions: Does the product promise rapid improvement in health or performance? Does it seem too good to be true? Does the manufacturer use the results of a single study or series of anecdotes to support its use?

And remember, supplements are just that — supplemental. They can't replace a nutritious diet. To achieve and maintain good health, you need to build your "health pyramid" — don't smoke, eat nutritious foods, exercise every day, rest up, have a plan for dealing with stress, and make sure to have meaning in your life. Once you've created and maintained this foundation, adding specific supplements may provide the added edge you're looking for.

Promise and peril

Dietary supplements may be popular, but are they right for you? That depends on the product, your current health and your medical history.

Dietary supplements contain ingredients that affect how your body functions, just as nonprescription and prescription medications do. Some supplements may be beneficial, but in other instances herbal supplements may be risky. Their labels are often vague, and the supplement may pose more unwanted side effects than benefits.

If you're considering a dietary supplement, educate yourself about the product you intend to use before purchasing it, and talk to your doctor about the supplement you're considering taking.

It's wise to avoid dietary supplements if:

- **You're pregnant or breast-feeding.** As a general rule, don't take any medications when you're pregnant or breast-feeding unless your doctor approves. Medications that may be safe for you as an adult may be harmful to your baby or your breast-feeding infant.
- **You're having surgery.** Many herbal supplements can affect the success of surgery. Some may decrease the effectiveness of anesthetics or cause dangerous complications such as bleeding or high blood pressure. Tell your doctor about any herbs you're taking or considering taking as soon as you know you need surgery.

- **You're younger than 18 or older than 65.** Older adults may metabolize medications differently. And few herbal supplements have been tested on children or have established safe doses for children. While it's recommended that all individuals consult with a doctor before taking dietary supplements, it's especially important that you do so if:
- **You're taking prescription or nonprescription medications.** Some herbs can cause serious side effects when mixed with prescription or nonprescription drugs, such as aspirin. Talk to your doctor about possible drug interactions.

More information on supplement safety can be found in Chapter 9.

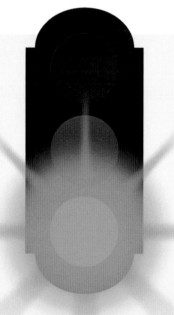

What a green light means

In upcoming pages, you'll find herbs and other supplements that have been given a green light. Remember that a green light doesn't mean it's OK to take the product for any condition or in any amount. Oftentimes, a product is given a green light because studies have found it beneficial for just one or two conditions. There may be other conditions for which it isn't effective. Always take the product according to directions. Don't take more than is recommended, and always discuss your use of supplements with your doctor. You'll note that we usually advise not to take the product for more than six months. This is because — with some exceptions — most products haven't been studied for longer than six months to determine their long-term effects.

Herbs and other botanicals

Acai berry

Acai berry is a reddish, purple fruit that comes from the acai palm tree, native to Central and South America.

Acai berry is generally sold as a juice but is also available in pill and capsule form. It's marketed for its weight-loss and anti-aging properties. The berry is believed to have a high antioxidant content — higher than cranberry, raspberry and blueberry, which are known as powerful antioxidants. Some cosmetics and beauty products also contain acai oil.

Research on the acai berry has been limited.

Our take

While this juice has become quite popular, there just isn't enough data to determine if it really offers something special beyond other, less costly fruit juices. Many manufacturers recommend very high doses or offer potent extracts of the berry. The safety of long-term use in such high doses is unknown.

What the research says

Although acai berry is touted as a weight-loss product, few studies have tested the benefit of acai berry in promoting weight loss. The juice is also used by some to treat osteoarthritis and high levels of cholesterol in blood (hypercholesterolemia), but, again, there's insufficient evidence to prove the berry is effective. The safety of acai berry is also unknown. More research is needed.

Andrographis

Andrographis (*Andrographis paniculata*) is an Indian herb known for its bitter properties. It has been used for centuries in India and other Asian countries as a treatment for digestive problems. More recently, the herb has become popular as a remedy for upper respiratory infections, including cold and flu.

Because of its potential immune-stimulating actions, the herb is also being studied as a possible treatment for many diseases, including cancer and HIV.

Pregnant women shouldn't use andrographis because it could terminate the pregnancy.

Our take

A specific product (andrographis combined with *Eleutherococcus senticosus*) may shorten the duration or lessen the symptoms of the common cold. Since there are few other potential remedies for a cold, we give andrographis a green light for short-term use to treat the common cold.

What the research says

There is reasonably strong evidence from clinical trials to suggest that andrographis effectively reduces the severity and duration of upper respiratory infections. Some research also suggests that regular use of andrographis might reduce your risk of getting a cold by up to 50 percent. The herb appears to be safe when used short-term, but more research is warranted.

Artichoke

Supplements containing artichoke extract are taken to relieve digestive symptoms and lower cholesterol. The extract comes from the plant's large, lobed leaves — not its fruit, the artichoke "heart."

The supplements appear to be safe when used as directed; however, they can cause flatulence. They may also cause an allergic reaction in people who are sensitive to ragweed or flowers such as chrysanthemums, marigolds and daisies. People with gallstones should avoid its use because it may worsen the condition.

Our take

Indigestion (dyspepsia) is a common problem and oftentimes it's not very responsive to conventional treatments. Short-term use of artichoke may help relieve this often vexing condition. Discuss its use with your doctor before you begin.

What the research says

Studies indicate artichoke leaf extract may reduce symptoms such as nausea, vomiting and abdominal pain associated with indigestion (dyspepsia). Artichoke extract may also mildly reduce cholesterol levels, especially in people with higher cholesterol levels. In both cases, it may take several weeks before you notice an improvement in symptoms.

Avocado

Avocado oil is available in capsule form and as a cream that you rub on your skin. Orally, avocado is taken to treat osteoarthritis and to reduce cholesterol levels. Topically, it's used to treat conditions such as hardening of the skin (sclerosis) and psoriasis. For the treatment of osteoarthritis, avocado oil is sometimes combined with soybean oil.

Avocados are naturally high in monounsaturated fatty acids, a healthy form of fat. They also have a high fiber content and contain many nutrients.

When consumed in amounts commonly found in food, avocado supplements appear to be safe. Topical preparations can cause itching, which typically improves with use.

Our take

While there are some preliminary studies supporting the use of avocado supplements, there aren't long-term studies to verify their safety over time. Since both arthritis and high cholesterol are chronic conditions that require daily treatment, we'd like to see safety data before giving avocado a green light.

What the research says

An avocado-enriched diet high in monounsaturated fats may lower total cholesterol and low-density lipoprotein (LDL, or "bad") cholesterol and increase high-density lipoprotein (HDL, or "good") cholesterol. Whether avocado supplements work as well as the real fruit is unproved. For the treatment of osteoarthritis, oral supplements that contain both avocado and soybean oils may improve pain and disability, especially for osteoarthritis of the hip. Preliminary evidence suggests the oils may slow cartilage degeneration and promote cartilage repair. For other conditions, there's less evidence avocado oil is effective.

Black cohosh

Black cohosh (*Actaea racemosa*), formerly known as *Cimicifuga racemosa*, is a member of the buttercup family. It's also called black snakeroot and bugbane.

Because it has effects similar to the female hormone estrogen, black cohosh is used to relieve premenstrual pain and symptoms of menopause. In the past, it was also used to treat rheumatic joint pain.

Black cohosh is generally well tolerated, but it can cause stomach discomfort. There is also some concern it may cause liver damage in some people.

Our take

Black cohosh may improve menopausal symptoms, especially hot flashes, if used in recommended doses. While recent studies have cast some doubt on its effectiveness, we continue to give it a green light because there are few other options for treating hot flashes. For other conditions, there's less evidence it may be beneficial, so be cautious. Don't take it for longer than six months or during pregnancy.

What the research says

Several controlled trials report that black cohosh improves menopausal symptoms such as hot flashes, headache and mood disorders. There are also indications it may relieve heart palpitations and sleep disturbances. However, many of the studies were small, poorly designed and didn't extend beyond six months.

Blond psyllium

The seed and outer covering of blond psyllium are used in medicinal products and processed foods. They contain the active ingredient mucilage, which swells and forms a thick mass as it absorbs liquid.

Blond psyllium is used as a laxative and for softening stools. It's also taken for conditions such as irritable bowel syndrome (IBS), high cholesterol and high blood pressure.

In food manufacturing, it serves as a thickener or stabilizer in some products. Some foods containing blond psyllium claim the food may reduce heart disease. While blond psyllium can lower cholesterol, there's no proof is reduces heart disease risk.

Our take

Many people find relief of symptoms of irritable bowel syndrome with this product. Side effects are minimal and generally easy to manage. As for high cholesterol, the effect of blond psyllium is usually modest, at best. However, it can be a useful ally as part of an overall treatment plan for managing cholesterol.

What the research says

Blond psyllium is effective as a bulk laxative for reducing constipation. It can also reduce cholesterol levels in people whose total and low-density lipoprotein (LDL, or "bad") cholesterol is mildly to moderately high. It may improve blood sugar levels in people with diabetes and reduce diarrhea associated with conditions such as irritable bowel syndrome. To reduce gastrointestinal side effects, start with a small dose and gradually increase the amount.

Butterbur

Butterbur (*Petasites hybridus*) is a shrub found along marshy meadows and riversides. Its name comes from its large, supple leaves that were used to wrap butter before the days of refrigeration.

There's evidence that butterbur may help prevent migraines and treat hay fever (allergic rhinitis). This may be due to its anti-inflammatory properties and its ability to relax blood vessel walls.

People who are allergic to ragweed, marigolds and daisies need to be especially cautious if taking this supplement.

Our take

Butterbur gets a green light because the herb appears to be relatively safe if taken for a short period to help prevent migraines or to treat symptoms of hay fever. Plus it's nonsedating. However, don't take butterbur for either of these conditions without first consulting with your doctor, to prevent possible drug interactions.

What the research says

Some studies indicate participants who took butterbur were able to significantly decrease the number of migraine attacks. Other studies suggest that butterbur may alleviate the stuffiness and nasal congestion of hay fever. However, due to the small sample sizes and short durations of these studies, the results can only be considered preliminary. Additional research is needed.

Cat's claw

Cat's claw (*Uncaria tomentosa*) is a woody vine from the tropical rainforests of Central and South America. Its name comes from hooked thorns that run along the vine's surface. The herb is available in tablet or capsule form and sold as a tea.

The plant was highly prized among various indigenous groups in the Americas for its medicinal properties. Today, it's used to boost the immune system and to treat inflammatory conditions as well as cancer.

Cat's claw may lower your blood pressure, so if you're taking antihypertensive drugs, talk to your doctor before taking the supplement.

Our take

Preliminary studies suggest a possible role for cat's claw in treating ailments such as rheumatoid arthritis and osteoarthritis. So far, the trials have been small. Large studies are needed to confirm the full potential of its medicinal qualities and determine its safety. There's less evidence cat's claw can help boost the immune system or treat cancer.

What the research says

Studies indicate modest benefits for easing joint pain from rheumatoid arthritis, as well as osteoarthritic knee pain during physical activity (but not during rest). The herb is thought to have immune-stimulating and anti-inflammatory effects.

As for its role as an immune system booster, a few small studies have produced conflicting results.

Cayenne

Originating in the Americas, the hot, fiery cayenne pepper (*Capsicum annuum*) is known in kitchens around the world as red pepper or chili pepper.

The bright red fruit of the plant contains an ingredient called capsaicin, which has been found to deplete nerve cells of a chemical that helps transmit pain messages.

Applied as a cream, capsaicin can relieve joint and muscle pain. Make sure to keep the cream away from your eyes, nose and mouth and wash your hands after application. Capsaicin is also taken in tablet form to relieve gastrointestinal problems.

The Food and Drug Administration has approved use of capsicum in over-the-counter topical pain relievers.

Our take

We give cayenne a green light because it can be an effective topical pain reliever for rheumatoid arthritis and osteoarthritis, as well as for nerve damage caused by the complications of diabetes. Follow label directions. For other conditions, be cautious. The evidence still isn't there to support its use.

What the research says

Several studies support the use of topical capsaicin for pain relief, especially to joints located close to the skin's surface, such as fingers, knees and elbows. There have been fewer studies done on capsaicin taken in pill form. It may have some therapeutic benefit for gastrointestinal problems, but there are no studies supporting its effectiveness.

Chasteberry

Chasteberry (*Vitex agnus-castus*) is the peppery fruit of a tree that's native to the Mediterranean region. Long thought to inspire chastity, it earned the name "monk's pepper" in the Middle Ages. Monks supposedly chewed chaste tree parts to make it easier to maintain their celibacy.

Today, chasteberry is used primarily to treat menstrual conditions. Evidence that it can treat infertility in women is weak. There's no evidence it reduces sexual desire.

Our take

Early research suggests chasteberry may be an effective treatment for symptoms of premenstrual syndrome (PMS) and premenstrual dysphoric disorder (PMDD). While the herb appears relatively safe, its full effects aren't known, so use it with caution.

What the research says

In clinical trials, chasteberry reduced menstrual-related symptoms including breast pain or tenderness, swelling, cramps, food cravings, irritability, and depressed mood. Though generally well tolerated, chasteberry can cause gastrointestinal upset, headache and itching.

Cinnamon

In addition to a kitchen spice, cinnamon is used in traditional medicine. There are many different types of cinnamon. The variety *Cinnamomum cassia* is the one most often used in natural remedies.

People take cinnamon to help control type 2 diabetes. It's also taken for digestive disorders, including preventing nausea and treatment of stomach cramps, and a variety of other conditions.

In addition, cinnamon is an ingredient in lotions, mouthwashes and toothpaste.

Our take

Cinnamon is safe when used appropriately, but it needs more study. The cinnamon sold for cooking and baking generally contains a mixture of different varieties. You don't know how much — if any — *Cinnamomum cassia* you're getting. Don't set aside proven diabetes medications for cinnamon. Use of cassia cinnamon for other conditions lacks reliable information.

What the research says

Most research suggests that cinnamon isn't an effective treatment for diabetes. In one preliminary study, cinnamon extract seemed to lower blood sugar and cholesterol in people with type 2 diabetes. However, other studies haven't confirmed these results. Another study found cinnamon ineffective at reducing blood cholesterol or triglyceride levels.

Devil's claw

Devil's claw (*Harpagophytum procumbens*) has been used in the traditional medicine of people of the Kalahari Desert in southern Africa.

The plant is also known as the "hook plant." It gets its name from the appearance of its fruit, which is covered with hooks. The hooks are designed to attach to animals in order to spread the seeds.

Devil's claw is used to relieve pain and inflammation in joints and to treat headache and back pain.

Our take

Devil's claw is used extensively in Europe and appears to be effective as an anti-inflammatory agent for treating osteoarthritis and low back pain. Side effects appear to be minimal. Initially, some people experience diarrhea, but it usually goes away after a short while. There's no known benefit for rheumatoid arthritis.

What the research says

Studies suggest devil's claw helps to decrease osteoarthritic pain. Separate trials indicate that it may also help alleviate low back pain. The medicinal ingredients in the plant's roots are thought to contain anti-inflammatory properties. However, additional study is needed before more definitive recommendations can be made.

Echinacea

You may know echinacea by its common name, the coneflower. It belongs to the same plant family as the sunflower, thistle and black-eyed Susan.

The roots and herbs from three echinacea species are prepared for medicinal use as pills, applications and teas. The most popular is *Echinacea purpurea*, or the purple coneflower.

Echinacea traditionally has been used to treat everything from skin wounds to dizziness to cancer. In the 20th century, it became an extremely popular remedy for colds and flu.

Recent interest in echinacea is due to its purported ability to boost the immune system — in particular, its ability to fight colds and upper respiratory tract infections.

The use of echinacea is popular and growing. In the United States, sales of echinacea may represent about 10 percent of the dietary supplement market.

Because the active ingredient hasn't been identified, there's often a problem with quality control. Some products may contain very small amounts of echinacea, if any at all.

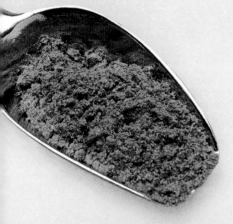

Our take

Unfortunately, there's still no cure for the common cold. Despite all of the claims, latest study results suggest echinacea isn't an effective method for cold prevention or treatment, as once thought. If you have a cold, it won't hurt you to try echinacea for a few days, but there's no guarantee that it will help. Don't use it for more than eight weeks at a time. As for other claims, the research isn't there yet. It's unclear whether echinacea can boost the immune system.

What the research says

Here's what some studies of echinacea have found:

Cancer

There's no clear evidence that echinacea has an effect on any type of cancer in humans.

Immune system booster

Echinacea has been studied alone and in combination with other ingredients for its effect on the immune system — including people receiving chemotherapy for cancer. It's still unclear if there are any significant benefits. Definitive conclusions will require additional studies regarding safety and effectiveness.

Upper respiratory tract infections

Numerous human trials have found echinacea can reduce the duration and severity of upper respiratory infections, particularly when the herb is taken at the earliest onset of symptoms. Some studies have also found echinacea may reduce your risk of getting a cold. However, many of the trials have been small or of weak design. And some studies have found echinacea to be of no benefit.

Vaginal yeast infection

Some studies have found that taking echinacea orally in combination with a topical antifungal cream seems to help prevent recurrent vaginal yeast infection.

Ephedra

Ephedra sinica, or ma-huang, is an evergreen shrub native to the Central Asian desert. It contains the alkaloids ephedrine and pseudoephedrine, which stimulate the central nervous system.

Ephedra was once a popular remedy for weight loss and obesity (it's frequently combined with caffeine in medications) and to enhance athletic performance. It's also been used for asthma, allergies, colds and headache.

Because of its serious side effects, the sale of dietary supplements containing ephedra is no longer allowed in the United States. The herb can cause severe life-threatening or disabling conditions in some people, including heart attack, seizure and stroke. However, ephedra products are still available on the Internet.

Our take

We don't recommend ephedra for treatment of obesity or any other condition because it can be dangerous. Serious cardiovascular side effects may occur if the herb is taken at higher doses.

What the research says

Ephedra is most commonly taken for weight loss. It also was once a popular treatment for asthma, colds and other respiratory illnesses.

Asthma

Ephedra became a popular treatment for childhood asthma in the 1920s because of its ability to relax the bronchial air passages. Since then, better asthma medications have been developed. Ephedra also is considered too risky because it can cause serious side effects, and commercial products may contain variable concentrations of the herb — either too much or too little.

Weight loss

Ephedra used in combination with caffeine appears to promote weight loss. But studies to date have been small and not of good quality, and they raised serious concerns about the safety of ephedra.

Herbs to watch out for

Some herbs may pose serious health risks. Here is a listing of herbs considered to be dangerous, either because of their potential for serious side effects or because overdoses can be fatal. This list isn't complete — there may be others.

Alpine ragwort	Ephedra	Lobelia
Belladonna	Germander	Pennyroyal
Bitter orange	Golden ragwort (life root)	Scotch broom
Chaparral	Goldenseal	Skullcap
Coltsfoot	Kava	Yohimbe
Comfrey	Licorice	Herbs containing aristolochic acid (such as wild ginger)

Keep in mind that dangerous herbs may be mixed into products that contain a combination of herbs. That's why it's important to read the label on all products so that you know what you're taking. For information on safe use of

Herbal weight-loss products: Do they work?

The appeal of quick weight loss with the help of over-the-counter weight-loss pills is often hard to pass up. But are they a safe option for weight loss? And do they do anything but lighten your wallet?

The chart below lists some herbs and other compounds used in over-the-counter weight-loss pills and what they will — and won't — do for you.

Dietary supplements and weight-loss aids aren't subject to the same rigorous standards as are prescription drugs or medications sold over-the-counter. Therefore, they can be marketed with limited proof of effectiveness or safety.

Many weight-loss pills contain a cocktail of ingredients — some with more than 20 herbs, botanicals, vitamins, minerals or other

add-ons. Some over-the-counter weight-loss products even include unapproved prescription medications — ingredients such as sibutramine, fenproporex, fluoxetine, bumetanide, furosemide, phenytoin and cetilist.

How the ingredients in many "herbal" products interact within your body is largely unknown. Using them can be a risky venture.

Supplement	The claims	What you need to know
Bitter orange	Decreases appetite	• Touted as an "ephedra substitute" but may cause health problems similar to those of ephedra • Long-term effects unknown
Chitosan	Blocks absorption of dietary fat	• Relatively safe, but unlikely to cause weight loss • Can cause constipation, bloating and other gastrointestinal complaints • Long-term effects unknown
Chromium	Reduces body fat and builds muscle	• Relatively safe, but unlikely to build muscle or cause weight loss • Long-term effects unknown
Conjugated linoleic acid (CLA)	Reduces body fat, decreases appetite and builds muscle	• Might decrease body fat and increase muscle, but isn't likely to reduce total weight • Can cause diarrhea, indigestion and other gastrointestinal problems
Country mallow (heartleaf)	Decreases appetite and increases the number of calories burned	• Contains ephedrine, which is dangerous • Likely unsafe and should be avoided
Ephedra	Decreases appetite	• Can cause high blood pressure, heart rate irregularities, sleeplessness, seizures, heart attacks, strokes and even death • Banned because of safety concerns
Green tea extract	Increases calorie and fat metabolism and decreases appetite	• Limited evidence to support claim • Can cause vomiting, bloating, indigestion and diarrhea • May contain a large amount of caffeine
Guar gum	Blocks absorption of dietary fat and increases the feeling of fullness, which leads to decreased calorie intake	• Relatively safe, but unlikely to cause weight loss • Can cause diarrhea and other gastrointestinal problems
Hoodia	Decreases appetite	• No conclusive evidence to support claim

Feverfew

Feverfew (*Tanacetum parthenium*), also known as bachelor's button or midsummer daisy, is a member of the daisy family. It has been used for centuries to fight migraines, fever, rheumatoid arthritis and menstrual irregularity.

Generally, the feverfew leaf is prepared as a powder or tablet. The active ingredient is parthenolide. For the treatment of migraines, parthenolide seems to make the cerebral blood vessels less reactive to chemicals that may cause headaches.

The herb has been used safely in studies lasting up to four months.

Our take

If you experience migraines and aren't helped by medication, you may want to give feverfew a try to see if you notice any benefits. However, do so only under a doctor's supervision, don't take more than the recommended amount and don't take it for more than a few months. Be aware that feverfew may cause an allergic reaction in people sensitive to flowers such as daisies and marigolds.

What the research says

Studies indicate that feverfew, taken at the recommended daily amount, can reduce the frequency of migraine attacks. It may also reduce pain and nausea. Because these were short-term studies, the effects of long-term use remains unknown. More evidence is needed from longer term studies.

Evidence that the herb is beneficial in the treatment of rheumatoid arthritis is inconclusive.

Flaxseed

Flaxseed is available in many forms. Whole or crushed flaxseed can be mixed with water or juice and taken by mouth. Flaxseed is sold in a powder form, as meal or flour. And flaxseed oil is available in liquid and capsule form.

Flaxseed and flaxseed (linseed) oil are rich sources of the essential fatty acid alpha-linolenic acid, which is similar to some heart-healthy fatty acids in fish oil.

Flaxseed — but not flaxseed oil — is also high in soluble fibber and rich in lignans, which may have anti-cancer properties. Lignans are a type of fiber containing a chemical (a phytoestrogen) similar to the human hormone estrogen.

Flaxseed is taken to treat constipation, reduce cholesterol and blood sugar, relieve symptoms of menopause and prevent cancer. Because it may have anti-inflammatory properties, some people also take it to treat inflammatory diseases such as lupus or rheumatoid arthritis.

While considered safe, consuming flaxseed in large amounts may lead to bloating, gas and diarrhea — or constipation if seed or powder forms aren't taken with enough water. Because it may lower the body's ability to absorb medications, it's best not to take flaxseed at the same time as medications or other dietary supplements.

Gamma linolenic acid

Gamma linolenic acid (GLA) is an omega-6 fatty acid. It's necessary for good health, but it isn't produced in the body.

The body obtains GLA from the breakdown of certain foods during digestion. GLA supplements are available from seed extracts of black currant, borage and evening primrose.

GLA is converted in the body to compounds with anti-inflammatory properties. It's used to treat a wide range of conditions, including rheumatoid arthritis, inflammation of the skin (dermatitis), nerve damage due to diabetes and ulcerative colitis.

Our take

We give gamma linolenic acid a green light because it appears to help prevent nerve damage (peripheral neuropathy) from diabetes. There really is no better alternative treatment for this condition, and GLA appears to be relatively safe. But make sure to follow label directions.

For treatment of other conditions, such as rheumatoid arthritis, there's not enough evidence that it works.

What the research says

Two good-quality studies indicate that GLA may help prevent nerve damage in people with diabetes. Additional larger studies are needed to confirm this result.

There's some evidence that GLA may be useful in the treatment of rheumatoid arthritis but, again, more study is needed. Benefits are not apparent for the treatment of dermatitis.

Our take

When flaxseed is consumed as part of a healthy lifestyle approach — an approach that also includes daily exercise and following a low-cholesterol diet — it can be helpful in controlling cholesterol levels.

What the research says

Studies show that flaxseed — about 40 to 50 grams a day — can reduce total cholesterol and low-density lipoprotein (LDL, or "bad") cholesterol levels. There's also some indication that it may lower blood sugar levels in people with type 2 diabetes. However, because most of the studies haven't been well designed, additional research is needed to determine flaxseed's benefits.

For the treatment of menopausal symptoms, results have been mixed, but in some women with mild symptoms, flaxseed reduced hot flashes and night sweats.

Most of the evidence relating to flaxseed's potential anti-cancer properties comes from laboratory research. Researchers have found that a diet supplemented with flaxseed may reduce formation and spread of prostate cancer, breast cancer and melanoma in mice. More research in humans is needed.

Garlic

Garlic (*Allium sativum*) is a member of the lily family and a close relative of the onion. It's been used for centuries to treat conditions ranging from high blood pressure to tumors to protection from snake venom.

Researchers believe the compound allicin, which gives garlic its aroma and flavor, is responsible for garlic's health benefits. Allicin is thought to be a powerful antioxidant.

Garlic's most common uses are for high cholesterol, heart disease and high blood pressure. It's also used to prevent certain cancers, including stomach and colon cancers. It's most effective when you eat it raw and in large amounts, but it can also be purchased dried or powdered, and in tablet or capsule form.

Garlic is safe for most adults. Side effects include breath and body odor, heartburn and stomach upset. You shouldn't use garlic if you're taking anti-clotting drugs because garlic can reduce the ability of blood to clot, thereby increasing the risk of bleeding.

Our take

Garlic gets a green light because studies suggest that garlic and garlic supplements may help lower low-density lipoprotein (LDL, or "bad") cholesterol, and the supplements appear to be of low risk, except in individuals taking anti-clotting medications.

If you take garlic tablets, make sure they contain allicin, the active ingredient in garlic. Odor-free preparations may not include allicin.

What the research says

Here's what some studies have found:

Cancer

Some studies suggest consuming garlic as a regular part of your diet may lower the risk of certain cancers, including gastric and colon cancers. However, no clinical trials have examined this.

Cholesterol

Several studies have reported small reductions in total blood cholesterol and in low-density lipoprotein (LDL, or "bad") cholesterol from garlic use. Well-designed and longer studies are needed to gather more information.

Heart

Preliminary research suggests garlic may slow hardening of the arteries (atherosclerosis), a condition that can lead to heart disease. Research also suggests garlic may reduce blood pressure in people with hypertension and in those with normal blood pressure.

Ginger

Ginger (*Zingiber officinale*) is an aromatic spice from Asia. The product you buy in grocery stores is the underground stem (rhizome) of the plant. It's also available as a powder, tablet, extract, tincture and oil.

Traditionally, ginger has been used to relieve nausea from pregnancy (morning sickness), as well as nausea related to motion sickness, chemotherapy and use of anesthesia during surgery. Ginger may also be used to treat pain associated with arthritis.

Few side effects are linked to ginger when it's taken in small doses. However, ginger is not recommended for nausea during pregnancy if you have a history of bleeding disorders or miscarriages.

Our take

Ginger gets a green light because it's been shown to be somewhat effective in reducing morning sickness and in delaying motion sickness and in speeding recovery from it. It's generally considered safe when taken in small amounts and for a short term. High doses can cause abdominal discomfort.

Before taking ginger to prevent nausea associated with pregnancy, talk with your doctor. Avoid ginger if you take anticoagulant medications because it may increase bleeding risk.

What the research says

Here's what some studies have found:

Arthritis

It is unclear whether ginger is effective in treating osteoarthritis, rheumatoid arthritis, or joint or muscle pain. Results of a few small studies have been mixed.

Nausea

A limited number of studies suggest that ginger may help ease nausea from pregnancy when used for short periods. However, it takes a few days for ginger to work. Study results on the effectiveness of ginger to prevent or relieve nausea from motion sickness, chemotherapy and anesthesia have been mixed.

Avoid Internet misinformation: Check the three D's

Although the Internet offers an ideal way to discover the latest in alternative medicine treatments, it is also one of the greatest sources of misinformation. To weed out the good information from the bad, use the three D's:

Dates. Check the creation or update date for each article. If you don't see a date, don't assume the article is recent. Older material may be outdated and not include recent findings.

Documentation. Check the sources. Are qualified health professionals creating and reviewing the information? Is advertising clearly identified? Look for the logo from the Health on the Net (HON) Foundation, which means that the site follows HON's principles for reliability and credibility of information.

Double-check. Visit several health sites and compare the information they offer. If you can't find supporting evidence to back up the claims of an alternative product, be skeptical. And before you follow any advice you read on the Internet, check with your conventional doctor for guidance.

Ginkgo

Ginkgo (*Ginkgo biloba*) is one of the oldest living species of tree. Its fan-shaped leaves as well as seeds have both been used in traditional medicine, but today most ginkgo products are made with extract prepared from the dried leaves.

The beneficial components of ginkgo are believed to be flavonoids, which have powerful antioxidant qualities, and terpenoids, which help improve circulation by dilating blood vessels and reducing the "stickiness" of platelets.

Ginkgo has been used to treat circulatory disorders and symptoms associated with reduced blood flow to the brain, particularly in older adults. These symptoms include memory loss, dizziness, headache and ringing in the ears.

The herb is generally well tolerated but should be used cautiously if you're taking anti-clotting medication (including aspirin). You should also avoid the herb if you're taking a thiazide diuretic. Ginkgo may raise your blood pressure if used with this drug.

Our take

Studies have produced some encouraging results for the use of ginkgo as a treatment of certain circulation disorders and what are sometimes called cerebral insufficiencies — symptoms such as absent-mindedness and confusion — which may be associated with Alzheimer's disease. However, studies have found ginkgo isn't an overall "brain booster," and the safety and effectiveness of ginkgo haven't always been proved.

What the research says

Here's what some studies have found:

Claudication

A number of studies suggest that ginkgo causes small improvements in the symptoms of claudication, such as leg pain due to clogged arteries. However, ginkgo may not be as helpful for this condition as exercise or some prescription drugs.

Dementia

Some studies have suggested that ginkgo benefits early-stage Alzheimer's disease and certain dementias, and that it may be as helpful as some drugs. But more recent studies, which have been larger and well-controlled, indicate that ginkgo doesn't reduce the risk of Alzheimer's or other dementias.

Memory enhancement

Recent studies also suggest that ginkgo doesn't improve memory and brain function. Over the years, ginkgo has been touted as a remedy for reducing the effects of aging on the brain. However, there's not enough evidence to recommend ginkgo for this purpose. A 2009 study of 3,000 people found no difference in attention, memory and other cognitive functions between those who took ginkgo and those who didn't.

Other

Studies indicate possible benefits of ginkgo in the treatment of depression and seasonal affective disorder, glaucoma, macular degeneration, tinnitus, sexual dysfunction, and some symptoms of premenstrual syndrome (PMS).

Ginseng

The term *ginseng* generally refers to two species of the plant, Asian ginseng (*Panax ginseng*) and American ginseng (*Panax quinquefolius*). Siberian ginseng (*Eleutherococcus senticosus*) is a different type of plant, and it doesn't contain the same active ingredients as Asian and American ginseng.

The gnarled, brown ginseng root is the part of the plant that's used in supplements. The root sometimes resembles a human body because of stringy offshoots that look like arms and legs. Due to that resemblance, practitioners of traditional Chinese medicine often considered the herb a cure-all for most human ills: allergies, asthma, appetite stimulant, bleeding disorders, breathing difficulties, cancer, dizziness, headache, heart disorders, insomnia, liver disease, stroke, and many more.

It's best not to take ginseng for more than three months or to exceed the recommended maximum daily doses. Also don't take ginseng if you have uncontrolled high blood pressure, as the herb may raise blood pressure.

Our take

The sum total of evidence suggests that short-term use of ginseng may improve mental performance and that it produces few side effects when taken as directed, therefore we give it a green light. Never take ginseng for an extended period of time. More research is needed before specific recommendations regarding its use can be made.

More studies are also needed to determine ginseng's effectiveness against diabetes. Ginseng shouldn't be substituted for proven therapies.

What the research says

Here's what some studies have found:

Cancer

Studies report that ginseng may reduce the risk of certain cancers, but much of this work was undertaken by the same research group and is considered preliminary. A Mayo Clinic study did find that ginseng seemed to reduce fatigue in people with cancer. The results are being confirmed in an ongoing study.

Exercise performance

Athletes use ginseng to improve stamina, but it's unclear how much benefit it provides. Study results have been mixed.

Heart

Ginseng appears to have some antioxidant effects that may benefit people with heart disorders. However, better studies are needed to make a firm recommendation.

Mental performance and mood

Studies report that ginseng can modestly improve the performance of thinking and learning tasks, based on measurements of reaction time, concentration and logic. Ginseng may also improve mood and enhance sleep. Although this evidence is promising, most studies have been small and not of the best design.

Type 2 diabetes

Several studies report that ginseng may lower blood sugar levels in people with type 2 diabetes, both at fasting states and after eating. Limit daily amounts to no more than 3 grams. The glucose-lowering effect may vary among preparations because of variations in substances called ginsenosides.

Goji berry

Goji berries are orangish-red berries that come from a shrub native to China called the lycium shrub. In Asia, people have eaten goji berries for generations in hopes the berries will help them live longer.

Today people eat dried berries, take goji berry supplements or drink goji berry juice for a variety of conditions, including diabetes, high blood pressure and cancer. The berry is also thought to boost brain health, improve circulation and treat eye disorders.

Like other berries, such as blueberries or strawberries, goji berries are high in antioxidants. Antioxidants may slow aging by reducing damage to cells.

Our take

While this juice has become quite popular, there isn't enough data to determine whether it really offers something special beyond other, less costly fruit juices. Also, many manufacturers recommend very high doses or offer potent extracts of the berry. The safety of long-term use at such high doses is unknown.

What the research says

There's insufficient information available about goji berries to determine if they're effective. Studies to date have generally been done in the laboratory or in animals, and not in humans. Goji berry products appear to be safe; however, they may interact with some medications. Because of this, talk to your doctor before consuming goji berries.

Goldenseal

Goldenseal (*Hydrastis canadensis*) is a member of the buttercup family. It received its name from the gold scars on the base of the stem.

The plant's underground stem (rhizome) contains an ingredient called berberine, which may act as an antibiotic and mild laxative. Goldenseal is used to disinfect cuts and treat various inflammatory conditions, and it's prepared as a digestive aid. The herb is also combined with echinacea to treat upper respiratory tract infections.

Unfortunately, goldenseal can have serious side effects, especially when taken in high doses for long periods.

Our take

Although goldenseal has demonstrated certain antibiotic and anti-inflammatory qualities, studies regarding the effectiveness and safety of this herb have been of poor quality. Goldenseal gets a red light because it can produce serious side effects if used for longer periods, and there's insufficient evidence that it works.

What the research says

Several studies examined the use of goldenseal to treat infectious diarrhea. There are questions regarding the amount of active ingredient used and whether this amount was significant enough to have an effect.

Goldenseal may be combined with echinacea to treat colds and upper respiratory tract infections. Although the ingredient berberine may possess certain antimicrobial qualities, its effect in humans needs more study.

Green tea

Green tea is made from the dried leaves of *Camellia sinensis*, an evergreen shrub native to Southeast Asia. History dates its use in China as far back as 5,000 years ago. To this day, tea remains an integral part of daily life in many Asian societies, and consumption of green tea has become widespread throughout the world.

Processing the leaves of *Camellia sinensis* in different ways produces the different varieties of green tea, black tea and oolong tea. Tea contains polyphenols — compounds with strong antioxidant activity. Another active ingredient in tea is caffeine, which stimulates the nervous system and heart and acts as a diuretic.

People living in Asian countries, where green tea has been shown to have health benefits, have access to better quality green tea than do most Americans. Generally, the less processed the tea leaves are, the stronger the tea's antioxidant properties. To find the good stuff, check out Asian grocery stores or specialty tea shops.

Our take

Although all of the benefits of green tea still haven't been proved, it gets a green light because it does appear to have some medicinal qualities and it doesn't pose serious side effects. Drinking green tea possibly may help reduce the risk of various cancers. It's also linked to lower blood cholesterol and triglycerides. Research on the tea's benefits is continuing, and we hope to know more in the near future.

What the research says

Here's what some studies have found:

Cancer prevention

Drinking green tea is associated with reduced risk of bladder, esophageal and pancreatic cancers. There is also some evidence that women who regularly consume green tea may be at lower risk of developing ovarian cancer. Green tea in the form of an oral or topical preparation may also reduce cervical dysplasia, a condition that increases risk of cervical cancer.

Cardiovascular conditions

Green tea taken orally seems to lower cholesterol and triglycerides. Evidence suggests higher consumption is associated with significantly lowered total cholesterol, triglycerides, low-density lipoprotein (LDL, or "bad") cholesterol and increased high-density lipoprotein (HDL, or "good") cholesterol.

Genital warts

A specific green tea extract ointment (Veregen) can clear genital warts after 10 to 16 weeks. This prescription product is approved by the Food and Drug Administration.

Longevity

A 2006 study involving 40,000 people in Japan found the more green tea people drank, the longer they lived. Cardiovascular disease was significantly less common among those who drink more than five cups a day.

Obesity

Small trials have looked at the association between green tea consumption and weight loss. Study results are mixed. More research is needed.

Hawthorn

Hawthorn (multiple crataegus species) is a thorny shrub from the rose family. Historically, the fruit was used in traditional medicine, but today extracts from the flowers and leaves are more common.

It's a popular alternative medicine for cardiovascular health. Active ingredients include flavonoids, which are known to help dilate blood vessels, improve blood flow and increase heart rate. Other ingredients in hawthorn have powerful antioxidant effects.

Our take

Although hawthorn appears to have some positive benefits regarding cardiovascular health, not enough is known about its effectiveness and safety. Don't self-medicate with hawthorn. If you have a heart condition, talk with your doctor before taking the herb.

What the research says

Results from multiple studies indicate that hawthorn may be beneficial in the treatment of congestive heart failure. However, there's insufficient evidence regarding its effectiveness in treating coronary artery disease, angina and other cardiovascular disorders.

Hoodia

Hoodia (*Hoodia gordonii*) is a cactus native to the Kalahari Desert in southern Africa. The native San people have been known to eat hoodia to ward off hunger and thirst during long hunts.

The active ingredient has been identified as P57. This compound is believed to stimulate the hypothalamus, a portion of the brain's interior that turns off hunger signals. You end up thinking you're full even if you haven't eaten. This quality has made hoodia a popular ingredient in weight-loss products.

Our take

There's still too much that's unknown about hoodia to recommend its use. More research is needed to establish its potential effectiveness and long-term safety as an appetite suppressant. In addition, unregulated products claiming to contain hoodia may have little or none of the active ingredient.

What the research says

To date, no objective, long-term studies have been undertaken to demonstrate the effectiveness and safety of hoodia as an appetite suppressant. One small study — sponsored by a supplement manufacturer — suggests that the herb affects the part of the brain that controls hunger.

Kava

Kava comes from a pepper plant called *Piper methysticum* that's native to the South Pacific islands. The root of the plant is a source of extracts and powder. Kava is also commonly consumed as a beverage.

The active ingredient in kava acts as a sedative and a muscle relaxant. Therefore, it became popular as a stress and anxiety reliever. Some people use it to relieve insomnia.

Because of its sedating effects, kava should never be taken before driving or operating heavy machinery. And it shouldn't be mixed with alcohol or other sedatives.

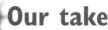
Our take

Kava appeared to be a promising treatment for stress and anxiety, but reports of serious liver problems — even with short-term use — caused the herb to lose its luster. A recent review of these reports has raised the possibility that the problems occurred because the users had underlying liver problems or used the herb incorrectly. We still advise avoiding kava until more information is available.

What the research says

Numerous well-conducted studies have found kava to be at least moderately effective in the treatment of anxiety. In fact, kava may be as effective as certain prescribed medications. However, reports of severe liver damage linked to its use have caused several European countries to pull it off the market. The Food and Drug Administration has issued warnings but not banned sales.

What makes a good study?

As you read through this publication, you'll find that quite often we say the product hasn't been "well studied," or it needs "more rigorous scientific study." So what constitutes a good study?

In general, the larger the study the better. When a study involves several hundred people or more — especially if the study lasts over several years — it gains more credibility.

How the study was performed also is key. Prospective double-blind studies that have been carefully controlled, randomized and published in peer-reviewed journals are the gold standard. What does that mean? Here's some information to help you out.

- **Clinical studies** are those that involve human beings — not animals. They're usually preceded by studies that demonstrate safety and effectiveness of the treatment in animals.

- In **randomized controlled trials,** participants are usually divided into two groups. The first group receives the treatment being studied. The second is a control group. People in this group receive standard treatment, no treatment or an inactive substance called a placebo. Participants are assigned to these groups on a random basis to help ensure all of the groups will be similar.

- In **double-blind studies,** neither the researchers nor the participants know who is receiving the active treatment or who is receiving the placebo.

- **Prospective studies** are forward-looking. Researchers establish criteria for study participants to follow and then measure or describe the results. Information from these studies is usually more reliable than that of retrospective studies. **Retrospective studies** involve looking at past data, which leaves more room for errors in interpretation.

- **Peer-reviewed journals** only publish articles that have been reviewed by an independent panel of medical experts.

Mangosteen

Mangosteen (*Garcinia mangostana*) is a tropical fruit native to Southeast Asia. Despite its name, mangosteen isn't related to the mango. The fruit is the size and shape of a tangerine, with a thick, dark rind and creamy flesh.

Mangosteen's rind and pulp can be blended together and sold as a drink. The juice typically consists of a mix of mangosteen and other fruit juices, such as apple, pear and blueberry — often with an undisclosed amount of mangosteen juice.

Mangosteen juice has become a popular drink that's often marketed with the name Xango Juice. Mangosteen products are also available in capsule and tablet form.

Like many fruits and vegetables, mangosteen is a rich source of antioxidants, natural compounds in foods that may protect against certain diseases, such as heart disease and cancer. Mangosteen also contains unique chemicals called xanthones, which appear to have potent anti-inflammatory effects.

Mangosteen is promoted to maintain the body's microbiological balance, help the immune system, improve joint flexibility, fight infections and inflammation, treat menstrual problems, improve mental health, and a host of other benefits.

Because the fruit isn't readily available in the United States, products made from mangosteen are generally expensive.

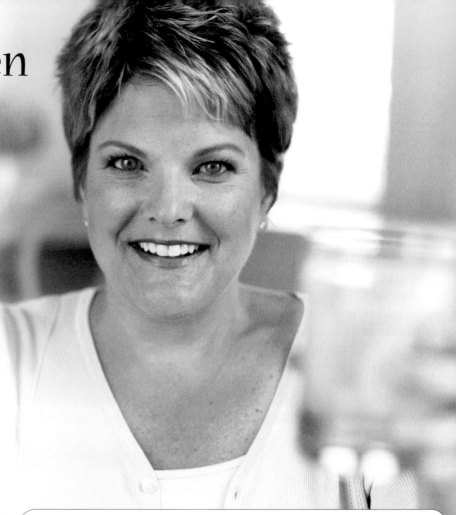

Our take

Mangosteen shows possible promise as an immune system booster, helping your body to fight off germs and infection. But it lacks quality evidence demonstrating that either the fruit or its juice is an effective treatment. At this time, don't expect much beyond the nutritional benefit of its fruit.

What the research says

At this point, there is insufficient reliable information available about the effectiveness of mangosteen. Of those studies that have been done, most have taken place in a laboratory and not in humans. In laboratory tests, mangosteen extracts were used to stop certain bacteria and fungi from growing. In the laboratory, mangosteen also slowed growth of certain cancer cells.

A large scale trial of mangosteen is currently under way at Mayo Clinic. The results of that trial should shed significant light on the ultimate role of mangosteen in human health.

Milk thistle

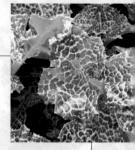

Milk thistle (*Silybum marianum*) is a member of the aster family and named from the white veins on its spiked, variegated leaves. It was commonly used in ancient Greece and Rome to treat disorders of the liver and gallbladder.

The active ingredient in milk thistle is silymarin, which is extracted from the plant's seeds. This flavonoid is believed to have antioxidant qualities. Milk thistle is considered safe to use within recommended amounts, and it typically doesn't produce any serious side effects.

Milk thistle supplements are available as a capsule, tablet, powder and liquid extract.

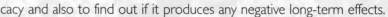

Our take

Milk thistle gets a green light because its active ingredients appear to protect the liver and block or remove harmful substances from the organ. More extensive research is still needed to determine the herb's efficacy and also to find out if it produces any negative long-term effects.

What the research says

Studies suggest milk thistle may reduce blood sugar levels when combined with conventional diabetes treatment. It also seems to improve symptoms of indigestion (dyspepsia). Milk thistle may also limit further liver damage in people with certain liver conditions, including alcohol-related liver disease, toxin-induced liver damage and hepatitis.

Because most studies have been small, and some poorly designed, more research is needed.

Mistletoe

Mistletoe (*Viscum album*) was a sacred herb in Celtic traditions and considered a "cure-all." The two major types of mistletoe are the European and American varieties.

Mistletoe has been used in Europe as an anti-cancer therapy, but it's not an accepted cancer treatment in the United States.

Mistletoe extracts are prescription drugs given by injection. It's important to note that you should never eat any part of the plant or drink the extract because mistletoe is poisonous.

Our take

In Germany, it's common for people with cancer to take mistletoe in addition to receiving chemotherapy or radiation. Despite its widespread acceptance in Europe, the herb lacks good data to back up its effectiveness and safety. While mistletoe may hold some promise as a cancer treatment, better research is needed before we feel comfortable recommending its use.

What the research says

An extensive body of literature exists regarding use of mistletoe to treat cancer, but the individual studies have been small or of poor design. Therefore, not enough is known about the herb. Although mistletoe extract has shown the ability to stimulate the immune system, there's no evidence that this bolstered immunity prevents or kills cancer cells.

Noni juice

Noni (*Morinda citrifolia*) is a small tree native to the Pacific Islands and Polynesia. It's also known as the Indian mulberry.

The juice from the foul-smelling, bitter-tasting noni fruit is used to treat a wide range of conditions, including arthritis, diabetes, high blood pressure, pain, diarrhea, cancer, AIDS, multiple sclerosis and bad breath. These claims are usually based on testimonials, often from the people who are attempting to sell noni products.

Noni juice is generally safe to drink, but it has been linked to a few cases of liver damage (hepatotoxicity).

Our take

When a product is advertised to treat almost every ailment, that's generally a good indication there's more "hype" than "help" at play. There's no convincing evidence that noni juice has any beneficial effect on your health. Orange juice and apple juice generally contains more antioxidants than does the juice from noni fruit.

What the research says

At least one clinical trial involving noni juice is under way — this one to study the effects of noni juice on people in the advanced stages of cancer. Some studies show that noni juice has antioxidant qualities, but likely no more than almost any other type of fruit. Despite the claims, there's no evidence that noni juice reduces cholesterol.

Passionflower

Passionflower (*Passiflora incarnata*) is a woody vine native to North America, but today it's mainly grown throughout Europe.

American Indians used the herb as a mild sedative. It has been used in traditional medicine for anxiety, insomnia, restlessness and any conditions with possible emotional or psychological origins.

Generally, passionflower is considered safe when used as a flavoring or taken within recommended amounts. In Europe, it's combined with other herbs as an over-the-counter sedative.

Topical preparations are used for hemorrhoids and burns.

Our take

As a folk medicine, passionflower has a long history, and though it lacks good evidence as to its effectiveness, small studies have shown it may reduce anxiety. The herb is generally considered safe to use, as long as you take it according to directions. Keep in mind that because it's a sedative it can cause drowsiness.

What the research says

Passionflower lacks quality clinical trials to show that it effectively treats anxiety or restlessness. Further complicating matters is the fact that passionflower is often combined with hawthorn and valerian in commercial products, making it difficult to distinguish the unique qualities of each herb.

Passionflower is generally considered safe. In some studies it was found to cause dizziness, confusion, sedation and a rapid heartbeat.

Peppermint

Besides being a popular flavoring, peppermint (*Mentha x piperita*) has a long history of use for digestive symptoms such as indigestion, nausea, cramps and diarrhea, as well as for colds and headaches.

The main active ingredient is the phytochemical menthol, which helps relax stomach muscles and improve the flow of bile, allowing food to pass through the stomach faster. Peppermint also has a soothing effect on skin irritations. The herb is generally considered safe for use with few side effects.

Peppermint is available in capsule and liquid forms.

Our take

Peppermint has some benefits in treating certain digestive disorders, such as irritable bowel syndrome and possibly heartburn. However, its muscle-relaxing qualities could worsen heartburn symptoms associated with gastroesophageal reflux disease (GERD), so take it under a doctor's supervision. There's insufficient evidence that peppermint can treat colds, nasal congestion and tension headaches.

What the research says

In some studies, the symptoms of irritable bowel syndrome improved significantly among people taking peppermint capsules. In others, there was no benefit. A combination of peppermint oil and caraway oil has also been shown to alleviate symptoms of heartburn (dyspepsia). More research involving larger, better designed studies is needed to fully determine its effectiveness.

Policosanol

Policosanol is a mixture of alcohol-based compounds derived from sugar cane or beeswax. It's used to protect against heart disease, by lowering cholesterol levels, and is taken to reduce the risk of blood clots.

It's unknown what the active ingredient in policosanol is or how it works, but the supplement is generally safe and well tolerated.

Most studies of policosanol have taken place in Cuba using Cuban sugar cane. Although more than 25 countries currently use policosanol, products are not always readily available in the United States.

Our take

Initial studies on the benefits of policosanol all were done in Cuba — where sugar cane is grown — and all were positive. More recent studies done outside of Cuba haven't produced the same benefits. This draws into question the plant's ability to reduce cholesterol, along with other heart-health claims. You could be wasting your money.

What the research says

A number of studies demonstrated that policosanol can reduce low-density lipoprotein (LDL, or "bad") cholesterol and triglyceride levels and raise high-density lipoprotein (HDL or "good") cholesterol levels. However, more recent studies found the product ineffective. There are also questions regarding optimal dose and long-term safety. Other studies have suggested that the plant may be effective in preventing blood from clotting.

Pycnogenol

Pycnogenol is a compound derived from the bark of the maritime pine tree (*Pinus pinaster*), native to the coast of southern France.

The compound has antioxidant qualities similar to those of green tea and grape seed. Antioxidants help neutralize highly reactive molecules known as free radicals that can damage your body's cells.

Pycnogenol is generally considered safe to use at recommended doses, with no significant side effects.

Our take

Pycnogenol may have a future role as an antioxidant. It should be noted, though, that Pycnogenol probably contains nothing that can't be gained from a diet rich in vegetables and fruits. Because the name is trademarked and patented to a single company, Pycnogenol is likely to be a more expensive option.

What the research says

Studies indicate Pycnogenol may improve breathing in people with asthma, reduce leg pain cause by chronic venous insufficiency, reduce retinal damage (retinopathy) caused by diabetes, and reduce systolic (upper number) blood pressure. However, more studies are needed to better determine how Pycnogenol works and what should be a standardized dose.

Red yeast rice

Red yeast rice is the product of yeast (*Monascus purpureus*) grown on white rice. The powdered yeast-rice mixture is a dietary staple in many parts of Asia and has been used in traditional Chinese medicine, primarily for heart problems.

Red yeast rice contains several compounds that appear to lower cholesterol levels. One of them is monacolin K, the same ingredient as in the prescription cholesterol drug lovastatin (Mevacor). This led to a legal and industrial dispute as to whether red yeast rice should be considered a drug or a dietary supplement.

Don't take red yeast rice if you're already taking cholesterol medication.

Our take

Red yeast rice is capable of lowering blood cholesterol levels and while the supplement is generally considered safe, it also carries the same potential side effects as statin cholesterol drugs. The only advantage of taking red yeast rice in place of a statin drug may be the cheaper cost. However, with a supplement, there's less assurance regarding quality and how much active ingredient is actually in the product you buy.

What the research says

A number of studies indicate that red yeast rice can lower your total blood cholesterol level, your low-density lipoprotein (LDL, or "bad") cholesterol level and your triglyceride level.

Cholestin was a well-known, nonprescription brand of red yeast rice extract until the Food and Drug Administration ruled it was an illegal, unapproved drug. The manufacturer has since reformulated Cholestin without the extract.

Saffron

Saffron is a spice derived from the flower of the saffron crocus (*Crocus sativus*). The dried stigmas of saffron are used to make saffron spice. It can take up to 75,000 saffron blossoms, harvested by hand, to make a pound of spice. That is why saffron is one of the world's most expensive spices.

There is interest in saffron for its anti-cancer effects. Saffron is also used for depression, premenstrual syndrome (PMS), asthma, insomnia and a host of other conditions.

Our take

While several small trials suggest saffron may have some beneficial effects on depression, most of the results come from a single group of researchers in Iran. Until the results are replicated by other researchers, it's probably best to be cautious.

What the research says

Studies suggest saffron may improve symptoms of depression and PMS. However, it may take weeks to notice the effects. Laboratory research and animal studies also indicate that saffron may inhibit growth and spread of cancer cells. Much more study is needed. Saffron seems to be well tolerated.

Saw palmetto

Saw palmetto (*Serenoa repens*) is a fan palm that thrives in the United States' warm southeastern climate. The dark purple berries were a staple food of American Indians and also used as an expectorant and antiseptic.

There are many products on the market today containing saw palmetto, frequently in combination with other ingredients. In Europe, saw palmetto is used to treat symptoms of an enlarged prostate gland, a condition called benign prostatic hyperplasia (BPH). Although saw palmetto is a popular treatment for BPH in the United States, it's not considered a standard treatment.

Saw palmetto is also used as a mild diuretic, a sedative and an antiseptic.

Our take

In some men, saw palmetto can be an effective treatment for managing symptoms of an enlarged prostate. Study results have been mixed. While some studies have found saw palmetto to be very effective for mild to moderate symptoms, others have found it to be of no benefit. Because saw palmetto is generally safe, it doesn't hurt to give it a try. But don't use it if you have a bleeding problem because it can increase bleeding. Talk to your doctor before using saw palmetto.

What the research says

A number of studies have suggested that saw palmetto can increase urine flow, diminish inflammation, reduce nighttime urination and improve the overall quality of life for individuals dealing with an enlarged prostate gland. One larger trial, however, found no significant benefits from saw palmetto use.

Some studies suggest that saw palmetto can be as effective as the anti-androgenic drug finasteride (Proscar). It's not clear if the herb actually reduces the size of the prostate gland or just improves symptoms.

The herb hasn't been found effective for other conditions.

'Herbal viagras' — Are they safe?

Prescription medications such as sildenafil (Viagra) treat erectile dysfunction by increasing blood flow to the penis when a man is sexually aroused. Some herbal products marketed as "natural versions" of these stimulants contain substances that improve blood flow, but are not as specific for blood vessels in the penis as are the prescription drugs. As a result, these herbal remedies may cause generalized low blood pressure and restrict blood flow to vital organs.

The Food and Drug Administration has identified several products sold as so-called "dietary supplements" for treating erectile dysfunction and enhancing sexual performance that are dangerous because they contain potentially harmful ingredients. The following supplements are on the FDA list. There may be more.

Actra-Rx	HS Joy of Love
Actra-Sx	NaturalUp
Libidus	Blue Steel
Nasutra	Erextra
Neophase	Super Shangai
Vigor-25	Strong Testis
Yilishen	Shangai Ultra
Zimaxx	Shangai Ultra X
4Everon	Lady Shangai
Liviro3	Shangai Regular
Lycium Barbarum L.	Hero
Adam Free	Naturale Super Plus
Rhino V Max	Xiadafil VIP tablets
V.Max	True Man
Energy Max	LibieXtreme
Y-4ever	Libimax X Liquid
Powermania	Herbal Disiac

The herb ginseng is widely believed to enhance sexual performance but, lacking significant quality control, it's often difficult to know what kind of product you're getting. Another popular herb called yohimbe can be dangerous if used in excessive amounts.

The bottom line: If you have erectile dysfunction, see your doctor to discuss proven treatment options.

Soy

Soy (*Glycine max*) is a member of the pea family and native to southeastern Asia. The soybean has been a dietary staple of Asian countries for thousands of years. Fermentation techniques allow soy to be prepared in more easily digestible forms such as tempeh, miso, tofu and tamari (soy) sauce.

Active ingredients in soy include isoflavones, weak forms of estrogen that mimic your own naturally occurring estrogen. For that reason, isoflavones are also known as phytoestrogens. How beneficial they are to your body is still being studied.

Interestingly — despite its broad popularity — no one has thoroughly tested the safety and effectiveness of soy as a supplement. Therefore, there's still a lot to learn.

Our take

Diets high in soy foods do have health benefits. For example, soy is a great source of dietary protein minus all of the fat and cholesterol found in meat. Soy also provides fiber, vitamins and minerals. But claims that soy can reduce blood cholesterol levels are uncertain.

Little is known about soy supplements. Although they appear to be safe, use them under your doctor's supervision and with the knowledge that they may be of limited benefit.

What the research says

Here's what some of the research suggests:

Cancer

A few studies attempted to determine the impact of a soy-based diet on hormone-related cancers such as breast, colon and endometrial cancers. Population studies suggest that eating a high-soy diet may slightly reduce a woman's risk of breast cancer. Most of the research has been conducted in Asian women. There's less evidence about the effects of soy in Western populations.

Cardiovascular disease

Studies suggest that soy doesn't affect long-term cardiovascular outcomes such as heart attack or stroke.

High cholesterol

The thinking used to be that adding soy to your diet produced a moderate decrease in cholesterol levels. This view changed after the American Heart Association, following an extensive review of research, concluded that soy-based foods don't significantly lower cholesterol. In addition, the reduction in low-density lipoprotein (LDL, or "bad") cholesterol came from eating large amounts of soy, not the amounts found in many food products.

Menopausal symptoms

Consuming 20 to 60 grams of soy protein daily seems to modestly decrease the frequency and severity of hot flashes in some women.

Osteoporosis

Most evidence suggests that soy protein can increase bone mineral density or slow the loss of bone mineral density.

St. John's wort

St. John's wort (*Hypericum perforatum*) is a flowering shrub that gets its name from the fact that it's often in full bloom on the traditional date of the birthday of the biblical John the Baptist. It has a long history as a treatment for depression, anxiety, insomnia and nervous disorders. It's also prepared as a salve for wounds and burns.

The flowers and leaves contain active ingredients such as hyperforin. But there are other, still unidentified but very active, components in the plant. It's available in tablet, powder and liquid form.

Although St. John's wort is believed to be safe for general use, some of its active compounds don't mix well with prescription drugs and other supplements. These include antidepressant medications, birth control pills, anticoagulant drugs, certain asthma medications and steroids.

Our take

St. John's wort is effective in treating mild to moderate depression and it's relatively safe. It's drawback — and the reason we give it a yellow light instead of a green — is that it interacts with many medications and has caused serious side effects. You shouldn't take St. John's wort if you take prescription medications. It's also important to talk to your doctor before taking St. John's wort. If you have a more severe form of depression, you may need a stronger medication.

What the research says

Studies have generally focused on depression and anxiety:

Anxiety

Results from studies examining the effectiveness of St. John's wort on symptoms of anxiety have been varied. In one case, St. John's wort was combined with the herb valerian. At this time, there's not enough evidence to make a recommendation.

Depression

Several studies support the therapeutic benefit of St. John's wort in treating mild to moderate depression. It's been shown to be as effective as some prescription antidepressants and with fewer side effects. Two studies reported no benefits for major depression. The greatest concern with using St. John's wort is the potential for serious interactions with various types of prescription drugs.

Choosing the right brand

With so many manufacturers of supplements to choose from, how do you know what's a good brand — and that the product actually contains what it says it does? Here are some suggestions:

- **Look for standardized supplements.** The U.S. Pharmacopeia's USP Dietary Supplement Verified seal on the label indicates the product has met certain manufacturing standards. Other groups that certify supplements include ConsumerLab.com, *Good Housekeeping* and NSF International. Although each group takes a slightly different approach, the goal of each is to certify the product meets a certain standard.

- **Look for a large, recognizable manufacturer.** While this isn't a guarantee that the product contains exactly what it says it does, chances are better that a well-known company with a good reputation will make the effort to produce a quality product.

- **Be cautious about supplements manufactured outside the United States.** Many European herbs and other dietary supplements are highly regulated and standardized. But toxic ingredients and prescription drugs have been found in some supplements manufactured in other countries.

Stinging nettle

Stinging nettle (*Urtica dioica*) has a long history of use. Its leaves and stem are covered with tiny hairs containing histamine, an irritating chemical when it comes in contact with the skin.

Stinging nettle is often used for treating an enlarged prostate, often in combination with the herb saw palmetto. It's also used to treat allergic rhinitis, arthritis and joint pain, and insect bites.

Our take

Stinging nettle is generally regarded as safe to use. It's even consumed as a vegetable or made into tea. But how effective it is in treating conditions such as enlarged prostate is uncertain.

What the research says

Several studies suggest that stinging nettle moderately improves symptoms of enlarged prostate. Stinging nettle also may have certain anti-inflammatory qualities for treating joint pain. In both cases, more research is needed.

Valerian

Valerian (*Valeriana officinalis*) is a tall, flowering grassland plant native to Europe and Asia. It is also found in North America. Valerian has long been used as a tranquilizer and to treat insomnia, anxiety and stress.

The roots and underground stems of valerian are used to make teas and supplements, including capsules, tablets and liquid extracts. Many chemical constituents of valerian have been identified, but it's not known which may be responsible for its sleep-promoting effects.

Valerian is generally considered safe to use for short periods of time. It can cause mild side effects such as headaches and dizziness.

Our take

Valerian appears to be beneficial for insomnia and anxiety and is generally safe at recommended doses. Don't take valerian for more than a few weeks at a time.

What the research says

Most research shows that valerian can help you fall asleep and may improve sleep quality. Take valerian an hour or two before bedtime.

There is contradictory evidence about the effectiveness of valerian for anxiety. In some studies, people who used valerian reported less anxiety and stress. In other studies, people reported no benefit.

Vitamin B-3 (niacin)

Vitamin B-3 (niacin) is one of the eight B complex vitamins that help the body convert food to energy. Niacin also helps improve blood circulation and cholesterol levels.

Food sources of niacin include lean meats, poultry, fish, peanuts and brewer's yeast. The recommended daily intake of niacin is 16 milligrams (mg) for men and 14 mg for women.

Seek your doctor's advice before taking a niacin supplement if you have diabetes, gallbladder or liver disease, or glaucoma. Larger doses can cause a flushing reaction.

Our take

Niacin may be used to help improve your cholesterol levels, but this should only be done under a doctor's supervision. Cholesterol-lowering effects typically require large doses (usually greater than 1,000 milligrams a day). In this respect, niacin should be considered a prescribed medication and not a vitamin.

What the research says

Niacin in high doses can reduce low-density lipoprotein (LDL, or "bad") cholesterol and triglycerides and raise high-density lipoprotein (HDL, or "good") cholesterol. Studies show that niacin may also slow the development of atherosclerosis when used with other cholesterol-lowering drugs, diet and exercise. Studies also suggest that niacin may help protect against Alzheimer's disease and age-related mental decline.

Vitamin B-6

Vitamin B-6 (pyridoxine) is an important vitamin for normal brain development and for keeping the nervous system and immune system healthy.

Food sources of vitamin B-6 include poultry, fish, potatoes, lentils, soybeans, whole-grain products, nuts, seeds, carrots and bananas. It can also be taken as a supplement.

There are medications, including certain antibiotics and birth control pills, that interfere with the metabolism of vitamin B-6, possibly causing a vitamin deficiency.

Our take

Vitamin B-6 supplements are effective for treating a hereditary form of anemia and for preventing an adverse reaction to the antibiotic cycloserine. They should be taken under medical supervision.

What the research says

Vitamin B-6 has been shown to work together with vitamins B-9 and B-12 to control blood levels of homocysteine. Elevated levels of homocysteine increase your risk of heart attack or stroke. There is also some evidence that vitamin B-6 may reduce symptoms of premenstrual syndrome (PMS). The larger the doses the greater the risk of side effects, including nerve damage.

Vitamin B-9 (folate or folic acid)

Vitamin B-9, also called folate, occurs naturally in certain foods. Folic acid is the synthetic form of folate. This vitamin is important in red blood cell formation and for healthy cell growth and function. This is especially important during periods of rapid cell division and growth, such as during pregnancy and infancy.

Food sources of folate include citrus juices and fruits, beans, nuts, seeds, dark green leafy vegetables and fortified grain products. Folic acid is found in supplements and in fortified breads and cereals.

The recommended dietary allowance for men and women is 400 micrograms daily.

Our take

There's solid evidence that folate or folic acid can prevent neural tube birth defects such as spina bifida in pregnant women. It may also prevent heart disease and possibly some cancers. If you don't get adequate folate in your diet, take a folic acid supplement or multivitamin. Don't take more than 1,000 micrograms of folic acid daily.

What the research says

Folic acid has been shown to work together with vitamins B-6 and B-12 to control elevated blood levels of homocysteine, reducing your risk of heart attack and stroke. Studies indicate that folate can help prevent anemia during pregnancy and reduce the risk of birth defects. Preliminary results suggest that folate may reduce the risk of breast, cervical and pancreatic cancers.

Vitamin B-12

Vitamin B-12 (cobalamin) plays essential roles in red blood cell formation, cell metabolism, nerve function and production of DNA.

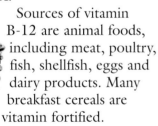

Sources of vitamin B-12 are animal foods, including meat, poultry, fish, shellfish, eggs and dairy products. Many breakfast cereals are vitamin fortified.

Your body is capable of storing several years' worth of vitamin B-12, so a deficiency is rare. However, vegetarians who completely eliminate meat from their diets are prone to a deficiency of this vitamin.

Our take

It's essential to get sufficient amounts of vitamin B-12 because of its importance to almost every body system. Most children and adults in the United States consume recommended amounts of vitamin B-12. Generally, older adults are at a greater risk of developing a deficiency. Supplements are important for vegetarians, as plant foods don't contain vitamin B-12.

What the research says

Studies show that a deficiency of vitamin B-12 can produce abnormal neurological and psychiatric symptoms, including anemia, fatigue, muscle weakness, dementia and mood disturbances.

Preliminary research reveals possibilities for vitamin B-12, in combination with other ingredients, for treating cardiovascular disease, high cholesterol, breast cancer and Alzheimer's disease.

Vitamin C

Vitamin C (ascorbic acid) is necessary for the body to form blood vessels, cartilage, muscle, and collagen in bones. It's also vital in the body's healing process. Vitamin C also has strong antioxidant properties.

The human body doesn't produce vitamin C, so it's necessary to include it in your diet. Food sources include citrus fruits, berries, tomatoes, peppers, broccoli and spinach. Vitamin C supplements come in the form of tablets, capsules and chewables.

Many uses for vitamin C have been proposed. Several studies are looking at the possible benefits of vitamin C, but only a few have produced effective results so far. Research does suggest, though, that higher intakes of vitamin C are associated with improved physical performance and muscle strength, especially in older adults.

Topical preparations containing vitamin C are used to help prevent sunburn and improve the appearance of wrinkled skin.

Most experts recommend getting antioxidants, including vitamin C, from a diet high in fruits, vegetables and whole grains, rather than from taking supplements. Foods provide many other health benefits you can't get from a supplement.

Our take

Vitamin C is important to your physical health and meeting the recommended dietary allowance (75 to 90 mg for adults) is considered essential. Few of the many purported medical uses of vitamin C supplements — to treat asthma, diabetes and cancer — have been proved in scientific studies. Using supplements to treat the common cold remains controversial; however, there's nothing else better and preliminary evidence suggests the supplements may be beneficial.

What the research says

Here's what some of the research suggests:

Age-related macular degeneration (AMD)

Taking vitamin C in combination with other vitamins and minerals seems to prevent AMD from worsening. The benefits tend to be more noticeable in people with more advanced disease.

Atherosclerosis

Studies suggest that vitamin C decreases the risk of atherosclerosis, narrowing of your arteries due to buildup of fatty deposits (plaques). Atherosclerosis increases your risk of a heart attack and other heart-related conditions.

Cancer

Vitamin C may decrease the risk of mouth and other cancers in some people, but more study is needed. Vitamin C appears to lower cancer risk more in men than in women. Researchers suspect that may be because men have a lower intake of antioxidants than do women and therefore may benefit more from supplementation. Studies on the protective effects of vitamin C against developing breast cancer are mixed.

Common cold

Many studies have examined the effect of vitamin C consumption on the prevention and treatment of the common cold. Most have failed to show significant benefits but research is ongoing.

Iron absorption

There's evidence vitamin C increases the body's ability to absorb iron.

Vitamin D

Your body manufactures vitamin D when direct sunlight converts a chemical in your skin into an active form of the vitamin (calciferol). Vitamin D is necessary for building and maintaining healthy bones. That's because calcium, the primary component of bone, can only be absorbed by your body when vitamin D is present.

You can also get vitamin D from certain dietary sources, including fortified milk, fortified cereal and fatty fish such as salmon, mackerel and sardines.

The amount of vitamin D your skin makes depends on many factors, including the time of day, season, latitude and your skin pigmentation. Depending on where you live and your lifestyle, vitamin D production may decrease or be completely absent during the winter months. Sunscreen used during the summer months also can decrease vitamin D production.

The current recommended dietary allowance for vitamin D developed by the Food and Nutrition Board (FNB) is 200 international units (IU) for people ages 19 to 49 years, 400 IU for people ages 50 to 70 years, and 600 IU for those older than 70. The National Osteoporosis Foundation feels those numbers should be higher. It recommends adults under age 50 get 400 to 800 IU daily and adults age 50 and older get 800 to 1,000 IU daily.

Our take

There's a lot of interest in vitamin D, and it's possible we may see a change in recommendations. If you don't get adequate vitamin D from your diet or being outside, supplements may be necessary.

What the research says

Here's what some of the research suggests:

Cancer

Laboratory and animal evidence as well as epidemiologic data suggest that vitamin D plays a role in the prevention of colon, prostate and breast cancers. Further research is needed.

Falls

Older adults who get adequate amounts of vitamin D on a daily basis experience fewer falls.

Inherited disorders

Inherited disorders resulting form an inability to absorb or process vitamin D, such as familial hypophosphatemia, may be treated with vitamin D supplementation.

Osteomalacia

Vitamin D supplements are used to treat adults with severe vitamin D deficiency, resulting in loss of bone mineral content, bone pain, muscle weakness and soft bones (osteomalacia).

Osteoporosis

Studies show that people with adequate amounts of vitamin D and calcium in their diets can prevent or slow bone mineral loss due to osteoporosis and reduce bone fractures.

Psoriasis

Applying a topical preparation that contains a vitamin D compound called calcipotriene to the skin can treat plaque-type psoriasis in some people.

Rickets

This rare condition develops in children with vitamin D deficiency due to lack of sunlight exposure or vitamin D in the diet. Vitamin D supplementation can treat the problem.

Vitamin E

Vitamin E has antioxidant properties, which protect body tissues from damage caused by free radicals — unstable molecules associated with degenerative processes brought on by aging and chronic disease. Vitamin E also protects red blood cells and is important in reproduction.

Vitamin E exists in eight different forms, and the most active form — typically found in supplements — is known as alpha-tocopherol. Food sources of vitamin E include vegetable oils, wheat germ, whole-grain products, avocados, green leafy vegetables and nuts, especially almonds.

For years, vitamin E was thought to offer protection against such conditions as heart disease, cancer, Alzheimer's disease and cataracts. As a result, many people began taking supplements in megadoses. But a recent analysis of clinical trials found more was not necessarily better when it came to this vitamin. Studies showed people who consume at least 400 IU of vitamin E daily for at least a year could be at an increased risk of premature death.

It should be noted that many of the study participants had chronic illnesses. And in many of the trials, the participants took supplements containing multiple antioxidants, masking the specific role played by vitamin E. Still, high daily intake may pose health risks and should be avoided.

Our take

It's known that getting plenty of vitamin E in your diet is good for you. Therefore, the belief was that vitamin E supplements would be beneficial, too. However, studies involving people who took alpha-tocopherol vitamin E supplements have produced negative results. This has led researchers to question if other forms of vitamin E might be better than alpha-tocopherol, including a "mixed" vitamin E supplement, which contains all eight forms. We don't know the answer yet. Or, it may be that you can't beat Mother Nature, and there aren't any supplements that provide the benefits of natural vitamin E in foods.

The Recommended Dietary Allowance is 22 international units (IU) a day from dietary sources or 33 IU from supplements. If you do decide to take a vitamin E supplement, don't take more than 400 IU daily, unless otherwise directed by your doctor.

What the research says

Here's what studies have found:

Age-related macular degeneration (AMD)

Taking vitamin E in combination with other vitamins and minerals seems to prevent AMD from worsening. The benefits tend to be more noticeable in people with more advanced disease.

Alzheimer's disease

Vitamin E may slow the decline of cognitive function in people with moderately severe Alzheimer's disease, but there's no evidence it's effective for mild symptoms or that it can prevent the disease.

Cancer

There's no scientific evidence that vitamin E is effective treatment for any type of cancer. High-dose antioxidants may reduce the effects of chemotherapy and radiation therapy.

Cardiovascular disease

Although research results conflict, recent studies show vitamin E supplements provide no benefits in the prevention of cardiovascular disease. The American Heart Association recommends obtaining antioxidants, including vitamin E, by eating a balanced diet rather than from taking supplements.

Multivitamins: Do you need one?

The best way to get your vitamins and minerals is through a balanced diet. However, there are times when a supplement containing a variety of vitamins and minerals — commonly referred to as a multivitamin pill — may be appropriate.

If you don't eat well — you don't eat the recommended servings of fruits, vegetables and other healthy foods — you may benefit from a vitamin and mineral supplement. In addition, if you have to limit your diet because of food allergies or intolerance to certain foods, a supplement may be appropriate. Multivitamins are also recommended for strict vegetarians who eat no animal products. These individuals may not get enough vitamin B-12, zinc, iron and calcium.

If you're over age 65, there are a variety of reasons why you may not get the nutrients you need. A multivitamin may make more sense than taking single-nutrient pills.

It's generally recommended that pregnant or breast-feeding women take additional vitamins, but you should discuss what to take with your doctor.

What to watch for

Consider these points when choosing a multivitamin:

- **Iron.** Although supplemental iron is advised during pregnancy and for iron deficiency anemia, too much iron can be toxic. For men and post-menopausal women, it's probably wise to take a pill with little or no iron — 8 milligrams (mg) a day or less. "Senior formulas" generally have less iron.

- **Vitamin B-6 (pyridoxine).** Adequate levels of this vitamin may help lower blood homocysteine, a possible risk factor for heart attack, and improve immune system function. Older adults who lack variety in their diets may not get enough vitamin B-6, so a multivitamin that contains about 2 mg is often a good idea. Avoid excessive doses. Too much vitamin B-6 can result in nerve damage to the arms and legs, which is usually reversible when supplementation is stopped.

- **Vitamin B-12 (cobalamin).** Adequate levels of this vitamin may reduce your risk of anemia, cardiovascular disease and stroke. Older adults often don't absorb this vitamin well. A multivitamin with at least 2 micrograms (mcg) may help.

- **Vitamin D.** This vitamin helps the body absorb calcium and is essential in maintaining bone strength and bone density. Many older adults don't get regular exposure to sunlight and have trouble absorbing vitamin D, so taking a multivitamin with 400 to 600 international units (IU) will likely help improve bone health.

- **Vitamin E.** A recent review of studies indicates that taking daily vitamin E supplements of 400 IU or more — and possibly as low as 150 IU — may pose health risks. Talk with your doctor before taking vitamin E supplements.

5 things you should know

1. Multivitamins don't need to cost much. Most generic products and store brands are fine.

2. Look for a third-party verification on the label, such as USP or NSF. This means the product has been tested in a laboratory and meets standards of quality.

3. Look for a multivitamin that contains a wide variety of vitamins and minerals in the appropriate amounts, usually 100 percent of the Daily Value (DV). Check the contents to make sure you're not getting too much of any nutrient, which can be harmful. In most cases, if the tablet doesn't exceed 100 percent of the DV, it's considered safe.

4. Take your multivitamin with food. If it contains iron, don't take a calcium supplement at the same time, since iron interferes with calcium absorption.

5. Claims such as "stress formula," "high potency," "natural" or "slow release" are often just marketing ploys and only add to the price.

Calcium

Calcium is the most abundant mineral in the human body. In addition to the support it provides to your skeleton, calcium is also needed for your heart, muscles and nerves to function properly. Your body also has built-in safeguards to maintain an adequate amount of calcium in your bloodstream.

Contrary to popular belief, need for the mineral actually increases with age. That's because the human body requires constant replenishment and, with age, the body becomes less efficient at absorbing calcium from the diet. For women, a drop in estrogen levels at menopause further reduces calcium absorption. In addition, some older adults tend to eat fewer dietary products that contain calcium.

Dietary sources of calcium include dairy products such as milk, cheese and yogurt, calcium-fortified cereals and juice, greens (spinach, bok choy, collards, kale, turnip), broccoli, green soybeans (edamame), and fish that are eaten with their bones (salmon, sardines).

Many people simply don't get enough calcium in their diets. American adults typically eat less than 600 milligrams (mg) daily, but the recommended daily intake ranges from 1,000 to 1,200 mg or more.

Our take

Dietary sources of calcium may be better for you than supplements because the foods contain other important nutrients as well. But if you struggle to get enough calcium in your diet, taking a supplement is fine. Calcium supplements are generally safe.

What the research says

Here's what some studies have found:

Calcium deficiency

Calcium supplements can ease the symptoms of mineral deficiency in people who don't get adequate amounts of the vitamin. A deficiency can cause low blood calcium levels, muscle spasms and low levels of parathyroid hormone.

High blood pressure

Calcium intake at normal recommended levels may help prevent or treat symptoms of moderate hypertension.

Osteoporosis

High calcium intake, through the use of supplements, helps reduce the loss of bone density in older adults and postmenopausal women, reducing the risk of osteoporosis. In people who have osteoporosis, calcium and vitamin D taken in combination with prescribed medications may be beneficial.

Premenstrual syndrome

Calcium intake at recommended levels may reduce some of the symptoms of premenstrual syndrome (PMS).

Chromium

Chromium is a trace mineral — trace meaning that, although essential, it's needed by the body in only small amounts. Dietary sources of chromium include whole grains, seafood, green beans, broccoli, potatoes and peanuts.

Although the exact role played by chromium isn't fully understood, it appears to assist in the cellular response to the hormone insulin. Because of this function, chromium is often associated with the treatment of diabetes and weight-loss products.

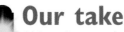

Our take

Although many American diets are low in chromium, it's rare to have a chromium deficiency. And be aware that diabetes is not a chromium-deficient disease. It's best to eat a balanced diet that includes sources of chromium and take supplements only under a doctor's supervision.

What the research says

Chromium interacts with insulin, so it's natural to think that supplements would have a positive impact on diabetes. Research results so far have been mixed. There's also no scientific evidence that chromium supplements have any benefit for weight loss. Some studies suggest that supplements may help control cholesterol levels, but there are better ways to accomplish this.

Iron

Iron plays an essential role in delivering oxygen to the body via the bloodstream. It also has many muscular and metabolic functions.

Dietary sources of iron include meat, seafood, poultry, whole grains, beans, peas and dark green leafy vegetables. The recommended dietary allowance for adult males and most women over age 50 is 8 milligrams (mg). Women of childbearing years should have 18 mg daily.

Lack of iron leads to anemia and reduces your resistance to infection. Too much iron can cause hemochromatosis, which can lead to diabetes and liver damage.

Our take

For most healthy men and postmenopausal women, iron deficiency is rare. To get enough iron, eat a balanced diet containing iron-rich foods. Women of childbearing age and people with conditions that cause internal bleeding, such as ulcers, may require iron supplements. Dieters, athletes and vegetarians who don't consume animal products also may require higher amounts of dietary iron.

What the research says

Studies show that iron supplements can prevent or treat iron deficiency anemia, a condition in which there are too few red blood cells to adequately carry oxygen to the body. This can result from too little iron in the diet. Research also has demonstrated that iron supplements may benefit women during menstruation or pregnancy.

Magnesium

Magnesium is involved in many biochemical reactions in the body, helping to maintain normal heart rhythm, immune system and muscle function.

Dietary sources of magnesium include legumes, whole grains, dark green leafy vegetables and nuts. Supplements combine the mineral with another substance, for example, magnesium citrate or magnesium gluconate. Your doctor may recommend supplements if necessary levels of magnesium can't be achieved through your daily diet.

Our take

It's uncommon for Americans to experience a deficiency in magnesium. Supplements are generally necessary only when a health problem or drug interaction causes excessive magnesium loss or limits absorption.

When taken with food, magnesium supplements are less likely to cause side effects such as diarrhea, nausea and abdominal cramps.

What the research says

Low magnesium levels are linked with a variety of conditions, including high blood pressure, heart disease, osteoporosis and poorly controlled diabetes. Use of certain medications, such as diuretics, and certain antibiotics also may affect magnesium levels. Studies suggest supplements may reduce some symptoms of premenstrual syndrome.

Selenium

Selenium is a trace mineral with antioxidant properties, especially when combined with vitamin E. It also helps maintain the body's immune system.

Dietary sources of selenium include milk, poultry, fish, organ meats and whole-grain products. The amount of selenium in these foods varies greatly, depending on amounts of the mineral in the soil.

Low selenium levels may contribute to atherosclerosis, hypothyroidism and certain cancers. Cigarette smoking and alcohol abuse both lower selenium levels.

Our take

The recommended dietary allowance of selenium is small — 55 micrograms (mcg) daily. If you take supplements, don't take more than 200 mcg a day. Selenium deficiency is rare and usually associated with severe gastrointestinal problems that affect absorption. There's insufficient evidence that selenium is beneficial for treating other conditions, including cancer and cardiovascular disease.

What the research says

Despite some earlier studies, recent research indicates that selenium does not significantly lower cancer or heart disease risk. There have also been preliminary studies involving selenium with respect to asthma, arthritis, infertility and the prevention of infection.

Zinc

Zinc is a trace mineral found in almost every cell in the human body. It's essential for normal growth, development and sexual maturation, and helps regulate appetite, stress level, and sense of taste and smell. Zinc plays an essential role in the immune system and also has antioxidant properties.

Zinc must be obtained through diet because the body doesn't produce enough of it. Dietary sources include meat, fish, poultry, liver, milk, wheat germ, whole-grain products and fortified cereals. The recommended dietary allowance for adult men is 11 milligrams (mg) of zinc and for adult women 8 mg.

Supplements may be needed for severe deficiencies resulting from malnutrition, alcohol abuse, liver cirrhosis and certain digestive disorders.

Avoid long-term high doses of zinc, which can lower high-density lipoprotein (HDL, or "good") cholesterol, suppress the immune system, and interfere with the absorption of copper, which may result in anemia.

⬤ Our take

Whether zinc can prevent or lessen a cold isn't clear. At this point, taking zinc tablets generally isn't recommended unless you have a severe deficiency. Vegetarians and some older adults may be able to correct mild zinc deficiencies with multivitamins containing zinc.

Zinc is important to your diet, but try to get the mineral through whole foods. Until more research becomes available, it's best not to exceed the Recommended Dietary Allowance.

What the research says

Here's what some studies have found:

Common cold

Studies conflict on whether zinc lozenges reduce the duration and severity of cold symptoms. Some studies indicate that taking a daily multivitamin-mineral supplement may increase the immune response in older adults while other studies suggest this may weaken the immune response.

Healing

Zinc deficiency can slow the healing process. Studies show that zinc supplements can help heal skin ulcers and bed sores in people with low zinc levels, but the supplements don't appear as effective when zinc levels are normal.

Other

Preliminary results suggest zinc may have some beneficial effects on sickle cell anemia, attention-deficit/hyperactivity disorder, Down syndrome and herpes simplex virus, but more research is needed.

Saving your eyesight

A large study called the Age-Related Eye Disease Study found that taking a combination of certain vitamins and minerals may slow the progression of age-related macular degeneration. Among people with macular degeneration who took a combination of vitamin C, vitamin E, beta carotene and zinc, advancement of the disease was reduced by up to 25 percent. Large doses were used in the study. Several commercial products are available that mimic the doses used in the study. Discuss with your doctor whether it makes sense for you to take one of these multi-ingredient preparations.

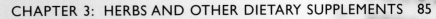

Coenzyme Q10

Coenzyme Q10 (CoQ10) is used to produce energy for cell development and maintenance. The compound also has strong antioxidant qualities.

CoQ10 is manufactured by the body, although it may be found in certain foods, such as meat and fish.

This supplement is taken to treat disorders such as heart disease, high blood pressure, asthma, migraines, Parkinson's disease and certain cancers. It's also believed to help prevent aging and memory loss, and to improve exercise performance. CoQ10 is used by millions in Japan for the treatment of cardiovascular disease.

Our take

There's some intriguing — though preliminary — evidence that CoQ10 may be beneficial for treating conditions such as congestive heart failure, high blood pressure and Parkinson's disease. It also may help prevent statin-induced myopathy, a condition that can arise from use of statin cholesterol medications. Take the supplements under a doctor's supervision.

What the research says

Preliminary studies suggest that CoQ10 may improve symptoms of Parkinson's disease. Other studies examining the effect of CoQ10 on Alzheimer's disease indicate generally positive results. Use of CoQ10 for treatment of cardiovascular conditions has produced mixed results. It may cause a slight decrease in blood pressure, and it may improve symptoms of congestive heart failure. CoQ10 is also being studied as a treatment for migraines.

Dehydroepiandrosterone (DHEA)

DHEA is a steroid advertised as an anti-aging hormone. It's taken to build muscle, reduce body fat, improve sex drive and sharpen memory.

DHEA supplements are produced in a laboratory from an extract taken from Mexican wild yams.

The steroid was banned from stores in 1985, but legislation in 1994 permitted it back on the shelves as a supplement. Its use is banned by many sports organizations.

Our take

Studies suggest DHEA may be effective in treating mild depression and systemic lupus erythematosus, but there's little to support its claims of an anti-aging tonic. Long-term use and high levels may cause serious side effects.

What the research says

A two-year Mayo Clinic study published in 2006 found that DHEA has no effect on anti-aging indicators such as endurance, muscle mass, fat mass and insulin sensitivity, and no effect on quality of life. DHEA may be useful for treating depression and lupus, but strictly under the guidance of a specialist.

Dimethyl sulfoxide (DMSO)

Dimethyl sulfoxide (DMSO) is an industrial solvent, similar to turpentine, that's sold in some health food stores as a treatment for arthritis and other conditions.

Some evidence suggests that DMSO can relieve pain and reduce swelling when rubbed on the skin. When used topically, DMSO may cause sedation, headache, dizziness, nausea, vomiting, diarrhea and skin problems.

It has been promoted as an alternative cancer treatment since the 1960s, but scientific evidence has not found it to be effective.

Our take

DMSO may be no more effective than other topical, over-the-counter pain relief products for arthritis symptoms. Furthermore, industrial-strength DMSO — the kind generally sold in stores — isn't medical grade and may contain poisonous contaminants. For these reasons, arthritis experts generally don't recommend using this solvent as a treatment for arthritis.

What the research says

Nearly 40 years of medical research on DMSO has yielded conflicting results. The only use of DMSO approved by the Food and Drug Administration is for treating interstitial cystitis, a rare bladder inflammation. Some studies using animals found that joints treated with DMSO actually developed more inflammation than did untreated joints.

5-hydroxytryptophan (5-HTP)

5-hydroxytryptophan (5-HTP) is an amino acid that the body converts into serotonin, a brain chemical that helps regulate sleep, appetite and mood.

Seed extract of *Griffonia simplicifolia*, a tree native to West Africa and Central Africa, is used to produce 5-HTP supplements.

5-HTP is used to treat a variety of conditions associated with low serotonin levels, including depression, anxiety and insomnia. The supplements are also taken for weight loss.

At higher doses, 5-HTP can be toxic. Don't take this product without a doctor's supervision.

Our take

In recent years, 5-HTP has become a very popular over-the-counter treatment for depression. But any supplement that affects brain chemicals carries the risk of adverse effects. Use of 5-HTP isn't advised until more extensive study is undertaken. Individuals taking prescribed antidepressant medications or any other drug affecting serotonin levels should avoid 5-HTP completely.

What the research says

Research indicates that 5-HTP may have value in the treatment of cerebellar ataxia, a condition in which the brain is unable to regulate limb movements and body posture. Preliminary studies also support the use of 5-HTP in treating depression and fibromyalgia, but larger, well-designed trials are needed before recommendations can be made.

Glucosamine and chondroitin

Glucosamine and chondroitin are natural compounds found in cartilage — the tough tissue that cushions joints. They're used to treat osteoarthritis, a painful condition caused by the inflammation, breakdown and eventual loss of cartilage. Since the late 1990s, sales of these products have exploded, reaching nearly $1 billion a year.

Glucosamine supplements are made from the skeletons of shellfish (chitin). There are several forms of glucosamine. The form considered best suited for cartilage repair is glucosamine sulfate. Chondroitin supplements are made from cow and shark cartilage, as well as from other sources.

The two compounds are often administered in combination to treat osteoarthritis. (Sometimes, the trace element manganese is also included.) It's not clear whether this combination works better than either supplement would alone.

Read product labels carefully. Avoid confusion with glucosamine sulfate and N-acetyl glucosamine. Glucosamine sulfate has been studied for treatment of arthritis; however, there's no clinical evidence to support the use of N-acetyl glucosamine in treating arthritis.

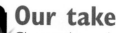 Our take

Glucosamine and chondroitin have become an extremely popular treatment for osteoarthritis. They appear to be safe and produce fewer adverse side effects than do medications such as NSAIDs. But how effective are they at treating arthritis? Many older studies gave very promising results. However, the results of a very large NIH-sponsored trial were mostly negative. The only individuals who appeared to receive some benefit were those with very severe symptoms.

While the studies may be conflicting, side effects from the supplements are few and far between. So far, no other treatments have shown promise in increasing cartilage. And it's still possible glucosamine and chondroitin may help. Therefore, they may be worth a try.

What the research says

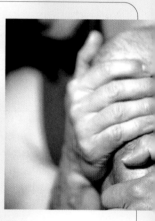

Results of more than 30 studies have produced enough mixed results that researchers aren't able to conclude that glucosamine and chondroitin improve pain and function in people with osteoarthritis of the knee. Glucosamine, though, has shown benefits for osteoarthritis in other joints. In some instances, it appeared to reduce joint pain and tenderness as effectively as did conventional medications and slow progression of the disease. Whether people taking glucosamine and chondroitin for longer periods have less joint damage compared with those taking an inactive pill (placebo) is uncertain and requires further study.

The National Institutes of Health (NIH) sponsored a four-year study in which glucosamine and chondroitin were used to treat people with osteoarthritis of the knee. Preliminary results of the study suggested that — when given separately or in combination — glucosamine and chondroitin generally weren't any more effective in treating pain than was a placebo. The study also found that a prescribed medication used for comparison was more effective than the placebo in relieving pain.

Meanwhile, a study conducted in Europe concluded that glucosamine was more effective than acetaminophen (Tylenol, others) in reducing joint pain from osteoarthritis.

Glucosamine and chondroitin haven't been well studied for treatment of rheumatoid arthritis.

Human growth hormone

Human growth hormone (HGH) is produced by the pituitary gland in the central brain. Human growth hormone stimulates and regulates childhood development, but levels of the hormone begin to decline around age 20.

Synthetic growth hormone, which must be injected, is used in some prescription medications such as somatropin. It's generally used for childhood conditions such as growth hormone deficiency.

Growth hormone stimulants, which claim to slow the aging process and keep you young and energetic, also are available in a variety of forms.

Our take

Human growth hormone levels decline naturally as a part of normal aging. Although human growth hormone products may provide some physical benefits, their ability to slow the aging process is unclear. Many of these benefits could be better achieved through regular physical exercise, and at a lot less expense. On the Internet, many products are sold as growth hormone stimulants. None of their claims has been proved, and the products should be avoided.

What the research says

Several small studies have shown that high doses of injected growth hormone can slightly reduce body fat and increase muscle mass and bone density. What's not certain is how these changes will affect overall strength, endurance and quality of life.

L-leucine

L-leucine is a branched-chain amino acid (BCAA), along with isoleucine and valine. BCAAs are used by athletes to increase endurance and energy levels during competition. BCAAs are also used to treat some forms of brain disease (encephalopathy), as well as anorexia in people with cancer and malnourishment in elderly individuals.

BCAAs can be found in any dietary source of protein, such as meat, legumes and dairy products. Supplements, ranging anywhere from 5 to 20 grams, are available as capsules, tablets and powder.

Our take

Study results so far are mixed on the benefits of BCAA supplementation in athletic competition. It should be noted that BCAAs would only have positive effects for endurance athletes, not for athletes competing in events of shorter duration. Nevertheless, BCAAs do appear safe to use, with no serious adverse reactions reported.

What the research says

The idea behind BCAA supplements in athletics is that physical performance, particularly in endurance events such as marathons, is hampered by mental fatigue. Supplements such as L-leucine delay fatigue by blocking the manufacture of serotonin in the brain. Some studies indicate that BCAA supplements taken right before exercise are effective, while others show little or no effect.

Melatonin

Melatonin is a hormone that controls the body's circadian rhythm, an internal system that regulates when you fall asleep and when you wake up. The synthesis and release of melatonin are stimulated by darkness and suppressed by light. Levels in the blood are highest just prior to bedtime.

Melatonin also helps control the release of female reproductive hormones, which determines the timing of menstrual cycles and menopause.

Supplements are synthesized from the amino acid tryptophan. The supplements are available as tablets, capsules, creams and lozenges.

Melatonin is used for a variety of medical conditions, most notably for disorders related to sleep, such as jet lag and insomnia. The hormone is a powerful antioxidant but at this point, no one knows exactly what it's capable of. Melatonin is advertised as a treatment for arthritis, stress, migraine, alcoholism, heart disease, cancer and symptoms of menopause.

Our take

Melatonin can promote sleep and appears to be safe for short-term use, but its long-term effects are unknown. It's likely that your body produces enough melatonin for its general needs, and taking supplements regularly isn't needed. Melatonin may be used occasionally, such as to overcome jet lag, for people who have difficulty making sleep adjustments. Treat melatonin as you would any form of sleeping pill, and use it under your doctor's supervision.

What the research says

Here's what some studies have found:

Insomnia

Research on older adults suggests that taking melatonin at least a half-hour or more before bedtime will decrease the amount of time required to fall asleep. However, most of these studies have been short-term and not of the highest quality. Little is known of the long-term effects, or how melatonin compares with insomnia medications.

Jet lag

Studies indicate that melatonin, when taken on the day of travel and continued for several days, will help reduce the time required to re-establish a normal sleep pattern in a new location. Best effects seem to occur when traveling eastward, and when crossing more than four time zones. However, the symptoms of jet lag are variable and not always easy to assess.

Other

Melatonin has been studied as a treatment for cancer, headache, seasonal affective disorder and smoking cessation. Small studies have also examined sleep disorders associated with irregular work shifts, menopause, depression and schizophrenia. More research is needed.

Sleep enhancement

Several studies indicate that healthy individuals taking melatonin before bedtime will feel "sleepiness" and fall asleep faster. It's unknown whether it will help people stay asleep.

Omega-3 fatty acids

Omega-3 fatty acids are derived from food. They cannot be manufactured in the body.

Omega-3 fatty acids have been shown to improve cardiovascular health, helping to reduce the risk of heart attack, stroke, high triglycerides and atherosclerosis. They also appear to improve symptoms of rheumatoid arthritis — studies haven't found a similar benefit for symptoms of osteoarthritis. There's some evidence omega-3s may help improve cognitive function later in life and improve weight loss.

Dietary sources of omega-3 fatty acids are cold-water fish such as salmon, mackerel, herring, sardines and trout. Fish oil contains both docosahexaenoic acid (DHA) and eicosapentaenoic acid (EPA). Other sources of omega-3s are canola and soybean oils, flaxseed, walnuts and wheat germ.

Omega-3 fatty acid (fish oil) supplements come in liquid, capsule and pill form. Most people can take 3 grams (3,000 milligrams) a day without adverse effects. Taking more than this amount increases the risk of bleeding and may lower your immune system response.

Our take

Omega-3 fatty acids are essential for good health, but try to get them from your diet by eating fish — broiled or baked, not fried. Omega-3 fatty acid (fish oil) supplements may be best suited for individuals with cardiovascular disease or an autoimmune disorder, such as rheumatoid arthritis. Fish oil supplements should be taken under a doctor's supervision.

What the research says

Here's what some studies have found:

Cardiovascular disease

Clinical trials of heart attack survivors found that daily omega-3 fatty acid supplements significantly reduced the risk of another heart attack, stroke or death. These benefits are less evident for people with no history of heart attack.

Depression

Epidemiologic research suggests eating fish lowers the risk of depression.

High blood pressure

Multiple studies report a small reduction in blood pressure in people who took fish oil supplements. Other approaches to lowering blood pressure, such as weight loss and salt reduction, may be more effective.

Lipids

There's strong evidence that omega-3 fatty acids can significantly reduce blood triglyceride levels. The benefits result from doses as low as 2 grams a day. Four grams a day provide even greater benefits. There also appears to be a slight improvement in high-density lipoprotein (HDL, or "good") cholesterol, although an increase in levels of low-density lipoprotein (LDL, or "bad") cholesterol also was observed.

Rheumatoid arthritis

Studies suggest fish oil supplements in combination with anti-inflammatory medications improve morning stiffness and joint tenderness for up to three months. More research is needed.

Probiotics

Probiotics refers to dietary supplements or foods that contain beneficial, or "good," bacteria similar to those normally found in the body. A common probiotic bacteria is *Lactobacillus acidophilus.*

These good bacteria compete with and inhibit harmful, disease-causing bacteria, helping to maintain a proper microorganic balance in your intestinal tract. Probiotic bacteria also help with digestion.

Probiotics come from food sources such as yogurt, cheese, miso, tempeh, and some juices and soy drinks, but they're also available as capsules, tablets, suppositories and powders.

Side effects, if they occur, tend to be mild. Gas and bloating are the most common.

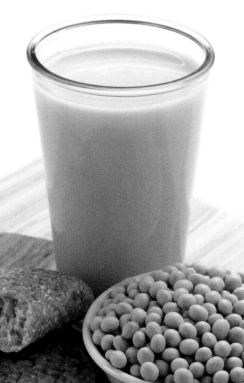

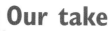

Our take

There's growing interest in probiotics, spurred by their potential to treat various gastrointestinal disorders, but more research still needs to be done. In the meantime, there appears to be little harm in taking supplements, although a good, balanced diet should provide you with sufficient "good" bacteria. Probiotics may help ease symptoms of lactose intolerance.

What the research says

Here's what some studies have found:

Cold and flu

There's good evidence that probiotics can reduce the risk of each and reduce the severity of symptoms in individuals who are afflicted.

Diarrhea

Probiotic supplements have been shown to manage diarrhea, especially following treatment with antibiotics, for example, treating a *Helicobacter pylori* infection. Probiotics may also reduce your risk of developing traveler's diarrhea.

Eczema

Probiotics seem to reduce the severity of eczema (atopic dermatitis) in infants and young children.

General health

A small study in Sweden found that a group of employees who were given the probiotic *Lactobacillus reuteri* missed less work due to respiratory or gastrointestinal illness than did employees who were not given the probiotic.

Irritable bowel syndrome

Research has found probiotics helpful in managing irritable bowel syndrome.

Yeast infections

Results of studies on use of probiotics for yeast infections is mixed. One study found that employees given probiotics missed less work due to illness than did employees not given probiotics.

S-adenosylmethionine (SAMe)

SAMe is a compound that occurs naturally in the human body. It's scientific name is S-adenosyl-L-methionine. Among other functions, SAMe helps produce and regulate hormones and maintain cell membranes. SAMe isn't found in food.

A synthetic version of the compound has become a popular dietary supplement in the United States, used for the treatment of depression, arthritis and liver disease. In other countries, such as Italy, Spain and Germany, SAMe is sold as a prescription drug.

SAMe may be administered orally, intravenously or intramuscularly. Generally, it's well tolerated. Side effects are more common with higher doses and include gas, nausea, diarrhea and headache.

Our take

SAMe has promise as an effective treatment for depression and osteoarthritis, but the long-term benefits and risks are still unknown. As with all supplements, it's best to consult your doctor before trying SAMe. Two drawbacks are the inconsistent quality and high price of various products. Furthermore, SAMe can interact with antidepressant medications you may be taking.

What the research says

Here's what some studies have found:

Depression

SAMe may be effective for treating major depression, although most of the studies were poorly designed. Large-scale, controlled studies are needed to clarify the benefit of SAMe in treating major depression.

Fibromyalgia

Two clinical trials indicated SAMe can improve symptoms of fibromyalgia.

Liver disease

Only preliminary tests have been conducted regarding its effectiveness for liver disease. SAMe may normalize levels of liver enzymes in people with liver disease; however, no conclusions can be made at this time.

Osteoarthritis

SAMe has been studied extensively in the treatment of osteoarthritis. Multiple trials indicate that SAMe can relieve pain from osteoarthritis as effectively as nonsteroidal anti-inflammatory drugs (NSAIDs), with fewer side effects. However, noticeable symptom relief may require up to 30 days. An optimal dose has yet to be determined.

Chapter 4
Mind-Body Medicine

A visit with Dr. Amit Sood

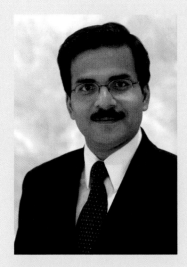

Amit Sood, M.D.
General Internal Medicine

❝ Approaches that at their core are based on the values of peace, forgiveness, compassion, selflessness, integrity and love will be the ones that will stand the test of time and continue to bring health and healing to this generation and the next. ❞

I welcome you to this section on mind-body medicine. Here you will learn about some of the commonly used mind-body approaches. While the precise techniques may seem different, the underlying theme is lucid and simple. Tai chi, yoga, meditation, progressive muscle relaxation and guided imagery all have in common a program that will help train your attention and refine your interpretations so your attention becomes focused and strong, and your interpretations are guided more by principles than prejudices.

It's desirable to approach the mind-body practices described here as a guide to a higher purpose. These practices are thus not an end in themselves. The purpose of achieving a perfect posture in yoga isn't limited to the posture itself. The real meaning behind yoga is to attain an optimal coordination of breath, body and mind that puts you in a state of "flow." This "flow" then might be a welcome fellow traveler with you for the rest of the day. Each of these practices are a means to unfold the deeper, kinder person that is within all of us — but sometimes is not able to manifest fully because of the daily trappings of life. Look at these skills as mentors that might help transform you into an embodiment of wisdom and love.

Why the growing interest in mind-body therapies in recent years? Impressive advances in neurosciences research have brought to our attention a startling and exciting discovery — the mind can change the brain. Software can indeed transform the hardware. Training our mind using mind-body approaches can soothe the limbic areas of the brain such as the amygdala, and engage areas of the brain such as the prefrontal cortex, whose activity enhances resilience and happiness, and trains executive functions. This literal rewiring of the brain by our recurring thought patterns and experiences is now popularly recognized as neuroplasticity. The concept of rewiring our brain by exercising our "free will" has brought a new generation of researchers into the field of mind-body medicine, particularly meditation. This has been a welcome phenomenon since healing practices can now be better structured and can be evidence-based to a greater level than previously imagined. However, it might be optimal to tread this path carefully lest our obsession to subject every aspect of our life to "evidence-based double-blind randomized controlled trials" be carried to an undesirable extreme.

As we learn newer and more refined mind-body techniques, it's important to recognize the simplicity of their underlying concepts. Approaches that at their core are based on the values of peace, forgiveness, compassion, selflessness, integrity and love will be the ones that will stand the test of time and continue to bring health and healing to this generation and the next. Embracing and popularizing such approaches is the legacy you and I will be proud to share with our children and grandchildren.

The science of the mind

Mind-body medicine refers to approaches that help us harness the power of the mind to prevent illness, decrease disease, enhance healing and promote well-being. The mind, often understood as a collection of thoughts and emotions, or more technically, as the infrastructure software of the brain, is a subtle yet powerful tool we use to conduct our daily lives. The health and vitality of the mind is extraordinarily important to maintain good health and live a balanced and satisfying life.

To better understand mind-body medicine, it helps to know how the mind operates. There are two simultaneous processes within the mind that together craft your everyday experiences — attention and interpretation. The process of attention helps you screen, select and absorb sensory information from the world. This information is then subject to interpretation, a process that relies on previous experience, preferences and a planned future course of life. Most of what you do is guided by the interaction of attention and interpretation.

Human attention has two basic characteristics that predispose you to stress, which can lead to illness. First, your attention has evolved to selectively focus on imperfections with an intention to correct them to your satisfaction. These imperfections could be either in the material world or within the contents of the mind.

In general, the memory or fear of imperfections (sometimes threats) that exists in your mind far exceeds those in the real world. Since it's in your instinct to solve problems and resolve issues, the load of imperfections in your mind predispose you to the second characteristic that leads to stress — the state of mindlessness.

In a state of mindlessness your attention is enslaved by the contents of the mind, away from the beautiful world. You become disengaged from the world, often surrounded by anxiety provoking excessive thoughts. This state not only invites stress, sleeplessness and decreased quality of life, but also may predispose you to multiple medical conditions, some of them potentially life-threatening.

The first promise of mind-body medicine is to help free you from excessive negative thoughts and the related state of mindlessness. The hope is to bring your attention to the splendor of the present moment in a state of acceptance that empowers you to engage in meaningful action.

Interpretation, the second process that contributes toward all of human experiences, depends on two key entities — principles and prejudices. The lessons you learn through your experiences help you live an efficient and productive life. However, some of the conclusions you make may become exaggerated and overgeneralized. Such conclusions, particularly when they're selfish, provide the fodder for human prejudices. Excessive prejudices can predispose you to a relatively rigid outlook and often an inability to see a situation from a more mature perspective that encompasses views and interests of the others. These prejudices contrive to push deeper into the human mind, increasing the risk of stress and illness.

The second promise of mind-body medicine is to help you free yourself from these prejudices and instead cultivate transformative principles. These are the principles of forgiveness, acceptance, compassion, a higher meaning to life, gratitude and interconnectedness. It's these principles that provide you balanced optimism and openness to experience, and can help you see the reality or lack thereof in our thoughts.

The mind and body connection

A simple definition of mind-body medicine reads like this: "positively influencing the mind to improve the health of the individual." The belief that mind and body are intricately connected goes back centuries. But with the development of Western medicine during the 17th century, this basic "connected" approach to health and wellness fell by the wayside. As scientists explored the inner workings of the human body, they discovered and introduced such fundamental concepts as germs as a source of disease, and medications and surgical techniques as a way to treat disease — practices that remain central components of modern medicine. The study of human biology paved the way for great strides in medicine and continues to inspire innovative treatments. However, treating disease strictly on a biological level has its limitations, as reflected by the growing number of individuals turning to treatments outside of modern medicine.

Today, we're faced with several diseases, such as fibromyalgia and irritable bowel syndrome, that aren't curable with potent drugs or surgical procedures. This recognition — combined with increasing scientific study implicating the mind as one of several factors in the development of disease — has led to a resurgence of mind-body medicine and to increased interest in "holistic" health and healing.

Mind-body practices have two core components. The first is to restore the mind to a state of peaceful neutrality. In this state, the mind achieves a state that's nonjudgmental, efficient and adaptive to the needs of the individual. To reach this state, the mind has to shed negative experiences acquired over the years. The second component of mind-body medicine is to use this "ready" mind in a manner to achieve beneficial health effects. This might be through spiritual intervention (prayer), spoken intervention (transcendental meditation), or practices involving breathing and posture (yoga) or soothing imagery (guided imagery).

The power and speed of the mind is phenomenal. And there's no reason to believe that a mind that can sample the soil of a distant planet would not have the capacity to initiate processes to heal its own body.

As we learn newer and more refined mind-body techniques, it's important to recognize the simplicity of their underlying concepts. Interventions that at their core are based on the values of peace, forgiveness, sharing, selflessness, integrity and love help us achieve the outcomes we seek.

Biofeedback

Biofeedback is designed to help you use your mind to control your body. With the assistance of a variety of monitoring devices, including those that measure heart rate, skin temperature and brain activity, you can learn to control certain involuntary body responses, such as blood pressure, muscle tension and heart rate.

Biofeedback has been shown to be helpful in treating about 150 medical conditions. You can receive biofeedback training in physical therapy clinics, medical centers and hospitals. A typical biofeedback session lasts 30 to 60 minutes.

During a biofeedback session, a therapist places electrical sensors on different parts of your body. These sensors monitor your body's response to stress — for instance, your muscle contraction during a tension headache — and then feed the information back to you via sound and visual cues. With this feedback, you start to associate your body's response — in this case, headache pain — with certain physical sensations, such as your muscles tensing.

The next step is to learn how to invoke positive physical changes, such as relaxing those muscles, when your body is physically or mentally stressed. Your goal is to produce these responses on your own, outside the therapist's office and without the help of technology.

Our take

Biofeedback is, for the most part, widely used and accepted. It has the potential to improve symptoms associated with many medical conditions. It has relatively few risks, and it's practiced in many medical centers. Provided you get proper instruction and supervision, biofeedback may be useful as part of a comprehensive treatment plan.

What the research says

Biofeedback is useful for treating many conditions. Studies indicate it has the potential to improve symptoms of asthma, Raynaud's disease, irritable bowel syndrome, constipation, nausea and vomiting associated with chemotherapy, incontinence, chronic pain, headache, anxiety, stress, high blood pressure, stroke, epilepsy and tinnitus. Research into its effectiveness in these and other areas is ongoing.

Devices to help you control your responses

Learning how to relax and decompress after a busy day or a stressful situation is possible, but it takes time.

Your doctor or a therapist may teach you how to do biofeedback, but to become good at it, you need to practice. A variety of products are available for purchase that can help you learn to activate your body's natural relaxation response.

Breathing sensor. This type of device monitors your breathing, helping you learn how to breathe more deeply and slowly. It's also been shown to reduce blood pressure.

To use the device, you put on headphones and attach a sensor around your chest. The sensor analyzes your individual breathing pattern and creates a personalized melody composed of inhaling and exhaling guiding tones. As you listen to the melody through the headphones, your body's natural tendency to follow external rhythms will enable you to easily synchronize your breathing to the tones.

By gradually prolonging the exhalation tone, the device teaches you to slow your breathing. As breathing slows, the muscles surrounding the small blood vessels in your body relax and blood flows more freely.

Heart rate variability monitor. These devices generally work in this way: From beat to beat, your heart rate naturally increases and decreases in a cycle or rhythm, known as heart rate variability.

Using a sensor that measures the pulse in your fingertip or earlobe, a device measures and displays your breathing and the time between your heartbeats. The display may be in a wave-like format. When you're stressed, your wave is jagged and spiky; when you're relaxed, the wave becomes smooth and consistent.

By controlling your breathing — breathing more slowly and deeply — you can control your heart rate variability, and actually watch the wave change in format.

There are a variety of these devices. Some hand-held models use tones and lights that give you feedback on your stress level. There are also

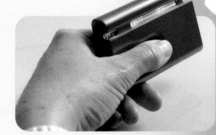

computer programs that use sophisticated imagery to enhance the feedback. Some programs even allow you to play "games" where the action on the screen is controlled by your level of relaxation.

Different approaches. Some people find biofeedback devices alone are sufficient enough to produce a deep state of relaxation. Others rely on meditation to reach relaxation, but they use biofeedback devices to assess their progress. Still others find biofeedback devices to be distracting, and they prefer not to use them. They rely on other methods to control their body responses. Regardless of which camp you fall into, the important thing is that you find something that works for you.

Guided imagery

Imagery is the thought process that invokes and uses the senses. You use it to see in your "mind's eye" a beautiful vista, or to conjure up aromas of your favorite foods. Guided imagery — sometimes referred to as visualization — has been used by cultures throughout the ages as a healing tool. It relies on memories, dreams, fantasies and visions to serve as a bridge between the mind and body.

Ancient Egyptians and Greeks, including Aristotle and Hippocrates, believed that images released spirits in the brain that aroused the heart and body. They also believed that a strong image of disease was enough to cause symptoms. Navajo Indians practice an elaborate form of imagery that encourages the person to envision himself or herself as healthy.

Evidence of peoples' ability to use their imaginations to assist in curing their ailments was documented by both Sigmund Freud and Carl Jung.

Modern research has shown that mental images produce physiological, biochemical and immunological changes in the body that affect health. Researchers have found that imagery can change specific immune system responses that affect such things as white blood cell count. Imagery has also shown a potential to improve quality of life in some people with cancer.

Guided imagery is even used to help improve a person's golf swing or piano performance.

Our take

Guided imagery gets a green light because it's an important tool in treating a variety of health problems. It provides benefits and it poses virtually no risk. Guided imagery is used in many medical settings to help manage an array of conditions and diseases from stress to pain to the side effects of cancer.

What the research says

Researchers using positron emission tomography (PET) scanning have found that the same parts of the brain are activated when people are imagining something as when they're actually experiencing it. For example, when someone imagines a serene image, the optic cortex is activated in the same way as when the person is actually seeing the beautiful vista. Vivid imagery sends messages from the cerebral cortex to the lower brain, including the limbic system, the emotional control center of the brain. From there the message is relayed to the endocrine and the autonomic nervous systems, which affect a wide range of bodily functions, including heart and respiration rates, and blood pressure.

Cancer care

Imagery has been used to reduce nausea, fatigue and hair loss, as well as reduce anxiety, prevent depression and create a sense of well-being among people with cancer.

Pre- and post-surgery

Research indicates that practicing guided imagery at least two to four times before surgery can reduce fear and anxiety and provide people with a greater sense of control. In a number of studies, individuals using imagery needed less pain medication and were discharged from the hospital one to two days earlier than were those who didn't use guided imagery.

Stress management

Imagery is considered an effective tool for turning on the relaxation response in people who are feeling stressed, overwhelmed or physically uncomfortable.

Stroke

Imagery is being explored as a means to improve motor skills in people who've had a stroke, what's called mental practice.

How to do it

Guided imagery can offer relief from symptoms such as anxiety and stress simply by closing your eyes to the outside world. Imagery can empower the mind to create healing.

When first learning imagery techniques, many people find listening to a CD with guided imagery coaching to be helpful. Others choose to work one-on-one or in a small group with an individual who is experienced in imagery. After you've received a bit of training, you can perform imagery on your own.

Four steps are important in making guided imagery work for you.

Step 1: Relaxation

To create a desirable image, the mind must be cleared of all chatter and ego-based distractions. Loosen tightfitting clothing and find a comfortable, quiet place. Once you are quiet and comfortable, begin taking slow, deep breaths and releasing all random thoughts as you exhale.

Step 2: Concentration

Focus attention on your breathing as a means to clear your mind. If your mind wanders, acknowledge the thoughts, release them easily and effortlessly as you exhale. Then refocus your attention on your breathing.

Step 3: Visualization

Now combine a desired image with an intention and for the next several minutes, focus on this image. You may find that your mind wanders — this may happen frequently, especially during the early stages of visualization. When it does, bring your focus back by using a slow, deep breath.

Step 4: Affirmation

A positive affirmation coupled with the image will help to create a positive message that will be stored and easily recalled at a later time. Combining an image with a word or phrase may help to engage both sides of your brain.

Hypnosis

Most of us have heard the term *mesmerize*. It comes from the name of an German physician, Franz Anton Mesmer, who is considered the founder of modern Western hypnotherapy. Mesmer held that illness was caused by an imbalance of magnetic fluids in the body, and that this imbalance could be corrected by transferring the hypnotist's own magnetism to the individual.

The word *hypnosis* comes from the Greek word *hypnos,* which means "sleep." Forms of hypnosis, trance and altered states of consciousness have been used by many cultures and civilizations throughout history.

There are three stages or phases to the process of hypnotism. They are pre-suggestion, suggestion and post-suggestion. The goal during pre-suggestion is to open the unconscious mind to suggestion. During the second phase, a specific suggestion is presented to the subject, questions may be asked or memories reviewed. Finally, in the post-suggestion stage, after returning to a normal state of consciousness, behavior that was suggested during hypnosis may be practiced.

The mechanisms by which hypnosis works are not well understood. Changes in skin temperature, heart rate and immune response have been observed. Some scientists believe that hypnosis activates certain mind-body pathways in the nervous system.

Our take

While hypnotism is often portrayed humorously on TV and in films, it can be an effective treatment for some people. Research indicates that some individuals are more susceptible to hypnotism than are others. Some practitioners hold that the more open you are to being hypnotized, the more likely it is that you'll benefit from the therapy. Hypnotism may be a reasonable choice if you need help dealing with a chronic condition. Since it poses little risk of harmful side effects, it may be worth a try.

What the research says

Hypnosis may offer relief to those with pain associated with a number of disorders, including cancer. It is also used in treating a number of behavioral problems. In addition, it may be used to reduce anxiety before a medical or dental procedure.

Anxiety

Several studies show that hypnosis reduces anxiety. Particularly, hypnosis has been shown to lower anxiety before certain medical and dental procedures, with the effect lasting up to three years.

Behavior change

Hypnosis has been used with mixed success to treat conditions including insomnia, bed-wetting, smoking cessation and some phobias. More study is needed to determine the long-term effectiveness of treating these disorders with hypnosis.

Hot flashes

Hypnosis may help relieve symptoms of hot flashes associated with menopause.

Pain management

The National Institutes of Health has cited evidence that supports the effectiveness of hypnotherapy in the treatment of chronic pain associated with cancer, irritable bowel syndrome, fibromyalgia, temporomandibular problems and dental procedures.

Tension headache

Studies indicate that hypnosis can relieve the pain of a tension headache. Additional research is still needed to establish whether hypnotherapy is an effective treatment for tension headache.

Meditation

The term *meditation* refers to a group of techniques, many of which have their roots in Eastern religious or spiritual traditions. Today, many people use meditation for health and wellness purposes.

In meditation, a person focuses attention on his or her breathing, or on repeating a word, phrase or sound in order to suspend the stream of thoughts that normally occupies the conscious mind. Meditation is believed to lead to a state of physical relaxation, mental calmness, alertness and psychological balance. Practicing meditation can change how you relate to the flow of emotions and thoughts and may help you control how you respond to a challenging situation.

Meditation may be practiced on its own or as a part of another mind-body therapy, such as yoga or tai chi. Like other mind-body therapies, once you learn how to meditate, you can do it on your own.

Meditation is used to help treat a number of problems, including anxiety, pain, depression, stress and insomnia.

Experiment and you'll likely find out what types of meditation work best for you and what you enjoy doing.

Our take

Meditation may be the perfect complement to the rush of a busy, complicated life. As the evidence supporting the use of meditation grows, adding it to your daily schedule may be just the antidote you need to deal with a hectic routine. In addition, if meditation helps to lower your blood pressure and reduce stress in your life, so much the better. The long-term benefits of meditation continue to undergo study.

What the research says

Different forms of meditation have been tested in over 1,000 clinical trials. While many studies have been small and not conducted with the highest rigor, the overall evidence supports use of meditation for a variety of conditions.

Anxiety and stress

Various types of meditation are used to treat anxiety. Studies have included people with illnesses such as cancer and depression. Meditation has been shown to reduce anxiety, decrease anger and decrease stress in people with cancer.

Asthma

Preliminary research on the use of transcendental meditation in treating people with asthma has shown some positive results. More research is needed.

Fibromyalgia

Improvement in symptoms has been reported among people with fibromyalgia who practice mindfulness meditation.

High blood pressure

Several studies indicate a program of meditation effectively reduces blood pressure in people with hypertension.

Other

Meditation has also been shown to improve attention, decrease job burnout, improve sleep, decrease chronic pain and improve blood sugar control.

Different types of meditation

There are several different approaches to meditation. You may want to take a class to help you learn more about the various types and determine which approach is best for you.

Analytical meditation

The meditator tries to comprehend the deeper meaning of the object upon which he or she is focusing.

Breath meditation

This approach involves focusing on one's breathing. It involves the conscious observing of every inhalation and exhalation, and the rising and falling of the chest. Breathing that is deep, slow, diaphragmatic and smooth is maintained during this practice.

Mindfulness meditation

Mindfulness meditation is based on the concept of being mindful of — having an increased aware-ness and complete acceptance of — the present. One mindful meditation exercise is to bring all your attention to the sensa-tion of the flow of your breath in and out of your body. The goal is to focus on what's being experienced in the present, without reacting to it or making any judgments about it. This approach is used as a way of

> " The goal is to focus on what's being experienced in the present, without reacting to it or making any judg-ments about it. "

learning a more balanced response to the thoughts and emotions of daily life.

Transcendental meditation

Transcendental meditation (TM) teaches you to focus on a mantra — a sound, word or phrase — repeated over and over. You may repeat your mantra either aloud or silently to yourself. By doing so, you keep distracting thoughts out of your conscious awareness. A goal of TM is to achieve a state of relaxed awareness or alertness. TM originated in the Vedic tradition in India.

Visualization

Visualization involves focusing on a specific place or object (see "Guided imagery" on page 100.)

Walking meditation

This form of meditation — called kinhin in the Zen tradi-tion — focuses on the subtle movements used to stand and walk. You focus your attention on the soles of your feet, first as you stand, and then as you walk. Walking meditation requires that, for safety reasons, you pay greater attention to what's going on around you.

How meditation affects the body

Practicing meditation has been shown to induce some changes in the body, such as in the body's fight-or-flight response. The system responsible for this response is the autonomic nervous system — sometimes called the involuntary nervous system. It regulates many body activities, including heartbeat, perspiration, breathing and digestion. The autonomic nervous system is divided into two parts:

The sympathetic nervous system helps mobilize the body into action. When you're under stress, it produces the fight-or-flight response. Heart rate and breathing increase, blood vessels narrow and muscles become tense.

The parasympathetic nervous system response is opposite to that of the sympathetic system. It creates what has been called the "rest and digest" response. The parasympathetic nervous system prompts the heart to beat more slowly, the blood vessels to dilate, improving blood flow, and the digestive tract to increase activity.

Researchers studying the effects of meditation are focusing on the brain and how meditation may reduce the activity of the sympathetic nervous system and increase that of the parasympathetic system.

Getting ready

Most types of meditation require four elements.

A quiet place

Many people who meditate prefer a place with as few distractions as possible. This can be particularly helpful for those just starting to practice meditation. Those who have more experience may be able to meditate in places with more distractions.

A specific posture

Depending on the type of meditation being practiced, it can be done while sitting, standing, lying down, walking or in other positions.

Focused attention

Focusing your attention is an important part of meditating. For example, you may focus on a mantra — a specific word or set of words. You may also choose to focus on your breathing, or on an object such as a candle or an image.

An open attitude

Keeping an open attitude during meditation means letting distractions come and go without engaging them — without stopping to think about them. When distracting or wandering thoughts occur during meditation, they aren't suppressed. Rather, you gently bring your attention back to the focus.

In some types of meditation, the meditator learns to observe the rising and the falling of thoughts and emotions as they occur.

Adapt meditation to your needs at the moment. Remember there is no right way or wrong way to meditate.

The soothing effects of aromatherapy

Aromatherapy, as its name implies, uses fragrant (essential) oils from a wide variety of plants in an attempt to alleviate pain, reduce stress, treat depression and promote a greater sense of well-being.

There are about 40 oils commonly used in aromatherapy. During an aromatherapy session at a spa, the oils may be smelled or applied to the skin during a massage. At home, you may add the oils to your bath water, burn aromatic candles or smell the oils while performing relaxation exercises.

Aromatic oils are usually mixed with a base, or carrier, such as vegetable oil, or they may be mixed with alcohol.

Several small scientific studies have found that lavender oil aromatherapy appears to have some effect in relieving anxiety. The scent of lavender is thought to have a calming effect on the nervous system. Lavender may also help some people bothered by insomnia fall asleep.

Aromatherapy has been studied in connection with improving quality of life for people with serious illnesses, but no firm evidence exists to its effectiveness in such cases.

Step-by-step instructions: How to meditate

One of the best ways to learn meditation is from an instructor, or you can try an instructional video or audio recording. You can also learn to meditate on your own. Here's an example of how to perform meditation at one of its most basic levels. It takes about 10 to 15 minutes. Try it and see how you do.

1. If you're able, turn on some soothing music and keep it at a low volume. Get comfortable in your chair or on the floor. Loosen any tight clothing. Let your arms rest loosely at your side. Allow yourself a few minutes to relax (pause).

2. If your thoughts wander, just let them while gently moving your attention back to the relaxation.

3. To begin, focus your eyes on a specific object in front of you, such as a tree, a picture or a candle flame. Notice its simplicity and its beauty.

4. Take time to notice your breathing, gradually slowing down the rate of inhaling and exhaling as you become more comfortable (pause).

5. Now relax and enjoy the feeling (pause).

6. Close your mouth and relax your shoulders, easing any tension that's built up (pause).

7. Inhale slowly and deeply through your nose. Let the air you breathe in push your stomach out.

8. Hold your breath as you slowly count to four. Then breathe out slowly through your mouth as you continue counting up to six.

9. Breathe in (three, four, five, six).

10. Hold (two, three, four).

11. Breathe out (three, four, five, six).

12. Breathe in (three, four, five, six).

13. Hold (two, three, four).

14. Breathe out (three, four, five, six).

15. Breathe in (three, four, five, six).

16. Hold (two, three, four).

17. Breathe out (three, four, five, six).

18. Breathe in (three, four, five, six).

19. Hold (two, three, four).

20. Breathe out (three, four, five, six).

21. Breathe in (three, four, five, six).

22. Hold (two, three, four).

23. Breathe out (three, four, five, six).

24. Continue breathing in (four, five, six).

25. Hold (two, three, four).

26. And out (three, four, five, six).

27. Remember, if stray thoughts enter your mind, gently return your attention to the relaxation (pause).

28. Now, as you breathe, silently and calmly repeat to yourself:

29. My breathing is smooth and rhythmic (pause).

30. My breathing is easy and calm (pause).

31. It feels very pleasant (pause).

32. Once you become familiar with how basic meditation works, you may want to close your eyes and focus on the music, or you can continue to look at the object you were concentrating on.

33. Continue to repeat to yourself:

34. My breathing is smooth and rhythmic (pause).

35. My breathing is smooth and rhythmic (pause).

36. I am peaceful and calm.

37. I am peaceful and calm.

38. Continue to take deep, rhythmic breaths. Let the tension fade away each time you breathe out. Let the music soothe you (pause).

39. If you've closed your eyes, gently open them and gaze at the object in front of you (pause).

40. Return to your day — peaceful, more focused and relaxed.

Meditation at Mayo Clinic

Mayo Clinic offers meditation as a treatment for various medical conditions. Meditation can relax and rejuvenate the mind and body, and helps many people refocus and gain happiness and inner peace. Hundreds of individuals have participated in meditation treatment at Mayo Clinic, and their responses have been overwhelmingly positive.

Meditation may help relieve such conditions as anxiety, depression, pain, stress and insomnia. Combined with conventional medicine, meditation may also improve cardiovascular health, rheumatologic conditions and digestive problems.

Individuals are usually referred by their doctor to the meditation program. Your symptoms, medical history and mental health will be assessed by a physician with experience in meditation practice. The meditation method often taught at Mayo Clinic is paced-breathing meditation.

A physician instructs the individual to relax and follow directions in order to focus on deep diaphragmatic breathing. Then, the person views a 25-minute DVD on paced-breathing meditation. During the first 10 minutes, the meditation method is explained with the assistance of visual imagery and sounds. After becoming comfortable with the practice, the individual is then guided during the next 15-minute segment of the DVD to do paced-breathing meditation.

The individual receives a copy of the DVD to use during daily practice at home. The DVD was developed at Mayo Clinic based on results of several research studies involving meditation. Almost all individuals say the experience is very positive and relaxing, and most report reduced stress and anxiety levels.

In addition to the DVD, Mayo Clinic has also developed a meditation application that can be used on an iPhone or iPod touch. The application begins with a short video that introduces key concepts. It then uses musical chords and visuals to teach you slow, paced breathing. You can choose a five-minute or 15-minute meditation program to help you clear your mind of daily distractions.

MAYO CLINIC
Meditation

Training
Learn Mayo Clinic Meditation

Meditation
15 Minutes

Meditation
5 Minutes

HEALING THOUGHTS   SHARE

Do not postpone joy.

Muscle relaxation

Progressive muscle relaxation is designed to reduce the tension in your muscles. Your goal may be to reduce anxiety and stress, which may be related to conditions such as panic disorder, high blood pressure and depression. Progressive muscle relaxation may also be used simply to improve concentration.

Our take

Muscle relaxation is easy to do. It can be done just about anywhere, and it offers a way to reduce stress and clear the mind within just a few minutes. It's a tool that you can use after a difficult meeting, or to unwind at the end of the day. You might decide to use muscle relaxation by itself, or to combine it with another mind-body approach, such as guided imagery or meditation, to get an even greater effect. The great thing about mind-body medicine is that you can choose therapies that best fit your needs and style.

How to do it

First, find a quiet place where you'll be free from interruption. Loosen tight clothing and remove your glasses or contacts if you'd like. Progressive muscle relaxation is performed either seated or lying down.

Beginning with your feet and working up through your body to your head and neck, tense each muscle group for at least five seconds and then relax the muscles for up to 30 seconds. Repeat before moving to the next muscle group.

It's recommended that you perform progressive muscle relaxation at least once or twice each day to get the maximum benefit. Each session should last about 10 minutes.

What the research says

There's a growing body of evidence that supports the effectiveness of muscle relaxation in the treatment of some conditions.

Anxiety and stress

Various relaxation techniques, including progressive muscle relaxation, have been shown to reduce anxiety, work-related stress, and symptoms related to panic disorder. However, because studies tend to employ more than one relaxation technique and often have too few participants, more research on progressive muscle relaxation is needed to verify its effectiveness.

Headache

Some studies have shown promising results of relaxation techniques in reducing the symptoms of tension headache.

High blood pressure

In several clinical studies, relaxation techniques have been shown to lower blood pressure in people with hypertension.

Music therapy

While music has been used in healing rituals throughout human history, the modern, formal profession of music therapy was first recognized in the 1950s. It was during that time that musicians were called on to treat injured military personnel in the United States. Also during this time, various creative arts were used to treat psychiatric disorders.

Music can influence both physical and mental health. One aspect of music therapy involves listening to and then discussing a piece of music in order to help people express themselves. Music therapy may also be used in an individual setting to achieve a state of relaxation.

In addition to its effect on health, studies have shown that music therapy improves sleep quality in students and reduces anxiety prior to exams.

Music therapists are professionally trained and certified. They work in many settings, including hospitals, prisons, drug and alcohol treatment programs, long term care facilities and hospices.

Our take

For many people, music occupies a central role in their lives. It revives their spirits, gets them moving and, in some cases, eases pain and suffering. Whether you listen to music simply for the joy and comfort that it brings, or you actively work with a trained music therapist as part of an overall treatment plan, music can be an important part of the healing process.

What the research says

There's scientific evidence that structured music therapy is effective in treating a number of conditions and disorders. Music therapy is sometimes combined with other approaches, including guided imagery, to achieve desired treatment goals.

Alzheimer's disease

Older adults with Alzheimer's disease and other memory disorders have been successfully treated with music therapy to reduce their aggressiveness and to improve their mood and willingness to cooperate in daily activities.

Autism

People with autism often show an increased interest in music, which may help in learning communication skills.

Depression

Evidence exists that music therapy can increase the effectiveness of some antidepressant medications.

Mood enhancement and well-being

Structured music therapy programs have been shown to improve mood in people facing burnout in their jobs and in people undergoing the rigors of cancer treatment, such as chemotherapy.

Relaxation and stress reduction

Music therapy has been shown to reduce heart rate, blood pressure and tension in a variety of study subjects, including surgery patients, heart bypass patients, individuals recovering from a heart attack, and in babies being treated for lung and breathing problems.

Pilates

With its recent surge in popularity, you might think that Pilates is a hot new exercise fad. In fact, Pilates is a low-impact fitness technique developed in the 1920s by Joseph Pilates.

Designed specifically to strengthen the body's core muscles by developing pelvic stability and abdominal control, Pilates exercises also help improve flexibility, joint mobility and strength. They can help you develop long, strong muscles, maintain a strong back and improve your posture.

Many Pilates exercises are done with special machines. The earliest Pilates machine, called the Reformer, was a wooden contraption outfitted with cables, pulleys, springs and sliding boards. Using their own body weight as resistance, exercisers used the Reformer to perform a series of progressive range-of-motion exercises that worked the muscles of the abdomen, back, upper legs and buttocks.

Although machines are still used, many Pilates programs offer floor-work classes as well, designed to stabilize and strengthen the core back and abdominal muscles.

Instead of emphasizing quantity, Pilates focuses on quality, meaning that exercisers do very few, but extremely precise, repetitions. Exercises can be adapted according to a person's own flexibility and strength abilities.

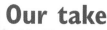 **Our take**

While Pilates is commonly practiced to enhance and maintain physical fitness, very little research has been done on the effectiveness of Pilates in reducing disease symptoms.

Getting proper instruction from a qualified Pilates teacher may cost more than some other mind-body therapies. However, doing so can increase the chances that you'll get the benefits that you desire and that your Pilates workouts will achieve the desired effect.

What the research says

Research shows that when practiced regularly, Pilates can increase strength. It can also help to lengthen muscles and increase their flexibility.

Obesity and low back pain

Very preliminary research suggests that practicing Pilates regularly may help with weight loss when included in a well-planned weight-loss program. Pilates may also help reduce low back pain.

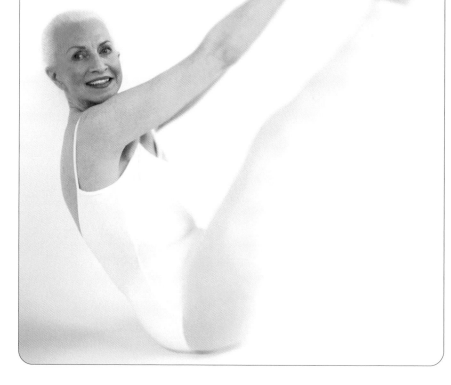

Relaxed breathing

Have you ever noticed how you breathe when you're stressed? Stress typically causes rapid, shallow breathing. This kind of breathing sustains other aspects of the stress response, such as rapid heart rate and perspiration.

If you can get control of your breathing, the spiraling effects of acute stress may automatically become less intense. Relaxed breathing, also called diaphragmatic breathing, can help you do that.

How to do it

Practice this basic technique twice a day, every day, and whenever you feel tense. Follow these steps:

- **Inhale.** With your mouth closed and your shoulders relaxed, inhale as slowly and deeply as you can to the count of six. When you breathe in, your abdomen should expand. Allow the air to fill your diaphragm.

- **Hold.** Keep the air in your lungs as you slowly count to four.

- **Exhale.** Release the air through your mouth as you slowly count to six.

- **Repeat.** Complete the inhale-hold-exhale cycle three to five times.

Our take

As with other relaxation techniques, relaxed breathing is easy to do, it can be done just about anywhere, and it's an easy way to reduce stress and anxiety without any expense.

Relaxed breathing can be learned through formal instruction, or you can follow the simple instructions on this page to get started. As with other mind-body therapies, relaxed breathing may be combined with guided imagery or meditation. There's little risk in giving it a try.

What the research says

There's evidence that relaxed breathing can help in the treatment of some diseases and conditions.

Angina

Preliminary research in people with angina suggests that some relaxation techniques may help reduce the frequency of angina attacks, reducing the need for medication. Additional studies are needed to confirm these findings.

Anxiety and stress

Relaxation techniques including relaxed breathing have been shown to help reduce anxiety and stress in people with panic disorder, work-related stress and some phobias.

High blood pressure

Relaxation techniques, such as relaxed breathing, may be combined with conventional therapy to reduce blood pressure and heart rate in people with high blood pressure.

Nausea and vomiting

Early research suggests that relaxation techniques may help reduce nausea and vomiting related to cancer chemotherapy.

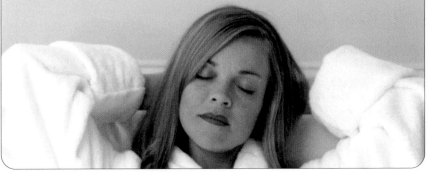

Spirituality and prayer

Spirituality has many definitions, but at its core it helps to give our lives context. Spirituality isn't necessarily connected to a specific belief system or even religious worship. Instead, it arises from your connection with yourself and with others, the development of your personal value system, and your search for meaning in life.

For many, this takes the form of religious observance, prayer, meditation or a belief in a higher power. For others, it can be found in nature, music, art or a secular community. Spirituality is different for everyone.

Spirituality begins with your relationship with yourself, is nurtured by your relationships with others, and culminates in a sense of purpose in life.

Realizing this, two of the best ways to cultivate your spirituality are to improve your self-esteem and to foster relationships with those important to you. This can lead to a deepened sense of your place in life and in the greater good.

Many people use prayer for their own health concerns and for those of others. In many religious institutions, prayer groups pray for members of their community who are sick.

Scientific investigation of the effectiveness of prayer in health settings has just begun. Evidence to date is inconclusive. However, there is some reason to believe that religious affiliation and practices are associated with better health and longer life.

Our take

We are complex beings with mind, body and spirit intertwined. For many of us, our busy lives mean that spirituality sometimes gets neglected until we're confronted by a major illness. But it doesn't matter so much what brings us back to our spirituality. It's just important that we nurture all aspects of our being in our quest to stay healthy. Find ways to energize your spirit, as well as your mind and body. Doing so can bring a healthy balance to your life.

What the research says

Several hundred studies have been conducted using spirituality and prayer, and they've produced mixed results. It's sometimes difficult for researchers to define various spiritual practices because they have different meaning for different people.

Cancer

Some studies of people with cancer report a change in the progression of the disease when prayer was used. Combining spirituality with other interventions improved the quality of life in people with cancer. More research is needed in this area.

Immune function

There is a small body of evidence linking immune function to spiritual well-being.

Spirituality: What's in it for you?

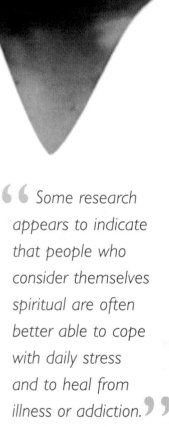

You may get many benefits from incorporating spirituality into your life. Spirituality can help you:

Focus on personal goals. Cultivating your spirituality may help uncover what's most meaningful in your life. By clarifying what's important, you can eliminate stress by focusing less on unimportant things that can sometimes consume you.

Connect to the world. The more you feel you have a purpose in the world, the less solitary you feel — even when you're alone. This can lead to an inner peace during difficult times.

Release control. When you feel part of a greater whole, you realize that you aren't responsible for everything that happens in life. You can share the burden of tough times as well as the joys of life's blessings with those around you.

Expand your support network. Whether you find spirituality in a church, mosque or synagogue, in your family, or in walks with a friend, this sharing of spiritual expression can help build strong relationships.

Lead a healthier life. Some research appears to indicate that people who consider themselves spiritual are often better able to cope with daily stress and to heal from illness or addiction.

Becoming more spiritual

If you want to strengthen your spirituality but aren't sure how to do it, here are some suggestions you might try:

- Practice prayer, meditation and relaxation techniques to access your inner wisdom and help you focus your thoughts.

- Keep a journal to help you express your feelings and record your progress.

- Seek out a trusted adviser or friend — preferably someone who has had similar life experiences — who can help you discover what's important to you in life.

- Read inspirational stories or essays to help you evaluate different philosophies of life.

- Talk to others whose spiritual lives you admire. Ask questions to find out how they found their way to a fulfilling spiritual life.

- Be open to new experiences. If you are exploring organized religion, remember to consider a variety of different faith traditions. If your spirituality is more secular, you might consider expanding your horizons with new experiences in the arts.

Some research appears to indicate that people who consider themselves spiritual are often better able to cope with daily stress and to heal from illness or addiction.

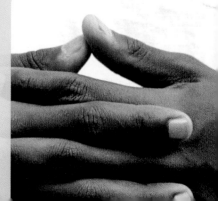

Nurturing relationships

Relationships provide many benefits. To expand your social network:

- Develop effective listening and communication skills.

- Make relationships with friends and family a priority, and stay in touch.

- Share your spiritual journey with loved ones.

- Seek out others with similar beliefs, and engage in conversation to learn from each other.

- Volunteer within your community.

- See the good in people and in yourself.

Tai chi

Tai chi (TIE-chee) is sometimes described as "meditation in motion." Originally developed in China as a form of self-defense, this graceful form of exercise has existed for about 2,000 years. It's becoming increasingly popular around the world, both as a basic exercise program and as a complement to other health care methods. Health benefits include stress reduction, greater balance and increased flexibility — especially for older adults.

To do tai chi, you perform a defined series of postures or movements in a slow, graceful manner. Each movement or posture flows into the next without pausing.

If you're trying to improve your general health, you may find tai chi helpful as part of your program. Tai chi is generally safe for people of all ages and levels of fitness. Studies show that for older adults tai chi can improve balance and reduce the risk of falls. Because the movements are low impact and put minimal stress on your muscles and joints, tai chi is appealing to many older adults. For these same reasons, if you have a condition such as arthritis or you're recovering from an injury, you may find it useful.

Tai chi appears to offer both physical and mental benefits no matter what your age. It's used to reduce stress, increase flexibility, improve muscle strength and definition, and increase energy, stamina and agility.

Our take

When learned correctly and practiced regularly, tai chi appears to be a very positive form of exercise. It's self-paced and noncompetitive. You don't need a large physical space or special clothing or equipment. You can do tai chi anytime, anyplace. It's easy to do in groups or by yourself. Because tai chi is slow and gentle, it has virtually no negative side effects. You could strain yourself when first learning, but with proper instruction, this shouldn't be a problem.

What the research says

Tai chi can reduce stress and increase balance and flexibility. Some studies suggest tai chi may be helpful in managing a number of conditions, including high blood pressure and depression.

Balance

Tai chi has been studied for its effect on improving balance and reducing risk of falling in older adults. Research is ongoing.

Cardiovascular disease

There's some evidence to indicate that tai chi may play a role in lowering blood pressure and cholesterol levels. It may also improve symptoms of congestive heart failure.

Depression

Using tai chi in combination with other therapies may treat depression and anxiety. Initial findings are encouraging, but more research is needed.

Exercise

Tai chi has been shown to improve aerobic capacity.

Pain

Tai chi may improve joint pain.

Sleep

Tai chi may improve sleep.

Yoga

If stress is getting the best of you, you might want to try yoga. This series of postures — sometimes named for mammals, fish or reptiles — along with controlled-breathing exercises, has become a popular means of stress reduction.

Though the practice of yoga has been around for thousands of years in India, its popularity in the United States has grown steadily only over the last 100 years or so. Today yoga classes teaching the art of breathing, meditation and posture are offered nearly everywhere from health clubs in big cities to community education classes in small towns.

Yoga represents one of the oldest health practices. The ultimate goal of yoga is to reach complete peacefulness of mind and body. While traditional yoga philosophy requires that students adhere to this mission through behavior, diet and meditation, chances are you aren't looking for a complete change in lifestyle but rather increased flexibility, relaxation or stress relief.

Yoga offers a good means of relaxation and stress relief. Its quiet, precise movements focus your mind less on your busy day and more on the moment as you concentrate on moving your body through specific poses.

There are several types of yoga. In the West, hatha yoga is the type most often practiced.

Our take

Yoga is rapidly gaining popularity in the United States. It's an excellent way to counteract stress and anxiety and to relieve the hunched posture that can come from sitting for hours in front of a computer. Practicing yoga regularly can improve your flexibility, balance, strength and posture. It's one of those activities that you can do alone or with a group, and it doesn't require a big investment to get started. The risks of yoga are low, which is all the more reason for giving it a try.

What the research says

According to the National Institutes of Health, yoga can help reduce stress, slow breathing, lower blood pressure, alter brain waves and assist your heart to work more efficiently.

Anxiety

Several studies have shown that practicing yoga several times a week can reduce the stress of daily living.

Asthma

Researchers have found that practicing yoga can reduce the need for medication in people with mild to moderate asthma.

Back pain

Yoga decreased symptoms of back pain in a well-designed study, with the improvement lasting for several months.

Depression

Some clinical research shows that yoga can improve some measures of cognitive function and decrease symptoms of depression.

High blood pressure

Practicing yoga regularly can help lower blood pressure, but it's unclear if yoga is more effective than other forms of exercise.

Osteoarthritis

People with osteoarthritis of the hands who took yoga had less finger pain than did those who didn't take yoga classes.

Other

Yoga has also been found to improve binge eating, chronic headaches, rheumatoid arthritis and diabetes.

Yoga cautions

Yoga, overall, is considered safe if you're generally healthy. Some yoga positions can put significant strain on your lower back and on your joints. See your doctor first if you have any joint problems or a history of low back or neck pain. You might want to avoid certain yoga positions depending on your condition.

Also see your doctor before you begin a yoga class if you have any of the following conditions, as complications can arise:

- High blood pressure that's difficult to control
- A risk of blood clots
- Eye conditions, including glaucoma
- Osteoporosis

If you're pregnant or nursing, yoga is considered generally safe. But avoid any poses that put pressure on your uterus, such as those that require you to twist at the waist. Some yoga classes are specifically tailored for pregnant women. Check with your obstetrician if you have any questions whether yoga is right for you and your baby.

Hatha yoga: A popular form of yoga

Hatha yoga focuses on physical poses and controlled breathing. Several versions of hatha yoga exist. The version you choose depends on your personal preferences. But all varieties of hatha yoga include two basic components — poses and breathing.

Poses

In a typical hatha yoga class, you may learn anywhere from 10 to 30 poses. More experienced yoga students might know many more, including more-advanced poses that require advanced stretching and twisting. Poses range from the seemingly easy, such as the corpse pose, which involves lying on the floor, completely relaxed, to the most difficult poses that take years of practice to master.

Remember that you don't have to do every pose your instructor demonstrates. If a pose is uncomfortable, or you can't hold it as long as the instructor requests, don't do it. Good instructors will understand. Spend time sitting quietly, breathing deeply until your instructor moves the class on to another pose that's more comfortable for you.

Breathing

Controlling your breathing is an important part of yoga. In yoga, breath signifies your vital energy. Yoga teaches that controlling your breathing can help you control your body and gain control of your mind.

You'll learn to control your breathing by paying attention to it. Your instructor may ask you to take deep, regular breaths as you concentrate on your breathing. Other techniques involve paying attention to your breath as it moves into your body and fills your lungs, or breathing through alternate nostrils.

Mind-body therapies and cancer treatment

Most people with cancer who use alternative practices don't expect the treatments to cure their cancer. They may use alternative therapies to treat the pain associated with their cancer and control the side effects of treatment, such as nausea and weakness. Your doctor might recommend conventional medications or alternative therapies, such as acupuncture or massage, for these signs and symptoms.

In general, these treatments aren't invasive, making them quite safe. Still, talk to your doctor about these therapies before using them.

Acupuncture. In this treatment, tiny needles are inserted into your skin to stimulate your body's natural energy, or qi (pronounced "chee"). By restoring the natural flow of qi, acupuncture is supposed to help your body heal itself. Acupuncture is effective in treating pain and nausea in some people with cancer.

Aromatherapy. Proponents believe that fragrant oils from plants can affect your mood. About 40 oils are commonly used in aromatherapy. You can experience aromatherapy at home or at a spa, or apply oil during a massage. Aromatherapy is said to help pain, depression and stress, and promote a general sense of well-being.

Healing touch. Touch therapy practitioners claim to use their hands to transmit "energy forces" that can improve the energy flow that runs through you. By moving their hands back and forth across your body, practitioners claim to be able to locate and remove energy force disturbances. Practitioners believe this reduces pain and encourages relaxation.

Hypnosis. This relaxation method effectively relieves some chronic pain, and it may also reduce nausea and vomiting in people with cancer. Although you may look like you're asleep during hypnosis, you actually go into a state of deep concentration. While you're under hypnosis, your practitioner may suggest you focus on goals, such as controlling your pain and reducing your stress.

Massage therapy. During a massage, your practitioner kneads your skin, muscles and tendons in an effort to relieve muscle tension and stress and promote relaxation. If you're currently receiving conventional chemotherapy, check with your doctor before undergoing massage. If you have a low platelet count because of chemotherapy, deep massage can cause bleeding or bruising. Certain types of massage and spinal manipulation can also be unsafe if the bones in your back or neck have been weakened by cancer.

Meditation. Meditation can produce a state of physical relaxation, mental calmness, alertness and psychological balance. Practicing meditation can change how you relate to the flow of emotions and thoughts and may help you control how you respond to a challenging situation, such as cancer.

Yoga. Yoga can help reduce stress, slow breathing, lower blood pressure, and produce peacefulness of mind and body. This can be especially helpful as you cope with cancer treatment.

Many other therapies including spirituality and prayer and art and music therapy have been tested in people with cancer and produced favorable results.

A note of caution: Giving up on conventional cancer treatment that has been proved repeatedly in clinical trials to help people with cancer can be risky and even deadly. Avoid alternative therapists who pressure you to forgo the treatment your doctor recommends for a treatment that's unproved. Work with your doctor on a therapy regimen that's right for you.

Chapter 5
Energy Therapies

A visit with Susanne Cutshall

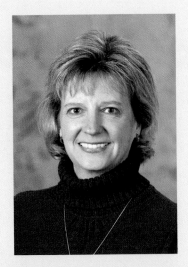

Susanne Cutshall, R.N., C.N.S.
Integrative Health Specialist,
Surgery

❝ *Those that practice energy medicine are looking to heal the body by activating its natural energies and restoring energies that have become weak, disturbed or out of balance.* ❞

Energy-based therapies (energy medicine) are a form of complementary and alternative medicine based on the belief that imbalances in the body's energy fields result in illness, and that re-balancing these energy fields can restore health and allow healing to occur. Those that practice energy medicine are looking to heal the body by activating its natural energies and restoring energies that have become weak, disturbed or out of balance. Energy-based therapies include a variety of practices such as acupuncture, therapeutic touch, magnetic therapy, qi gong and reiki.

Energy-based therapies have been in general use since the founding of the non-profit International Society for the Study of Subtle Energies and Energy Medicine in the 1980s. The National Center for Complementary and Alternative Medicine distinguishes between two types of energy fields. Veritable energy is that which can be measured, while putative energy cannot be measured or is of an unclear nature.

Veritable energy therapies utilize mechanical vibrations, such as sound, and electromagnetic forces, such as magnetism, to treat illness. Those practices that involve putative energy fields are based on the concept that human beings are infused with a subtle form of energy. Energy is believed to flow through the human body, and practitioners claim they can work with this subtle energy and effect changes in the physical body, influencing health. The goal for individuals seeking these therapies is to clear, balance and stimulate the human energy system and promote holistic healing of the body, mind and spirit.

Energy-based therapies may be among the most controversial practices because of the difficulty in convincingly using any biophysical means to measure the effects of some of the therapies. However, active investigations are being conducted at academic medical centers, including Mayo Clinic, and energy medicine, in general, is gradually gaining popularity.

Of all of the energy-based therapies, the most well-known and well-studied is acupuncture. Acupuncture, according to traditional Chinese medicine, uses fine filiform needles inserted and manipulated into specific points on the body, along energy fields known as meridians, where qi, the vital life energy, flows. Insertion of the needles into these specific points is done to relieve pain or for specific therapeutic purposes. As the needles are inserted, the person receiving treatment may feel a tingling sensation as the life force energy is accessed and cleared.

Further studies involving energy-based therapies are being developed to help confirm the existence of these subtle energies. In the meantime, the therapies are increasingly being integrated into patient care practices at medical centers across the United States.

Acupuncture

Acupuncture involves the insertion of very thin needles to various depths at strategic points on your body. Acupuncture originated in China thousands of years ago, but over the past two decades its popularity has grown significantly within the United States. Although scientists don't fully understand how or why acupuncture works, some studies indicate that it may provide a number of health benefits — from reducing pain to helping manage chemotherapy-induced nausea.

Acupuncture seems to be useful as a stand-alone treatment for some conditions, but it's also increasingly being used in conjunction with conventional medical treatments. For example, doctors may combine acupuncture with medication to control pain during and after surgery.

Numerous past studies of acupuncture have been proved inadequate because of the difficulty of conducting valid scientific studies. Therefore, it's difficult to create a definitive list of the conditions for which acupuncture might be helpful. However, preliminary studies indicate that acupuncture may help relieve symptoms associated with a variety of diseases and conditions, including low back pain, labor pain, headaches, osteoarthritis and fibromyalgia.

In the 2007 National Health Interview Survey, an estimated 3.1 million U.S. adults reported recently using acupuncture.

Our take

Acupuncture has been used at Mayo Clinic since the 1970s. Mayo Clinic also has licensed acupuncturists on staff. When performed properly by trained practitioners using sterile needles, acupuncture has proved to be a safe and effective therapy. A review of acupuncture by the World Health Organization found it was an effective treatment for 28 conditions and there was evidence to suggest it may be effective for several more.

What the research says

Research shows that acupuncture is effective in treating a number of medical problems.

Fibromyalgia

In a 2006 Mayo Clinic study, acupuncture significantly improved symptoms of fibromyalgia.

Headaches

Studies suggest acupuncture may help treat headaches of unknown cause. Several trials also indicate individuals with migraines may benefit from acupuncture.

Nausea and vomiting

Acupuncture can help reduce nausea and vomiting in people who are receiving chemotherapy. It may also help reduce nausea and vomiting from other causes, including pregnancy. A 2008 Mayo Clinic study found it decreased the incidence of severe nausea following cardiac surgery.

Osteoarthritis

Acupuncture has shown mixed benefits when used to treat osteoarthritis of the knee, hip and back. Some studies suggest it may provide considerable pain relief and improve joint function, while other studies show little or no benefit.

Pain management

A number of studies have shown that acupuncture is effective in treating postoperative dental pain, pain related to endoscopic procedures, low back pain and some forms of chronic pain, including fibromyalgia pain. Acupuncture has also been effective in reducing pain related to tennis elbow.

How does acupuncture work?

Traditional Chinese medicine is based on the belief that the body contains a vital life energy, called qi (chee), which runs along pathways within the body. Imbalances in the flow of qi are thought to cause illness.

These life-energy pathways are called meridians and are accessible at approximately 400 different locations, or points, on the body.

Practitioners of acupuncture attempt to rebalance your energy flow by inserting extremely fine needles into these points in various combinations. This allows your body's natural healing mechanisms to take over.

A typical session

Acupuncture therapy usually involves a series of weekly or biweekly treatments in an outpatient setting. It's common to have up to 12 treatments in total.

Each visit typically includes an exam, an assessment of your current condition, insertion of the needles and a discussion of self-care tips. A typical visit usually lasts 30 to 60 minutes.

During a session, the practitioner should use sterilized, individually wrapped stainless steel needles that are used only once and then thrown away. You may feel a brief, sharp sensation when the needle is inserted, but generally the procedure isn't painful.

It's common to feel a deep aching sensation when the needle reaches the correct spot. After placement, the needles are sometimes gently moved or stimulated with electricity or heat.

Some people are energized by the treatment, while it makes others feel relaxed.

Inside the body

According to the National Institutes of Health, researchers are studying at least three possible explanations for how acupuncture may work:

- **Opioid release.** During acupuncture, endorphins that are part of your body's natural pain-control system may be released into your central nervous system — your brain and spinal cord. This reduces pain much like taking a pain medication.

- **Spinal cord stimulation.** Acupuncture may stimulate the nerves in your spinal cord to release pain-suppressing neurotransmitters. This has sometimes been called the "gate theory."

During a session, the practitioner should use sterilized, individually wrapped stainless steel needles that are used only once and then thrown away.

- **Blood flow changes.**
  Acupuncture needles may increase the amount of blood flow in the area around the needle. The increased blood flow may supply additional nutrients or remove toxic substances, or both, promoting healing.

Pros and cons

As with most medical therapies, acupuncture has benefits and risks. It's safe when performed properly, and it has few side effects. It can be useful as a complement to other treatments. It may also be an alternative to controlling pain if you don't respond to or don't want to take pain medications.

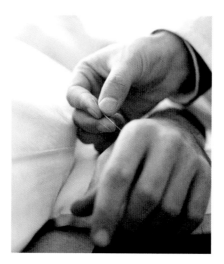

Acupuncture may not be safe if you have a bleeding disorder or if you're taking blood thinners. The most common side effects of acupuncture are soreness, bleeding or bruising at the needle sites and dizziness. Rarely, a needle may break or an internal organ might be injured. If needles are reused, infectious diseases may be accidentally transmitted. These risks are low in the hands of a competent, certified acupuncture practitioner.

Cost

Acupuncture is a form of complementary and alternative medicine that is increasingly covered by insurance. However, you should check with your insurance company before you begin treatment to see whether acupuncture will be covered for your condition. Some insurance companies require pre-authorization for acupuncture.

Acupuncture and cancer therapy

Clinical studies have shown that acupuncture is effective in reducing symptoms, including pain, in people with cancer. In one study, most of the people treated with acupuncture were able to stop taking medication for pain relief or take smaller doses.

However, because of the design and size of the studies, the findings aren't considered extremely reliable. Studies with stricter scientific controls are needed.

The strongest evidence as to the effectiveness of acupuncture is in the area of relieving nausea and vomiting associated with chemotherapy. In addition, several clinical trials are studying the effects of acupuncture on cancer and other symptoms caused by treatment, including weight loss, cough, chest pain, fever, depression, night sweats, hot flashes, dry mouth and swelling in the arms and legs. Studies have shown that, for many people, acupuncture either relieves symptoms or keeps them from getting worse.

Some studies also suggest acupuncture helps enhance or rejuvenate the body's immune system.

Acupuncture at Mayo Clinic

Experienced physicians and licensed acupuncturists at Mayo Clinic perform acupuncture to treat various conditions. Acupuncture can be helpful as a stand-alone treatment to provide pain relief or to treat nausea, or it may serve as an encompassing therapy to maintain good health and well-being, increase energy, and improve mood.

Specialists at Mayo Clinic recognize that treatments such as acupuncture work on many levels. They help promote mental, physical and spiritual health — creating a healthy balance of mind, body and spirit.

Mayo Clinic offers these acupuncture techniques:

- **Manual stimulation.** Needles are gently twisted by hand after placement.
- **Heat and electrical stimulation.** Needles are gently stimulated with a safe, low current of electricity, heat or both after placement.

Acupuncture usually is done in a series of weekly or biweekly treatments. Each visit typically includes an examination and assessment of the person's condition, insertion of the acupuncture needles, and a discussion of self-care tips. A visit generally lasts from 30 to 60 minutes. Sessions are tailored to the person's needs, concerns and diagnosis.

Mayo Clinic is involved in several acupuncture studies.

Healing touch

Healing touch, also known as therapeutic touch, draws on ancient healing practices from a number of cultures, including Indian, Asian and American Indian. Healing touch may be combined with deeply held religious beliefs and practices.

During a healing touch session, the practitioner first moves his or her hands a few inches above the recipient's body. This is done to assess the recipient's energy condition. Then the practitioner gently touches the recipient at various energy points on the body in a way that's designed to move energy through the practitioner to the recipient, strengthening and reorienting the recipient's energy flow within and surrounding the body. The goal is to promote the body's self-healing processes by opening blocked or congested flow of energy.

Some people who have undergone healing touch have responded that the treatment resulted in having a more positive mood, lowered pain, reduced anxiety or an improved sense of well-being. A typical session lasts 20 to 30 minutes.

Proponents of healing touch claim that it's effective in treating stress-related problems, allergies, heart conditions, high blood pressure and chronic pain. So far, there's no hard data to confirm this.

Our take

We recognize that people perceive health benefits from healing touch. Some people find the therapy to be relaxing, and certainly relaxation is good for your health. However, beyond relaxation, there's limited scientific evidence that healing touch improves health. Because there's little risk in healing touch, whether to try the therapy is up to you, based on how closely it fits with your personal beliefs.

What the research says

Many small studies of healing touch have suggested it's effective in treating a variety of conditions. These include wound healing, osteoarthritis, migraine and anxiety in burn patients. A review of 11 controlled studies on the effects of healing touch showed that participants in seven studies had positive outcomes, while those in three other studies showed no effect. In another study, the control group fared better than those who received healing touch therapy.

There is some impressive anecdotal evidence that healing touch works. However, more study is needed to confirm these findings. The National Institutes of Health is sponsoring some research looking at the possible effects of healing touch in treating symptoms such as pain, fatigue, depression and stress.

Magnetic therapy

Magnets have been used for centuries in an attempt to cure a number of disorders. During the Middle Ages, they were used to treat gout, arthritis, poisoning and baldness. In more recent times, magnets have been used to treat fibromyalgia, respiratory problems, high blood pressure and stress, among other conditions. By some estimates, people worldwide spend more than $1 billion a year on various forms of magnet therapy.

Magnetic therapy involves the application of a magnetic field to the body — using an electromagnet or a static magnet — for health benefits.

There are numerous theories about how magnets might work to treat symptoms. One theory is that static magnets — made of solid metal — change how cells in the body function. Another is that magnets alter the balance between cell growth and cell death. And yet another is that because it contains iron, blood may be a conductor of magnetic energy. None of these theories has been proved correct.

The Food and Drug Administration (FDA) has approved the use of electromagnetic therapy for treating some types of bone fractures and certain cases of depression. In addition, electromagnets have been studied for use in treating knee pain, chronic pelvic pain, bone and muscle problems, and migraines. The FDA still considers electromagnetic therapy as experimental for these uses.

Our take

Magnets are popular. Many people wear them thinking they can help reduce pain and other symptoms associated with conditions such as arthritis and fibromyalgia. What's important to know is there's a big difference between electromagnets and static magnets. Most of the current research involves electromagnets, which may hold some potential for treating conditions such as depression. Studies of static magnets — used in bracelets, shoe inserts, mattress-pad covers, and so forth — have generally produced negative results, indicating no benefit.

What the research says

Research into the effectiveness of magnetic therapy is under way on a number of fronts. While this approach has shown promise, evidence as to its effectiveness is still evolving.

Arthritis

Several studies have looked at magnetic therapy applied to osteoarthritic areas or areas of degenerative joint disease to see if the therapy can reduce pain. Much of the research has focused on knee arthritis. Most studies have been small or not well designed, and the effectiveness of magnetic therapy is unclear.

Bone fractures

Several studies report that pulsating electromagnetic therapy may help speed healing of bone fractures, especially those fractures that don't heal well, called nonunion fractures.

Depression

Transcranial magnetic stimulation (TMS) is used to treat people with depression who don't respond to medications (see page 126).

Fibromyalgia

A small Mayo Clinic study suggests TMS may be beneficial for treatment of pain associated with fibromyalgia.

Other

Pulsating electromagnetic therapy has been used to treat migraines, multiple sclerosis and sleep disorders. Further research is needed.

Types of magnets

There are two types of magnets used in magnetic therapy.

Static magnets

Static — or permanent — magnets are the kind with which we're most familiar. They come in different shapes and sizes, but they all have a couple of things in common. They're made of iron, steel, rare earth elements, or alloys, and they produce energy called a magnetic field. This field attracts iron, and is strongest — and opposite — at each end of the magnet. Thus, each magnet has a north and south pole — a property known as polarity.

Unlike electromagnets, the strength of the magnetic field of a static magnet remains constant (static) and can't be varied.

Static magnets are the type most often marketed for health purposes. They're incorporated into shoe inserts, mattress pads, belts, bracelets and other jewelry, and head wear. The theory is that the magnetic field from a static magnet interacts in some way with your body to correct imbalances or reverse negative trends.

Electromagnets

Electromagnets consist of a metal core that's wrapped with a wire coil. When an electrical current flows through the coil, a magnetic field is induced in the core.

Pulsating electromagnetic therapy has been used for several decades to enhance healing of some types of bone fractures. More recently, researchers have begun to experiment with electromagnetic energy for the treatment of depression, chronic pain, ringing in the ears and migraines.

Biological effects

There's growing evidence that magnetic fields can affect various biological processes. Recent research has shown that some blood vessels that are normally dilated will constrict when exposed to a field from a static magnet, and that vessels that are normally constricted will dilate. This may lead to treating some kinds of tissue swelling and vessel blockages. However, there's no good evidence yet that magnetic therapy is effective in treating these conditions.

Treating depression with magnetic fields

Transcranial magnetic stimulation (TMS) involves using brief powerful electromagnetic pulses to alter brain activity. The therapy has received approval from the Food and Drug Administration for use in individuals who have depression that isn't responding to drug therapy.

A typical TMS appointment lasts about an hour. It involves sitting in a reclining chair as a large electromagnetic coil is held against the scalp near the forehead, often on the left side. An electric current creates a magnetic pulse, or field, that travels through the skull. Those currents stimulate nerve cells in the region of the brain involved in mood regulation and depression.

You may feel a slight tapping or knocking sensation on your head during a TMS session. Although the procedure is generally painless, it may cause the muscles of your scalp or jaw to contract.

TMS doesn't involve surgery, and requires no anesthesia. You also don't need to be hospitalized. It can be done on an outpatient basis in a doctor's office.

In addition to the United States, TMS has been approved for use in Europe, Canada and Australia as a treatment for depression.

When TMS is performed on appropriate candidates, total remission of depression symptoms is possible, and about a 50 percent improvement in depression symptoms is common. One limitation of TMS is that you can't have it if you have a metal implant or device in your head or chest — such as a stent or pacemaker.

Reiki

Reiki (RAY-kee) is made up of the Japanese words *rei*, which means universal spirit, and *ki* (or qi), which means life force energy. As with other energy therapies, practitioners of reiki believe that disturbances in the body's energy systems can cause illness, and that by improving the flow and balance of energy, disease can be treated and health maintained.

The practitioner delivers reiki therapy through his or her hands with the goal of raising the amount of ki in and around the recipient. There are many forms of reiki. The two most common are traditional Japanese reiki and Western reiki.

During a session, which typically lasts 30 to 90 minutes, the fully clothed recipient either sits or lies down. The practitioner's hands are placed either on or a few inches above the recipient's body. There are between 12 and 20 different reiki hand positions. Each position is held until the practitioner feels that the flow of energy has slowed or stopped, usually between two to five minutes.

Recipients sometimes describe a deep sense of relaxation after a session, accompanied by a feeling of well-being. They also report sensations of warmth, tingling and sleepiness, and feelings of refreshment.

Reiki is used to treat stress, chronic pain and nausea from chemotherapy, to speed recovery from anesthesia, and to enhance well-being.

Our take

Similar to healing touch, the benefits associated with reiki may come from its ability to help promote relaxation. There's little, if any, health risk from the therapy. But there's also little evidence that it can effectively treat specific conditions. It's up to you if you think it's worth your money to give it a try.

What the research says

Reiki is touted for the treatment of many diseases and conditions. One study suggests that reiki may have some effect on blood pressure and heart and respiration rates.

The practice hasn't been well researched and is lacking in scientific evidence. A review conducted in 2008 did not find reiki effective and did not recommend its use for the treatment of any condition. Studies to date have not found any significant adverse effects from the use of reiki.

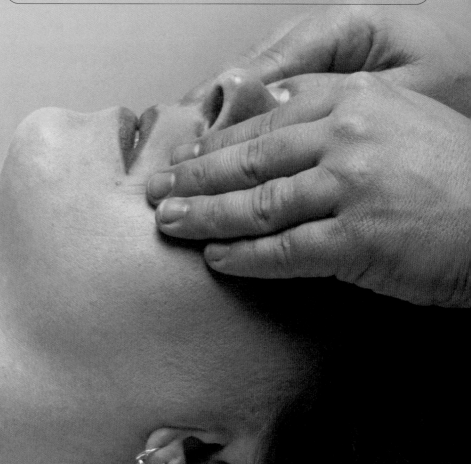

Chapter 6
Hands-on Therapies

A visit with Dr. Ralph Gay

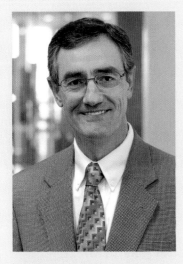

Ralph Gay, M.D., D.C.
Physical Medicine
and Rehabilitation

" Surveys show that about 8 percent of U.S. adults currently use chiropractic care and more than 7 percent seek massage therapy each year. "

Hands-on therapies — practices such as massage and manipulation — have been used to relieve pain and illness for centuries. This group of treatments includes some of the most commonly used complementary therapies, used most often to treat musculoskeletal conditions such as back pain, neck pain, headache and arthritis. As a group, the providers of these therapies represent the largest contingency of organized complementary care practitioners in the United States and Canada, with the chiropractic profession alone having more than 60,000 members and performing approximately 95 percent of manipulative therapy in the United States.

Although once popular, hands-on therapies fell out of favor with the rapid growth of modern (Western) medicine during the last century. For years, the osteopathic and chiropractic professions in the United States struggled for acceptance, while in other parts of the world hands-on therapies became part of organized medicine. Gradually, these therapeutic tools experienced renewed growth in North America. Surveys show that about 8 percent of U.S. adults currently use chiropractic care and more than 7 percent seek massage therapy each year.

Hands-on treatments — often called manual therapies — work by way of physical forces applied to the body. They have traditionally included massage, manipulation (joint movement caused by a thrusting procedure) and mobilization (joint movement without thrusting). As our understanding of the relationship between body structure and function has evolved, other therapies have been developed to help correct abnormal or inefficient motion. Movement therapies are thought to optimize the interplay between the nervous system and the musculoskeletal system and improve physical functioning. The Feldenkrais method and the Alexander technique are two examples of commonly used movement therapies.

Although not without risk, most hands-on treatments have limited potential for harm. When used appropriately, the most common side effect is local discomfort, which is generally short-lived. More serious complications can happen, though. Probably the most controversial treatment is neck (cervical spine) manipulation, which in rare instances can cause stroke (approximately 1 time in 1 million treatments). Fortunately, providers who use spinal manipulation — chiropractors, osteopaths and physical therapists — are some of the most highly educated complementary therapy practitioners.

The evidence supporting the use of hands-on therapies is growing. Some practices, such as spinal manipulation and mobilization and massage, have a significant body of scientific evidence supporting their use for conditions such as low back pain. Yet others are less well known and are only beginning to undergo scientific scrutiny. Ongoing research is necessary to establish the appropriate place for hands-on therapies in today's health care system.

Alexander technique

The Alexander technique is named for F.M. Alexander, an Australian-English actor who believed in a link between posture, body movement and physical problems. Using the Alexander technique, you learn to become more aware of your posture and body movements. But unlike other approaches to movement, such as yoga or Pilates, the Alexander technique isn't a set of exercises. Instead, it's a way to heighten awareness of how you move, to improve your coordination and help you become a more intelligent exerciser. The Alexander technique is used to relieve pain, prevent injury and improve function.

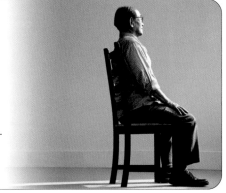

Our take
The Alexander technique is quite popular. Though there are limited data available as to its effectiveness, the risks are minimal. If you think it may help improve your coordination or relieve symptoms such as chronic pain, it's worth a try.

What the research says
Areas that have been studied include balance, low back pain, chronic pain from the temporomandibular joint (TMJ), Parkinson's disease, and lung function in musicians. Better designed studies are necessary to determine the effectiveness of the Alexander technique in treating these and other disorders.

Feldenkrais method

The Feldenkrais method uses gentle movements to develop increased flexibility and coordination. Though similar to yoga, the Feldenkrais method doesn't strive for correct positions, but instead aims for more dexterous, painless and efficient body movements. The goal is to create an awareness and quality of movement through body feedback rather than predefined postures. In group classes, which may be part of a physical or occupational therapy session, the instructor leads you through a sequence of movements — sitting in a chair, lying down or standing — that progress in range and complexity.

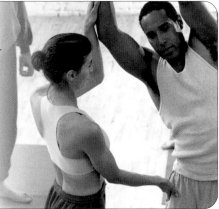

Our take
Similar to the Alexander technique, this form of movement therapy poses little risk. If you think it may help improve a musculoskeletal problem or symptoms of another condition, go ahead and give it a try. As to its effectiveness, there's not enough research to reach any definitive conclusions.

What the research says
The Feldenkrais method has been used to treat a variety of illnesses and disorders, including anxiety and depression, various musculoskeletal problems, and multiple sclerosis. In all cases, more research is needed to verify whether it's effective.

Massage

You might think of a massage as a luxury found in exotic spas and upscale health clubs. But did you know that massage, when combined with traditional medical treatments, is used to reduce stress and promote healing in people with certain health conditions?

During a massage, a therapist manipulates your body's soft tissues — your muscles, skin and tendons — using his or her fingertips, hands and fists. Massage can be performed by several types of health care professionals, such as a massage therapist, physical therapist or occupational therapist. Several versions of massage exist, and they're performed in a variety of settings.

A massage may make you feel relaxed, and most people use if for relaxation. But it isn't likely to cure everything that ails you. And, if performed incorrectly, it could hurt you. Learning about massage before you try one can help ensure that the experience is safe and enjoyable (see "What to expect during a massage" on page 132).

Massage can relieve tension in your muscles, and most people use it for relaxation, relief of stress and anxiety, or to reduce muscle soreness. Massage can also cause your body to release natural painkillers, and it may boost your immune system.

Our take

Massage is a great complementary and alternative treatment. Almost everyone feels better after a massage. The treatment has been shown to help relieve pain and soreness and reduce anxiety. There are different types of massage. If you find one that works for you, you may be surprised at how quickly it can become a regular part of your weekly routine! While generally safe, there are some instances in which a massage may not be recommended (see page 133).

What the research says

Here's what some studies have found:

Anxiety and stress

Massage reduces anxiety in depressed children and anorexic women. It also reduces anxiety and withdrawal symptoms in adults trying to quit smoking. People report it reduces stress.

Cancer treatment

People with cancer who receive regularly scheduled massage therapy during treatment report less anxiety, pain and fatigue.

Children with diabetes

Children who are massaged every day by their parents are more likely to stick to their medication and diet regimens, which helps reduce their blood glucose levels.

Immune system

People with HIV who participated in massage studies showed an increased number of natural killer cells, which are thought to defend the body from viral and cancer cells.

Pain

Pain was decreased in studies of people with fibromyalgia, migraines and recent surgeries. Massage may also help relieve low back pain.

Sports-related soreness

Some athletes receive massages after exercise, especially to the muscles they use most in their sport or activity. A massage might help increase blood flow to your muscles and reduce soreness.

What to expect during a massage

No matter what kind of massage you choose, you should feel calm and relaxed during and after your massage. When you have a massage, expect to:

Answer a few questions. Your massage therapist will want to know what you want from your massage. Are you looking for help with a pulled muscle? Massage therapists will also want to know about any medical conditions you may have, so they can decide if massage is safe for you or how to make it safer.

Disrobe. You'll be asked to remove your clothes, or at least most of them. Your massage therapist should give you privacy while you take your clothes off and provide a robe or a towel to cover yourself. A good massage therapist will understand your modesty and keep you covered as much as possible throughout the massage.

If taking your clothes off doesn't sound relaxing or if you're pressed for time, try a chair massage. These massages are conducted while you sit in a special chair that slopes forward so the massage therapist can work on your back. It's often done in the open, rather than in a private room.

Be asked to lie down. Most massages will require you to lie on a padded table. Pillows or bolsters might be used to position you during the massage.

This allows you to relax completely during the massage. Music usually plays softly while you're massaged.

Have oils and lotions used on your skin. Some massage therapists use oils or lotions to reduce friction while massaging your body. If you're allergic to any ingredients commonly found in body oils and lotions, tell your massage therapist. You may opt not to use oils and lotions if you prefer.

Never feel significant pain. Pain that's more significant than just momentary discomfort could indicate that something is wrong. If a massage therapist is pushing too hard, tell him or her to lighten the pressure. Your massage therapist will expect feedback from you to understand how best to massage you. Occasionally you may have a sensitive spot in a muscle that feels like a knot. It's likely to be uncomfortable while your massage therapist works it out. But if it becomes painful, speak up.

Spend about an hour. Most table massages last about an hour, though some may be shorter and others up to 90 minutes long. It's generally your preference.

Chinese massage

Chinese massage, called tui na, is the oldest known system of massage. It's been used in China for thousands of years, dating back to the Shang dynasty.

Unlike other forms of massage therapy, tui na is more closely related to acupuncture in its use of the meridian system. Through the application of massage and manipulation techniques at specific points on the body, tui na seeks to establish harmonious flow of the body's vital life energy — called "qi" — allowing the body to naturally heal itself. Qi is believed to run along an intricate system of channels, called meridians.

The term *tui na* translates into "push and pull" in Chinese. It's a series of maneuvers that include pressing, kneading and grasping, which range from light stroking to deep-tissue work. The maneuvers involve use of hand techniques to massage the body's soft tissues (muscles and tendons), acupressure techniques to affect the flow of qi, and manipulation techniques to realign the musculoskeletal system.

Unlike most other forms of massage, Chinese massage generally isn't a light, relaxing massage. It can be quite powerful and some people find portions of the massage to be a bit painful.

Tui na is generally used to treat injuries, joint and muscle problems, chronic pain, and some internal disorders. It shouldn't be used for conditions such as a bone fracture or external wound or open sores. It's also not recommended for life-threatening conditions such as a cancerous tumor.

Avoiding potential risks

Massage is generally safe as long as it's done by a trained therapist. But massage isn't for everyone. And for some people it can even be dangerous. Discuss massage with your doctor before making an appointment if you're pregnant or if you have:

- Burns or open wounds on the area to be massaged

- Had a recent heart attack

- Cancer — you'll want to avoid direct pressure on the tumor area

- Deep vein thrombosis

- Unhealed fractures

- Rheumatoid arthritis in the area to be massaged

- Severe osteoporosis

Massage done properly rarely leads to severe injuries. Ask your massage therapist about his or her training and qualifications — some states require licensing. And if any part of your massage doesn't feel right or is painful, speak up right away. Most serious problems come from too much pressure during massage. In rare circumstances, massage can cause:
- Internal bleeding

- Nerve damage

- Temporary paralysis

Talk to your doctor and your massage therapist if you have any concerns about your risk of injury. Asking questions can help you feel more at ease.

Massage at Mayo Clinic

Trained specialists at Mayo Clinic offer massage therapy for various conditions. Massage therapy techniques can decrease swelling and impaired joint mobility, ease muscle spasms and muscle tension, and increase circulation to promote healing. Massage can also reduce pain and improve muscle tone.

During a massage, a certified massage therapist or medical professional manipulates the soft tissues (muscles, connective tissue, tendons, ligaments and skin) of the body using varying degrees of pressure and movement after evaluating a person's needs. The massage strokes used depend on the injury or condition.

Specialists at Mayo Clinic recognize that many alternative medicine treatments, such as massage, can promote physical, mental and spiritual wellness. Mayo's Complementary and Integrative Medicine Program was developed to blend the best of both worlds — conventional medicine and evidence-based alternative practices.

Doctors and massage therapists at Mayo Clinic work together to coordinate a massage therapy treatment plan for an injury or condition as part of an individual's overall plan of care. Massage therapy may be recommended for conditions as such:

- Neck and back pain

- Headaches

- Temporomandibular joint (TMJ) pain and dysfunction

- Muscle and joint pain

- Numbness and tingling sensations (paresthesias) and nerve pain

- Fibromyalgia

- Myofascial pain syndrome

- Anxiety

- Stress-related insomnia

- Digestive disorders

- Sports injuries

- Soft tissue injuries

The benefits of massage therapy include reduced stress, anxiety and pain, improved circulation, improved levels of alertness, enhanced sleep patterns, release of the body's natural painkillers (endorphins), relaxation, and increased oxygen supply. Massage also can reduce heart rate and blood pressure and increase energy and immune system activity.

Massage may be a means to help you feel more relaxed and less anxious and to reduce pain. It's one of several useful tools for managing your health, but it doesn't take the place of standard medical treatment and exercise.

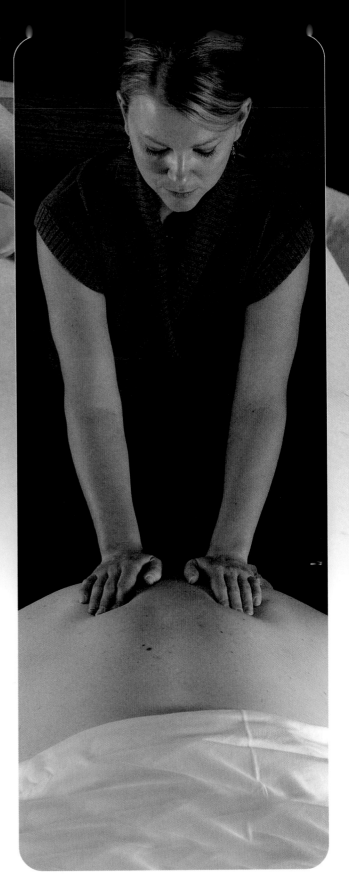

Ongoing research

Mayo Clinic has been involved in several studies involving massage therapy.

In two studies, Mayo researchers measured the effect of massage therapy on reducing pain, anxiety and tension in individuals undergoing cardiac surgery. The studies found that massage helps reduce feelings of pain and helps decrease anxiety. Because massage can reduce tension in the body, patients often feel better and may need less pain medication during recovery. Massage can be particularly beneficial to individuals who have open-heart surgery and the related back pain after surgery due to the rib cage being opened for access to the heart.

Researchers have also been exploring the effects of music on cardiac patients. Listening to music helps people relax and feel less tense; therefore, it helps decrease pain, improve the peoples' moods and promotes better sleep.

In another study at Mayo, staff receive seated chair massages in an effort to reduce stress. Researchers want to know if regular massage sessions can help improve job satisfaction and quality of life for those individuals involved in the study.

Still another study taking place at Mayo Clinic is focused on people with cancer. Researchers are evaluating the effects of massage in relieving pain and anxiety among individuals who receive chemotherapy.

Reflexology

The theory behind reflexology is that specific areas on the soles of your feet correspond to other parts of your body — such as your head or neck or your internal organs.

Reflexologists use foot charts to guide them as they massage, and then apply varying amounts of manual pressure to specific areas of the feet in an effort to influence a problem elsewhere in the body. Sometimes, reflexologists also use items such as rubber balls, rubber bands or sticks of wood to assist in their work. The practice was developed by William Fitzgerald, M.D., in the early 20th century.

Reflexology is practiced primarily as a form of treatment for a wide variety of problems. However, some reflexologists also claim to diagnose certain illnesses based on the condition of the soles of a person's feet.

Reflexology is sometimes combined with other hands-on therapies, and may be offered by chiropractors and physical therapists.

Our take

There's little risk involved in reflexology, and massaging the soles of your feet can feel good. But there's also not much evidence to indicate that the therapy can treat various diseases or symptoms, as its practitioners claim. Among most conventional doctors, the theory behind reflexology is a little difficult to grasp.

What the research says

Here's what some studies have found. All of the results require further research.

Anxiety

There is preliminary evidence that reflexology may be helpful in aiding in relaxation.

Menopause symptoms

Preliminary research suggests reflexology may reduce some symptoms of menopause, but the reduction wasn't significant.

Pain

Some research has shown that reflexology may reduce the pain of tension headaches and migraines, and cancer-related pain; however, the reduction in pain lasted only a short time.

Rolfing

Rolfing is a form of deep-tissue massage. It was developed by Ida Rolf, Ph.D., who called her work Structural Integration. It's based on the theory that the tissues surrounding your muscles become thickened and stiff as you get older. This affects your posture and how well you're able to move.

Rolfing practitioners use their fingers, knuckles, thumbs, elbows and knees to slowly manipulate muscles and the tissues surrounding muscles and joints in an effort to alter a person's posture and realign the body. The goal of Rolfing may be to relieve stress and anxiety, ease pain, improve posture and balance, or create more-refined patterns of movement so that you can make more efficient use of your muscles.

Because it involves manipulation of tissues deep beneath the skin, people with bleeding disorders or who are taking blood thinners should avoid Rolfing. Pregnant women and those with broken bones, advanced osteoporosis, rheumatoid arthritis or abdominal disorders should also avoid Rolfing. If you have questions about whether you might be at risk of potentially harmful side effects, talk with your doctor.

Our take

Some people find Rolfing to be very helpful, improving their posture or helping them to feel more limber. But the therapy can also be painful. If you have a specific underlying illness, such as advanced osteoporosis, the deep massage of Rolfing may also pose some risk. Therefore, it's best to talk to your doctor before embarking down the Rolfing path.

What the research says

Rolfing is used to treat many diseases and conditions. However, there is very limited research as to its effectiveness. It has been studied for the treatment of low back pain, cerebral palsy and chronic fatigue syndrome. The studies were small, and more reliable data are needed.

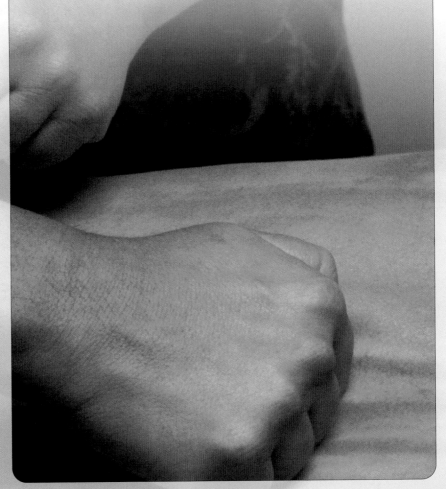

Spinal manipulation

Spinal manipulation is based on the premise that health and disease are directly related to the functioning of the body's neuromusculoskeletal system, and that with proper alignment of your bones, joints, muscles and associated nerves come health and healing.

Spinal manipulation — sometimes called spinal adjustment — is practiced by chiropractors, doctors of osteopathic medicine and physical therapists.

Spinal manipulation has been shown to be effective in treating certain musculoskeletal conditions, such as low back pain. It's generally considered to be safe, but it's not appropriate for everyone.

- Don't seek spinal manipulation if you have osteoporosis or symptoms of nerve damage, such as numbness, tingling or loss of strength in a limb, hand or foot.
- If you have a history of spinal surgery, check with your surgeon before a treatment.
- Manipulation may be hazardous if you've had a stroke related to vascular disease of the arteries in your neck.
- If you have back pain accompanied by fever, chills, sweats or unintentional weight loss, see a medical doctor to rule out the possibility of an infection or tumor.

Our take

Studies have found spinal manipulation to be an effective treatment for uncomplicated low back pain. For this condition, spinal manipulation has become an accepted practice and no longer is considered alternative. Studies also suggest spinal manipulation may be effective for headache and other spine-related conditions, such as neck pain. There's no evidence, though, to support the belief that spinal manipulation can cure whatever ails you.

Select a practitioner who's willing to work with other members of your health care team.

What the research says

Numerous, well-designed studies have shown that spinal manipulation is an effective treatment for mild to moderate low back pain.

Spinal manipulation is also used to treat other conditions. There's some evidence it may improve headache symptoms or help relieve neck pain. As for treatment of nonmusculoskeletal conditions, such as asthma or ear infections, studies either haven't been conducted or haven't found spinal manipulation to be effective.

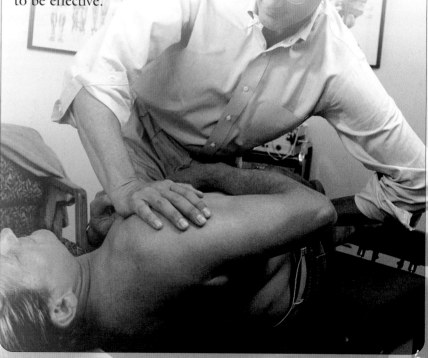

About chiropractic treatment

Chiropractic treatment is based on the concept that restricted movement in the spine may lead to pain and reduced function. Spinal adjustment (manipulation) is one form of therapy chiropractors use to treat restricted spinal mobility. The goal is to restore spinal movement and, as a result, improve function and decrease back pain.

During an adjustment, chiropractors use their hands to apply a controlled, sudden force to a joint. This maneuver often results in a cracking sound made by separation of the joint surfaces — not, as many people think, by "cracking joints." Although this sound is common, it doesn't have to occur for the treatment to be successful. Some chiropractors use instruments to adjust the spine. These methods have not been studied and are of uncertain value.

Chiropractors may also use massage and stretching to relax muscles that are shortened or in spasm. Many use additional treatments as well, such as exercise, ultrasound and electrical muscle stimulation.

As with any medical specialist, select a chiropractor who's willing to work with members of your health care team. It's becoming more common to see chiropractors practicing alongside other medical providers. Make sure you're comfortable with the recommendations, including how many sessions you'll need. For acute low back pain, four to six sessions are typically enough. Be questionable of chiropractors who ask to extend your treatment indefinitely.

When limited to the low back, chiropractic adjustment has few risks. However, manipulation of the neck has been associated with injury to the blood vessels supplying the brain. Rarely, neck manipulation may cause a stroke.

About osteopathic treatment

Doctors of osteopathy are known as D.O.s, and you can find them in medical institutions throughout the country, including Mayo Clinic. Doctors of osteopathy are fully trained in conventional medical care as well as osteopathic medicine.

Osteopathic medicine focuses on the whole person — the mind as well as the body — rather than solely on a set of symptoms. It combines conventional medicine — including the use of prescription medications — with spinal manipulation and attention to proper posture and body positioning. Osteopaths use specialized manipulative techniques to facilitate the return of the body to normal motion and function in order to allow the body to heal itself. Osteopathic manipulation is often more rhythmic and less abrupt than chiropractic techniques.

Osteopathic manipulation is designed to affect the whole person. Psychological changes are often observed after treatment, including changes in mood, altered nervous system activity and altered sensory experience. After an injury or illness, there's a natural tendency to focus on the part of the body that's injured or the origin of the illness, or to try to ignore it. Osteopathic manipulation attempts to put the individual back in touch with his or her entire body in order to aid in healing.

There's a growing body of research exploring the possible benefits of osteopathic treatment for a variety of health conditions.

Chapter 7
Other Approaches

A visit with Dr. Nisha Manek

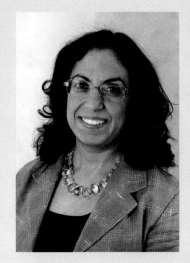

Nisha Manek, M.D.
Rheumatology

Treatments that comprise alternative medical systems focus on prevention and on achieving a healthy 'balance.' They promote diet, exercise, sleep and daily routines to maintain wellness and encourage healing.

This chapter takes a look at all-encompassing approaches to health and healing. Here you will find information about complete medical systems that are quite different from traditional Western medicine. The National Center for Complementary and Alternative Medicine refers to these practices as *whole medical systems.* Another term often used is *alternative medical systems.* This type of medicine is practiced by individual cultures and is largely based on traditional customs, many of which date back thousands of years.

Alternative medical systems originate from a variety of cultures. While some evolved in Western cultures, most originated elsewhere. Examples of systems that developed in Western cultures include homeopathic medicine and naturopathic medicine. Medical systems that evolved in non-Western cultures include ayurveda, which originated in India, and traditional Chinese medicine. Other alternative medical approaches in use today include American Indian, African, Tibetan and South American systems.

These all-encompassing approaches to health and healing are based on the beliefs that there is a powerful connection between mind and body and that the body has the power to heal itself. Treatments that comprise alternative medical systems focus on prevention and on achieving a healthy "balance." They promote diet, exercise, sleep and daily routines to maintain wellness and encourage healing. Ayurvedic medicine goes so far as to include daily care of the oral cavity, nasal passages, sinuses, eyes and skin.

One of the differing points between alternative medical systems and conventional medicine is that treatments are individualized. No two individuals with similar symptoms receive the exact same treatment. For example, two women who undergo menopause and experience hot flashes may see the same traditional Chinese medicine practitioner. However, they may receive different forms of acupuncture therapy and different herbs, depending on their individual "constitutional" diagnoses.

To date, research has generally focused on studying individual components of alternative medical systems and not the whole system, which is more complex. For example, there's research supporting the use of acupuncture in the management of osteoarthritis, postoperative nausea and vomiting. But acupuncture is only one component of traditional Chinese medicine. Likewise, there's research supporting the use of yoga for cancer fatigue and low back pain, but yoga is just one component of the ayurvedic system. Research on the effectiveness of whole medical systems is ongoing, and results are eagerly awaited.

Ayurveda

Ayurveda, which means "science of life," originated in India thousands of years ago and is thought to be the world's oldest system of natural medicine.

The basic theories on which ayurvedic medicine is based are that all things in the universe are joined together and that all forms of life consist of combinations of three energy elements: wind, fire and water. When these elements are balanced, a person is healthy. When they're unbalanced, the body is weakened and susceptible to illness.

To restore harmony and balance and treat illness, some of the therapies used by ayurvedic practitioners include:

- Enemas, fasting, or use of certain foods or metals to eliminate impurities and cleanse the body
- Breathing exercises, herbs or certain foods to reduce symptoms
- Massage of the body's "vital points," where life energy is stored, to reduce pain and fatigue or improve circulation
- Therapies such as yoga and meditation to reduce worry and anxiety and promote balance and harmony

In India, ayurvedic medicine is still practiced by the majority of the population, although it exists side by side with conventional Western medicine. According to a 2007 U.S. survey, more than 200,000 adults used ayurvedic medicine in the previous year.

Our take

Some treatments used in ayurvedic medicine, such as yoga, massage or meditation, appear to be safe and may be effective. There's likely little risk in giving them a try. However, good-quality scientific studies on ayurvedic practices are limited. Many therapies — especially those involving herbs or metals — lack sufficient scientific data to recommend their use. One study found 14 supplements to contain lead, mercury, arsenic or a combination of these contaminants. If you do use an ayurvedic supplement, do so only under a doctor's close supervision because some have the potential to be toxic.

What the research says

Here's what some preliminary studies have found:

Cardiovascular disease

The herbal and mineral formulation abana may reduce the frequency and severity of angina pain, improve cardiac function and reduce high blood pressure. A bark powder called terminalia (arjuna) may help angina. The traditional ayurvedic herbal remedies MAK-4 and MAK-5 may be useful in preventing atherosclerosis.

Cognitive function

The herb brahmi may improve memory and cognitive function, and the herbal formula MAK-4 may enhance attention capacity.

Diabetes

Studies using ayurvedic remedies have produced mixed results.

Hepatitis

The herbal preparation Kamalahar may improve liver function, as may root powder from the herb *Picrorhiza kurroa*.

Obesity

Diets based on ayurvedic practices may prove useful in promoting weight loss in some people. Controlled trials are needed to substantiate clinical observations.

Osteoarthritis

A formula containing roots of *Withania somnifera*, the stem of *Boswellia serrata*, rhizomes of *Curcuma longa* and zinc complex may improve arthritis symptoms.

Body elements

Ayurvedic medicine is based on some specific beliefs as to how the body functions.

Prana

An important concept of ayurvedic medicine is that the human body houses a vital life energy called *prana*. Prana — similar to "qi" in traditional Chinese medicine and "ki" in traditional Japanese medicine — is the basis of life and healing.

Doshas

As this vital life energy circulates throughout the body, it's influenced by elements called *doshas*. Doshas control the basic activities of the body, and they formulate important individual characteristics.

Each dosha is composed of a combination of basic elements: space (ether), air, fire, water and earth. These elements represent subtle qualities of life energy and how the energy expresses itself within the body.

Doshas are influenced by diet, activity and body processes and are continuously being formulated and reformulated. An imbalance in a particular dosha will produce symptoms related to that dosha, which are different from symptoms produced by an imbalance in another dosha.

Prakriti

Certain doshas are predominant in each individual and determine that person's "constitution." The ayurvedic term for constitution is prakriti.

Your constitution refers to your general health, how likely your body is to become out of balance, and your body's ability to resist or recover from illness.

Ayurvedic belief is that your constitution does not change over your lifetime.

The details on doshas

Doshas are known by their original Sanskrit names: *vata*, *pitta* and *kapha*. Each dosha has its essential physical and psychological characteristics.

- **Vata dosha.** The vata dosha is a combination of the elements of space and air. It's considered the most powerful dosha because it controls movement and essential body processes such as cell division, the heart, breathing and the mind. The vata dosha can be thrown off balance by things such as staying up late at night or eating before the previous meal is digested. People with vata as their main dosha are thought to be especially susceptible to skin, neurological and mental illnesses, such as anxiety and insomnia.

- **Pitta dosha.** The pitta dosha is a combination of the elements of fire and water. The pitta dosha is believed to control the body's hormones and digestive system. When the pitta dosha is out of balance, a person may experience negative emotions, such as anger or jealousy, or digestive symptoms, such as heartburn. The pitta dosha can be thrown off balance by eating spicy or sour food, by being angry, tired or fearful, or by spending too much time in the sun. People with pitta as their main dosha are thought to be susceptible to high blood pressure, heart disease and digestive disorders such as Crohn's disease.

- **Kapha dosha.** The kapha dosha combines the elements of water and earth. The kapha dosha is thought to help maintain strength and immunity and control growth. When the kapha dosha is out of balance, a person may experience nausea immediately after eating. Napping during the day, eating too many sweets, eating after you're full, and eating and drinking too many foods and beverages with too much salt and water also may aggravate the kapha dosha. People with kapha as their main dosha are thought to be vulnerable to diabetes, obesity, gallbladder problems, stomach ulcers and respiratory illnesses.

Homeopathy

Homeopathy is a medical system developed in Germany more than 200 years ago, which has been practiced in the United States since the early 19th century.

Homeopathy seeks to stimulate the body's ability to heal itself by giving small doses of highly diluted substances called remedies. Homeopathic remedies are derived from natural substances that come from plants, minerals or animals.

Homeopathic remedies are formulated according to two major principles:

- **The law of similars.** It is based on the theory that "like cures like." This law states that a disease can be cured by a substance that produces similar symptoms in healthy people. The same substance given to a sick person in much smaller doses can theoretically relieve the illness.

- **The law of infinitesimals.** Infinitesimal means too small to be measured. The belief is substances treat disease most effectively when they're highly diluted (often distilled in water or alcohol) to the point where none of the original substance remains.

Homeopaths treat each individual based on his or her health history, body type and physical, emotional and mental symptoms. Treatment may also include exercise and diet recommendations.

Our take

Homeopathic medicine is popular. However, it lacks good studies to prove its effectiveness. Studies that have been done have generally been small and have produced conflicting results. In general, the scientific community also finds the theories on which homeopathic medicine is based questionable and difficult to accept. These factors have kept it from being widely accepted into mainstream medicine.

Because homeopathic medicine mainly involves diluted substances containing little, if any, of their original formulas, the risk they pose is likely minimal. The risks you may be taking are spending money on something that may not work and forgoing proven conventional treatments for homeopathic therapies.

What the research says

A few studies on specific homeopathy treatments have been conducted, but they've been small or the quality and accuracy of the studies have been questioned.

Acute childhood diarrhea

Studies suggest homeopathic treatment may improve digestion and decrease duration of acute diarrhea episodes in children.

Allergies

For treatment of hay fever, one study found a homeopathic nasal spray may be as effective as the conventional spray cromolyn sodium. For treatment of perennial allergic rhinitis, one study found a homeopathic preparation may improve nasal airflow.

Influenza

The homeopathic remedy oscillococcinum has been studied for firstline treatment and prevention of influenza and flu-like syndromes. Current evidence doesn't support its use.

Pain

Homeopathic approaches to treat pain, including arthritic pain and muscle soreness, indicate possible benefits. The remedy arnica may reduce swelling and bruising.

Vertigo

Homeopathic therapies may work as well as conventional treatment in people with vertigo.

Naturopathy

Naturopathy is a form of health care based on the belief that the body has an innate healing power that can establish, maintain and restore health when it's in a healthy environment.

In naturopathy, the emphasis is on supporting health rather than combating disease. As such, naturopathic medicine relies on natural remedies, such as sunlight, air and water, along with "natural" supplements to promote well-being.

Early naturopaths often prescribed hydrotherapy — soaks in hot springs and other water-related therapies — to promote health. Today, naturopathic practitioners draw on many forms of alternative medicine, including practices such as massage, acupuncture, exercise and lifestyle counseling. Practitioners of naturopathy believe that health and healing should come in the most gentle, least invasive and most efficient manner possible.

Individuals who provide naturopathic care aren't all the same. A naturopath is a therapist who practices naturopathy. A naturopathic physician is a primary health care provider trained in a broad scope of naturopathic practices in addition to a standard medical curriculum. Both use the designation of N.D. — representing either naturopathic diploma or naturopathic doctor — which can cause confusion about the person's scope of practice, education and training.

Our take

Much of the advice of naturopaths is worth heeding: exercise regularly, practice good nutrition, quit smoking and enjoy nature. However, claims that treatments such as hydrotherapy detoxify the body and strengthen the immune system aren't backed up by scientific research. And just because a product or practice is considered "natural" doesn't mean it's safe. The best use of naturopathic medicine is to complement conventional medical treatment — naturopathy shouldn't be a complete substitute for conventional care. Be wary of practitioners who recommend that you avoid prescription drugs or surgery or other treatments known to be beneficial.

What the research says

Similar to homeopathy, there haven't been any quality research studies conducted on naturopathy as a whole — a complete system of medicine. There's no evidence that naturopathic medicine can cure cancer or any other disease, as some proponents claim.

A limited number of studies have been done on herbs used as naturopathic treatments. One study found that echinacea wasn't effective in treating colds in children, while another suggested an herbal extract containing echinacea may reduce ear pain associated with ear infections (acute otitis media). A study of another multi-ingredient naturopathic extract also indicated possible benefits in reducing ear pain associated with ear infection.

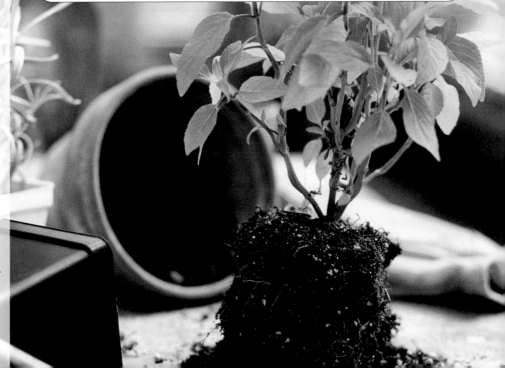

Traditional Chinese medicine

Traditional Chinese medicine is a system of medicine rooted in ancient Chinese philosophy (Daoism).

Traditional Chinese medicine is based on the belief that the body is a delicate balance of two complementary yet opposing forces: yin and yang. Yin represents the cold, slow or passive principle of life, while yang represents the hot, excited, active one. Health is achieved by maintaining an appropriate balance of the two.

An imbalance of yin and yang leads to blockage in the flow of blood and vital life energy (qi). To help unblock these pathways and restore health, practitioners of traditional Chinese medicine generally use one or a combination of treatments, which may include:

- Acupuncture, moxibustion or cupping
- Chinese herbs
- Massage and manipulation

Moxibustion is the application of heat from burning of the herb moxa at an acupuncture point. Cupping involves placing a heated cup over a part of the body. As the air inside cools, its volume decreases, creating a slight suction and stimulating blood flow.

Chinese herbs are usually processed as pills, capsules or powders — but the raw, dried forms common centuries ago are still used. There are more than 2,000 Chinese herbs.

Our take

In China, traditional Chinese medicine is integrated into the country's health care system and used side by side with modern medicine. In the United States people generally pick and choose certain components of traditional Chinese medicine and use them in isolation. Practices such as acupuncture, massage and manipulation can be of benefit in treating certain conditions. A few Chinese herbs also may be of use in treating conditions such as cardiovascular disease and side effects of cancer. However, Chinese herbs need to be approached with caution. They can be very powerful, and some are dangerous. Ephedra (ma-huang), the main active ingredient in many "natural" weight-loss products, is thought to have caused 22 deaths and 800 cases of toxicity.

What the research says

The individual component within traditional Chinese medicine that has received the most study is acupuncture. For more information on acupuncture, see page 120. For information on Chinese massage (tui na), see page 133. As for Chinese herbs, only a few good studies have been conducted. A challenge is that most Chinese herbs are used in combination, not alone.

Autoimmune and inflammatory disease

A small randomized trial of the Chinese herb thunder god vine showed a positive response in people with rheumatoid arthritis. A larger study found it to cause renal, cardiac and other toxicities.

Cancer

Studies suggest Chinese herbs may shrink tumors, reduce side effects and improve response to treatment. But the quality of the studies has been weak. Better studies are needed.

Cardiovascular disease

Chinese herb formulas are taken to reduce symptoms of angina, stabilize abnormal heart rhythms, and improve heart function and blood composition. While there's some evidence of potential benefits, the studies have been limited and of poor design.

Knee osteoarthritis

A recent study shows the Chinese therapy tai chi can effectively treat symptoms of knee arthritis in older adults.

The human 'ecosystem'

According to ancient Chinese belief, the laws that govern the natural world also apply to human life. A person is viewed as an individual ecosystem, related to a larger ecosystem.

The goal of traditional Chinese medicine is to maintain natural harmony. Harmony and disharmony — health and sickness — are determined according to concepts known as principles, elements and networks.

These concepts are all taken into consideration in determining the cause of illness and how to treat it.

8 principles

The eight principles are actually four pairs of opposites that describe patterns of disharmony.

- Interior/exterior refers to the location of the disharmony in the body — internal organs vs. skin or bones.
- Hot/cold refers to the symptoms of the disease, such as fever or thirst vs. chilliness or the desire to drink something warm.
- Excess/deficiency refers to whether the condition is acute or chronic, and whether the body's responses are strong or weak.
- The balance of yin/yang — the cold, passive principle of life vs. the hot, active one — is also a factor in determining disharmony and identifying disease.

5 elements

The five elements are fire, earth, metal, water and wood. The terms refer to dynamic qualities of nature and describe changes in the flow of life energy.

The five elements build upon one another and mutually reinforce each other. If one is out of balance, it can impair another.

The elements follow this sequence: wood creates fire, fire creates earth, earth creates metal, metal creates water and water creates wood.

5 networks

The body has five organ networks that each respond to a particular element:

- Heart/small intestine with fire
- Spleen/stomach with earth
- Lungs/large intestine with metal
- Kidneys/bladder with water
- Liver/gallbladder with wood

Acupressure: Benefits of putting on the pressure

Acupressure is a traditional Chinese medicine technique based on the same ideas as acupuncture. It involves placing physical pressure at specific points on the surface of the body by means of a finger, hand, elbow or various devices. The intent is to restore the flow of life energy (qi). Another term for acupressure is *shiatsu*.

Acupressure is used to treat a wide variety of conditions including musculoskeletal pain and tension, depression, anxiety, sleep difficulties, headache and nausea. Some people also use it as a relaxation technique.

One condition for which studies have shown acupressure to be effective is in treating nausea. Numerous scientific studies support the use of acupressure applied to a specific point (P6) on the wrist to prevent and treat nausea associated with surgery and chemotherapy, as well as nausea related to morning sickness that accompanies pregnancy. Some people have also found wrist acupressure effective in reducing motion sickness.

The P6 point is located about three finger-widths from the large crease in your wrist (see illustration).

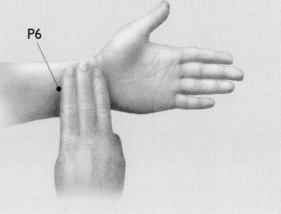

P6

Part 3

Your Action Plan

Choosing the best treatments for better health

The guiding philosophy of today's "new medicine" — integrative medicine — is to blend the best of complementary and conventional therapies to treat the whole person, not just the disease.

In Part 3, we take a look at 20 common conditions and offer advice on treatment and prevention, combining nontraditional therapies with conventional care to achieve optimal health.

We also discuss important information regarding safety. Complementary and alternative practices aren't regulated in the same manner as are prescription medications and other forms of conventional care. Therefore, it's important to be smart in how you approach complementary and alternative medicine, and not be fooled by fraudulent claims.

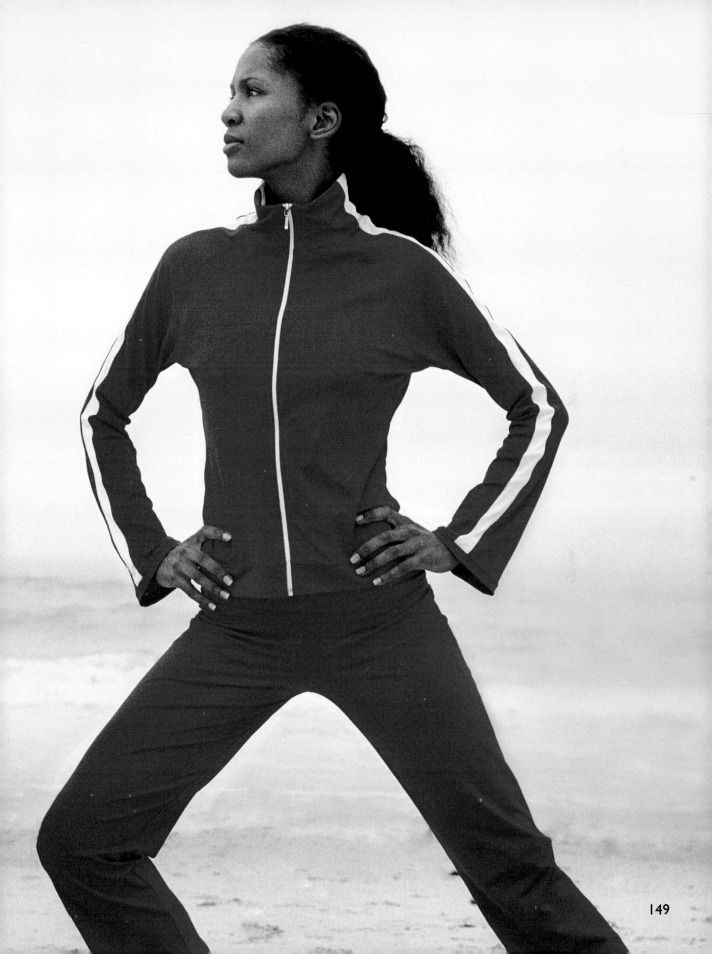

Chapter 8
Treating 20 Common Conditions

A visit with Dr. Dietlind Wahner-Roedler

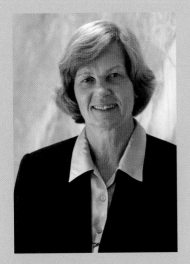

Dietlind Wahner-Roedler, M.D.
General Internal Medicine

" *The challenge for the coming decade will be to sift the 'wheat from the chaff' — incorporating those products and practices that are effective and safe, while avoiding those that aren't.* *"*

For much of the latter part of the 20th century, conventional medicine made amazing strides, from conquering polio to developing microscopic surgical techniques. It seemed that advancing research might be all that was needed to eradicate disease. In such a world, it's not surprising that some people took a casual approach to their health. After all, if smoking and poor diet led to a heart attack, medicine had a ready fix in bypass surgery or better yet, a stent. Why take the time to invest in your health if modern medicine could alleviate the consequences of bad choices? Unfortunately, modern medicine doesn't have all the answers.

What we've seen in today's medicine is a fabulous ability to "fix" things, once they're "broken" — treating heart attacks with coronary artery bypass surgery, kidney failure with kidney transplant or obesity with bariatric surgery. Yet the same degree of emphasis and expertise hasn't developed in regard to preventing these problems. Nor has as much focus been given to steps people can take when faced with a chronic condition that isn't amenable to a quick fix — such as high blood pressure, diabetes and arthritis. With the rapid aging of the U.S. population, it is becoming evident that self-care may be more important now than ever before.

Much of integrative medicine is focused on prevention — a heavy emphasis on diet, physical activity, stress reduction and maintaining connectedness — and on dealing with chronic issues more effectively. This might include using yoga in addition to medication to treat high blood pressure, or trying fish oil in addition to dietary changes to control high triglycerides. Sometimes, alternative medicine is a replacement to conventional medicine when a proven treatment isn't feasible because of side effects. An example is use of nonsteroidal anti-inflammatory drugs (NSAIDs) to treat arthritis. Though they control pain, they can also cause ulcers or high blood pressure. In this situation, glucosamine or devil's claw may be an alternative approach.

The difficulty incorporating more complementary and alternative therapies into the current health care regimen is that collective experience and knowledge regarding how to safely integrate such treatments is still largely in its infancy. While research is growing rapidly in this area, limited regulatory control has allowed ineffective and even dangerous alternatives to reach mass markets. The challenge for the coming decade will be to sift the "wheat from the chaff" — incorporating those products and practices that are effective and safe, while avoiding those that aren't.

To help with this challenge, the following chapter focuses on 20 common conditions and their conventional and complementary treatments. We look at the evidence for and against the most commonly encountered alternative treatments, giving recommendations where the evidence is strongest and more cautionary notes when the evidence is less or the risk is high. By following the same approach with other conditions as is outlined in these examples, you should be able to develop a sound approach to evaluating new therapies as they arise.

Arthritis

When you think of arthritis, you likely think of pain and stiffness in joints. And you'd be right on the money. Those are typical symptoms of osteoarthritis and rheumatoid arthritis, the two most common forms of arthritis (there are actually more than 100 forms).

Arthritis is the leading cause of disability in the United States. In fact, more than one-fourth of U.S. adults report ongoing pain or stiffness in their joints, and more than 45 million Americans have been diagnosed with some form of arthritis.

Osteoarthritis is commonly known as wear-and-tear arthritis. It involves the wearing away of the tough, lubricated cartilage that normally cushions the ends of bones in your joints. Rheumatoid arthritis results from an abnormal immune system response that causes inflammation of the lining of the joints.

Arthritis affects people of all ages, but it's most common among older adults. Women, possibly because of female hormones, are at higher risk of many forms of arthritis than are men.

Whites, blacks and American Indians are more likely to get arthritis than are Asians and Hispanics. In addition, people who are more than 10 pounds overweight are at increased risk, especially of arthritis of the knees. Past joint injury also can increase risk of osteoarthritis.

Conventional treatment for osteoarthritis

There's no known cure for osteoarthritis, but treatments can help to reduce pain and maintain joint movement. Conventional treatment typically involves a combination of therapies that may include medication, self-care, physical therapy and occupational therapy. In some cases, surgical procedures may be necessary.

Medications

Medications are used to treat the pain and mild inflammation of osteoarthritis and to improve the function of your joints. They include both topical medications and oral medications. Nonprescription topical pain relievers include Aspercreme, Sportscreme, Icy Hot, Bengay, and various formulations containing capsaicin, a cream made from hot chili (cayenne) peppers.

Nonprescription medications such as acetaminophen (Tylenol, others), aspirin, ibuprofen (Advil, Motrin, others) and naproxen sodium (Aleve) may be sufficient to treat milder osteoarthritis, but stronger prescription medications also are available. These include tramadol (Ultram), painkillers and various antidepressants.

Occasionally, your doctor may suggest injecting a joint space with a corticosteroid to relieve pain and swelling. Injecting hyaluronic acid derivatives into knee joints (visco supplementation) also can relieve pain from osteoarthritis.

Surgical or other procedures

Surgical procedures can help relieve disability and pain caused by osteoarthritis. Procedures include joint replacement, arthroscopic lavage and debridement to remove debris from a joint, bone repositioning to help correct deformities, and bone fusion to increase stability and reduce pain.

Self-care

Fortunately, you can relieve much of the discomfort associated with osteoarthritis through healthy-living strategies and self-care techniques.

These include exercising regularly to maintain mobility and range of motion, controlling your weight to reduce stress on joints, eating a healthy diet (to help control your weight), applying heat to ease pain and relax tense, painful muscles, and applying cold to dull the sensation of occasional flare-ups.

In addition, choosing comfortable, cushioned footwear is important if you have arthritis in your weight-bearing joints or back. And, it's important to take your medications as recommended to keep pain from increasing.

Complementary and alternative treatment

Several alternative therapies may help relieve the pain of osteoarthritis.

Common therapies

Glucosamine and chondroitin. Glucosamine sulfate is a dietary supplement derived from oyster and crab shells. It's a synthetic version of an amino sugar the body produces to preserve joint health. Chondroitin sulfate is a dietary supplement derived from cow and shark cartilage and other sources. The two are often used in combination.

More than 20 clinical studies lasting up to three years and enrolling more than 2,500 people have been conducted evaluating glucosamine for osteoarthritis — most often, osteoarthritis of the knee. When the findings of these studies are pooled, glucosamine appears to reduce pain scores by 28 to 41 percent, and improve functionality scores by 21 to 46 percent. The supplements can cause mild gastrointestinal effects but generally produce fewer side effects than do NSAIDs. If you're allergic to shellfish, don't take glucosamine until you talk with your doctor.

Acupuncture. Acupuncture may relieve pain from osteoarthritis in some individuals, especially knee pain. Find an experienced practitioner.

Tai chi and yoga. These movement therapies involve gentle exercises and stretches combined with deep breathing. Small studies have found they may reduce osteoarthritis pain. Avoid moves that cause pain.

SAMe. Commercially available SAMe is a synthetic version of a compound that occurs naturally in human tissue. The dietary supplement is thought to stimulate cartilage growth and repair, and increase cartilage thickness. You may need to take SAMe for several weeks before you experience relief from symptoms. Side effects can include flatulence, vomiting, diarrhea, headache and nausea. SAMe can negatively interact with antidepressant medications.

Ginger extract. A couple of small studies found ginger modestly reduced pain. Researchers speculate that compounds contained in ginger may have anti-inflammatory effects. More study is needed.

Cat's claw. Studies suggest cat's claw also may have anti-inflammatory properties. Additional research is needed to determine efficacy and safety.

Devil's claw. It has been used extensively in Europe and has a growing body of scientific evidence attesting to its ability to reduce arthritis pain.

Avocado and soybean oil. Researchers are looking at a specific extract in these oils that may inhibit cartilage breakdown and promote repair.

Little evidence

Although they remain popular, there's little evidence to support the use of magnets for arthritis. Side effects appear to be rare, but magnets can disrupt pacemakers and may harm babies during pregnancy.

Coping skills are important

Because osteoarthritis can affect your everyday activities and overall quality of life, coping strategies are an important element of dealing with the disease, whether you choose conventional or alternative treatments.

Coping strategies include keeping a positive attitude so you're in charge of your disease, rather than vice versa, knowing when to limit activities, using assistive devices, and avoiding grasping actions that can strain finger joints.

Strategies also include spreading the weight of an object over several joints when lifting, such as using both hands to lift a heavy pan, maintaining good posture to evenly distribute your weight, and using your strongest muscles and large joints (for example, leaning into a heavy door to open it rather than pushing it with your hands).

An occupational therapist can also help you in selecting the right assistive devices for daily living.

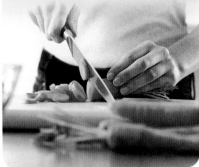

Conventional treatment for rheumatoid arthritis

Treatment typically involves a combination of self-care techniques similar to those used for osteoarthritis (see page 152) and medications. Sometimes, surgery or other procedures may be necessary.

Medication

Medications for rheumatoid arthritis can relieve its symptoms and slow or halt its progression. Medications used include nonsteroidal anti-inflammatory drugs (NSAIDs), such as aspirin and ibuprofen (Advil, Motrin, others), steroids such as prednisone and methylprednisolone, disease-modifying antirheumatic drugs (DMARDs), such as hydroxychloroquine (Plaquenil) and methotrexate (Rheumatrex).

Also used are immunosuppressants, such as leflunomide (Arava) and azathioprine (Imuran), TNF inhibitors, such as etanercept (Enbrel) and infliximab (Remicade), the interleukin-1 receptor antagonist anakinra (Kineret), and the drugs abatacept (Orencia) and rituximab (Rituxan).

Surgery and other procedures

If joint destruction is too severe, joint replacement can often help restore joint function, reduce pain or correct a deformity.

Complementary and alternative treatment

Evidence appears strongest that fish oil supplements offer the most promise as an integrative treatment.

Common therapies

Omega-3 fatty acids. Research shows that regularly taking omega-3 fatty acid (fish oil) supplements may improve morning stiffness and joint tenderness in people with rheumatoid arthritis. But the effect of the supplements has not been well studied beyond three months. Because high doses can cause bleeding, don't take more than 3 grams (3,000 milligrams) a day without consulting a doctor.

Gamma-linolenic acid (GLA). GLA is a type of omega-6 fatty acid that comes from plant oils, such as evening primrose and borage. Some studies indicate GLA may reduce pain and stiffness of rheumatoid arthritis. Talk with your doctor before taking GLA because some plant oils can cause liver damage or interfere with medications.

Tai chi. This movement therapy involves gentle exercises and stretches combined with deep breathing. Small studies have found that it may reduce arthritis pain, although more study is needed. Tai chi is safe but you should avoid movements that cause pain.

Chronic fatigue syndrome

Chronic fatigue syndrome is a complicated disorder characterized by extreme fatigue that doesn't improve with bed rest and may worsen with physical or mental activity.

Of all chronic illnesses, chronic fatigue syndrome is one of the most mysterious. Unlike infections, it has no clear cause. Unlike conditions such as diabetes or anemia, there's essentially nothing to measure. And unlike conditions such as heart disease, there are relatively few treatment options.

Chronic fatigue syndrome may occur after an infection such as a cold or viral syndrome. It can start during or shortly after a period of high stress or come on gradually without any clear starting point or any obvious cause. Chronic fatigue syndrome is a flu-like condition that can drain your energy and sometimes last for years. People previously healthy and full of energy may experience a variety of symptoms, including extreme fatigue, weakness and headaches as well as difficulty concentrating and painful joints, muscles and lymph nodes.

Women are diagnosed with chronic fatigue syndrome two to four times as often as are men. However, it's unclear whether chronic fatigue syndrome affects women more frequently or if women report it to their doctors more often than do men.

Conventional treatment

There's no specific conventional treatment for chronic fatigue syndrome. In general, doctors aim to relieve symptoms by using a combination of treatments, which may include:

Lifestyle changes. Your doctor may encourage you to slow down and to avoid excessive physical and psychological stress. This may save your energy for essential activities at home or work and help you cut back on less important activities. Get enough sleep.

Gradual but steady exercise. Often, with the help of a physical therapist, you may be advised to begin a graduated exercise program in which physical activity gradually increases. This can help prevent or decrease the muscle weakness caused by prolonged inactivity. In addition, exercise improves your energy level and sleep.

Treatment of psychiatric problems. Doctors can treat problems often related to chronic fatigue syndrome, such as depression, with medication or behavior therapy — learning to change your behavior to reduce the symptoms of a certain disease or condition — or a combination of the two. If you're depressed, medications such as tricyclic antidepressants and selective serotonin reuptake inhibitors (SSRIs) may help. Even if you are not depressed, antidepressants may still help improve sleep and relieve pain. Tricyclic antidepressants include amitriptyline (Limbitrol — a multi-ingredient drug that contains amitriptyline), desipramine (Norpramin) and nortriptyline (Pamelor). SSRIs include fluoxetine (Prozac, Sarafem), paroxetine (Paxil), sertraline (Zoloft) and bupropion (Wellbutrin).

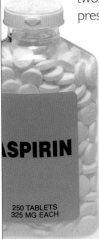

Treatment of existing pain. Acetaminophen (Tylenol, others) or nonsteroidal anti-inflammatory drugs (NSAIDs) such as aspirin and ibuprofen (Advil, Motrin, others) may be helpful to reduce pain and fever.

Treatment of allergy-like symptoms. Antihistamines such as fexofenadine (Allegra) and cetirizine (Zyrtec) and decongestants that contain pseudoephedrine (Sudafed, Dimetapp) may relieve allergy-like symptoms such as runny nose.

Treatment of low blood pressure (hypotension). The drugs fludrocortisone (Florinef), atenolol (Tenormin) and midodrine (ProAmatine) may be useful for certain people with chronic fatigue syndrome whose blood pressure drops far below normal levels.

Some medications can cause side effects or adverse reactions that may be worse than the symptoms of chronic fatigue syndrome. Talk to your doctor before starting any treatment for this condition. Because the causes of chronic fatigue syndrome

Complementary and alternative treatment

are not clear, an integrative approach to treatment involves addressing a variety of possible factors. These include diet, hormone balances, underlying infections, insomnia, pain and dysfunction of the body's energy-production system.

Diet. Poor dietary habits and nutrient deficiencies can lead to fatigue. Avoiding simple sugars and foods with a high glycemic index, such as white flour and potatoes, may help eliminate large fluctuations in blood sugar levels that can be associated with fatigue. Avoiding caffeine and addressing nutritional deficiencies such as low iron stores also may help.

Hormone balances. In addition to considering conventional therapies for hormone problems, an integrative approach might look at, for example, use of such alternative treatments as licorice, vitamin C or ginseng for adrenal issues. Licorice, however, may make heartburn symptoms worse, and high doses of vitamin C can cause loose stools. Ginseng can be stimulating and may worsen insomnia.

Underlying infections. Some alternative practitioners believe that people with chronic fatigue syndrome may be experiencing chronic infections, especially yeast infections and chronic sinusitis. Alternative treatment of a yeast infection might include use of probiotics, such as eating live-culture yogurt (see page 92). For chronic sinusitis, alternative treatment might include nasal irrigation with a neti pot (see page 173).

Insomnia. Although people with chronic fatigue syndrome are fatigued, many report difficulty sleeping. In addition to considering conventional sleep medications, an integrative approach might consider melatonin, valerian, or calcium and magnesium at bedtime. Some people, though, find valerian overstimulating rather than sleep-inducing.

Pain. An integrative approach to pain management might include — in addition to conventional therapies — massage, yoga and tai chi to improve posture problems, and acupuncture to reduce pain and fatigue. Some research has found natural D-ribose supplements may decrease pain an improve energy. D-ribose, a form of sugar, is an essential cellular energy source.

Energy. Fatigue could indicate a problem at the cellular level where the chemical reaction that releases energy takes place. Alternative approaches might include use of potassium, magnesium, vitamin C and B vitamins, if deficiencies exist. Coenzyme Q10, the coenzyme NADH, and the amino acid L-carnitine are under study.

Primary signs and symptoms of chronic fatigue syndrome

In addition to persistent fatigue not caused by other known medical conditions, chronic fatigue syndrome has eight possible primary signs and symptoms. These include:

- Loss of memory or concentration
- Sore throat
- Painful and mildly enlarged lymph nodes in your neck or armpits
- Unexplained muscle soreness
- Pain that moves from one joint to another without swelling or redness
- Headache of a new type, pattern or severity
- Sleep disturbance
- Extreme exhaustion after normal exercise or exertion

According to a Centers for Disease Control and Prevention (CDC) study group, a person meets the diagnostic criteria of chronic fatigue syndrome when unexplained persistent fatigue occurs for six months or more with at least four of the eight primary signs and symptoms also present.

Chronic pain

If you have a condition such as a broken bone, you recognize discomfort as a symptom and trust that treatment will help. After surgery, pain medication provides relief while your body heals. Chronic pain is different.

Sometimes, chronic pain follows an illness or an injury that appears to have healed. It can also be related to long-standing conditions such as arthritis. Other times, chronic pain develops for no apparent reason.

Whatever the cause, the emotional fallout of chronic pain can make you hurt even more. Anxiety or depression can magnify unpleasant sensations, and disrupted sleep may leave you feeling fatigued and helpless.

Conventional treatment

Chronic pain is a challenge, but there are a variety of conventional treatment options. They include:

Medication. Sometimes, over-the-counter pain relievers or medicated creams or gels are effective. For more severe pain, your doctor may prescribe an opioid medication or tramadol (Ultram). Some people find relief with tricyclic antidepressants such as nortriptyline (Pamelor) or amitriptyline. Anti-seizure drugs such as gabapentin (Neurontin) or carbamazepine (Tegretol) may relieve some types of chronic pain as well.

Injection therapy. Instead of prescribing pills to control chronic pain, your doctor might inject medication directly into the affected area. Such injections are usually a combination of a numbing agent (local anesthetic), which provides immediate relief, and a corticosteroid, which reduces inflammation.

Nerve stimulation. Various devices use electric impulses to help block or mask the feeling of pain. With transcutaneous electrical nerve stimulation (TENS), a portable, battery-powered unit delivers an electric impulse through electrodes placed on the affected area. Spinal cord and peripheral nerve stimulators are implanted beneath the skin with electrodes placed near the spinal cord. A hand-held unit allows you to control the level of stimulation.

Medication pumps. An implantable medication pump supplies pain medication directly into the spinal fluid. To replenish the pump, drugs are injected through the skin into a small port at the center of the pump.

Physical and occupational therapy. Stretching and strengthening exercises can improve your strength and flexibility. Sometimes learning new ways to handle daily activities can minimize the pain.

Counseling. A counselor can help you manage your emotional response to chronic pain, as well as identify patterns of thought or behavior that may aggravate your pain.

Exercise. Exercise can prompt your body to release endorphins, chemicals that block pain signals from reaching your brain. It can also help you build strength, increase flexibility, improve sleep quality and boost your energy level. In addition, it can improve mood and protect your heart and blood vessels. If you have chronic pain, talk to your doctor before starting an exercise program.

Complementary and alternative treatment

Various complementary therapies, including acupuncture, guided imagery, hypnosis and music therapy, may offer relief from chronic pain.

Common therapies

Acupuncture. This traditional Chinese therapy involves the insertion of fine needles into the skin at certain points to restore proper energy flow in the body. Research indicates that it may relieve pain from osteoarthritis, especially knee pain. It's generally a low-risk treatment, but make sure to find an experienced practitioner.

Guided imagery. This can refer to a number of therapies, including visualization, game-playing and storytelling. The goal is to help people visualize positive outcomes for issues they're dealing with. Guided imagery may alter breathing, heart rate and blood pressure. With pain, it's been shown to reduce postoperative pain and pain from laparoscopic surgery. It may also reduce cancer pain.

Guided imagery is generally considered safe. However, theoretically it could interact with certain mental conditions, so use it only with professional guidance if you have mental health issues.

Massage. A growing body of literature is beginning to validate the many benefits of massage therapy. Studies suggest it can help decrease headache pain, fibromyalgia pain and, possibly, back pain.

Biofeedback. Studies show it may improve symptoms — including pain — of headache, anxiety, stress, and irritable bowel syndrome.

Hypnosis. There's evidence that hypnosis can reduce chronic pain associated with cancer. It may also help with chronic pain from irritable bowel syndrome, tension headaches and certain other conditions.

Music therapy. Music can influence your physical and emotional states. Music therapists are trained to adapt the therapy to meet specific needs of individuals. It's been shown to raise pain thresholds, improve mood and provide relaxation, and has been effective in reducing pain from cancer, burns, osteoarthritis and surgery, among other conditions.

Meditation. Meditation may reduce pain by helping to treat anxiety, depression, stress and insomnia.

Tai chi. It may help relieve some types of pain by strengthening muscles and improving joint flexibility.

Conflicting or unclear evidence

In healing (therapeutic) touch, practitioners hold their hands close to a person to supposedly sense and manipulate the person's energy field. There's very little proof that it actually works, but many people report that they feel very relaxed after a healing touch session. Pending more studies, it falls into the category of "may not help but probably doesn't hurt."

Similarly, magnet therapy is popular but has very little in the way of scientific evidence to support its use as a pain treatment. Risks are mostly financial — although magnetic bracelets can cost only a few dollars, mattresses can cost hundreds or thousands of dollars.

Back pain

The back is a well-designed structure made up of bone, muscles, nerves and other soft tissues. You rely on your back to be the workhorse of the body — its function is essential for nearly every move you make. Because of this, the back can be particularly vulnerable to injury and back pain can be disabling.

Four out of 5 adults have at least one bout of back pain sometime during life. In fact, back pain is one of the most common reasons for health care visits and missed work.

On the bright side, you can prevent most back pain. Simple home treatment and proper body mechanics will often heal your back within a few weeks and keep it functional for the long haul. Surgery is rarely needed to treat back pain.

Treating back pain

Most back pain gets better with a few weeks of home treatment and careful attention. A regular schedule of pain relievers and hot or cold therapy may be all that you need. A short period of bed rest is OK, but more than a couple of days actually does more harm than good. If home treatments aren't working, your doctor may suggest:

Physical therapy and exercise. A physical therapist can apply treatments, such as heat, ice, ultrasound, electrical stimulation and muscle release techniques, to back muscles and soft tissues to reduce pain.

Prescription medications. Your doctor may prescribe nonsteroidal anti-inflammatory drugs or in some cases, a muscle relaxant.

Cortisone injections. For pain from a "pinched nerve," your doctor may prescribe cortisone injections — an anti-inflammatory medication — into the space around your spinal cord (epidural space).

Electrical stimulation. Transcutaneous electrical nerve stimulation (TENS) uses a unit that sends a weak electrical current through points on the skin to nerve pathways. This is thought to interrupt pain signals.

Back schools. These programs, available in many communities, focus on managing back pain and preventing its recurrence.

Additional treatments. For chronic back pain, treatment may also include antidepressant medications, which can relieve pain independent of their effect on depression, opioid medications, such as codeine or hydrocodone, or medications administered through a pump.

Surgery. Few people ever need surgery for back pain. There are no effective surgical techniques for muscle- and soft tissue-related back pain. Surgery is usually reserved for pain caused by a herniated disk.

Beyond the basics

Some more popular complementary and alternative therapies include chiropractic manipulation, hydrotherapy and massage.

Chiropractic manipulation. Spinal adjustment may help uncomplicated low back pain, especially when performed shortly after the pain begins. Evidence doesn't support its use for severe back pain. Manipulation of the neck may be unsafe for people with vascular problems or an aneurysm. Use caution if you have osteoporosis.

Hydrotherapy. For low back pain, hot whirlpool baths, combined with standard therapy, may help. Be cautious of high temperatures, and avoid intense water jets if you have blood clots, bleeding disorders, fractures, open wounds, severe osteoporosis or are pregnant.

Massage. This is a relatively safe way to relax tense muscles and help ease pain. Avoid if you have phlebitis, deep vein thrombosis, open wounds, inflamed or infected tissue, or an infectious disease.

Other treatments. Benefits are unproved but the risks appear low for use of meditation and yoga for back pain.

Common cold

A common cold is an infection of your upper respiratory tract. It's relatively harmless — but it sure doesn't feel that way when you have one. If it's not a runny nose, sore throat and a cough, it's watery eyes, sneezing and miserable congestion. Or maybe all of the above. In fact, because any one of more than 200 viruses can cause a common cold, symptoms tend to vary greatly.

Unfortunately, if you're like most adults, you're likely to have a common cold two to four times a year. Children, especially preschoolers, may have a common cold as many as eight to 10 times annually.

The good news is that you or your child should be feeling better in about a week. If symptoms aren't improving in that time, see your doctor to make sure you don't have a bacterial infection in your lungs, larynx, trachea, sinuses or ears.

Conventional treatment

There's no cure for the common cold. Antibiotics are of no use against cold viruses, and over-the-counter cold preparations won't cure a common cold or make it go away any sooner. However, over-the-counter medications can relieve some symptoms.

For fever, sore throat and headache, try acetaminophen (Tylenol, others) or other mild pain relievers. Don't give aspirin to children, because it may have a role in causing Reye's syndrome, a rare but potentially fatal disease.

For runny nose and nasal congestion, you can take an antihistamine or decongestant. Don't use decongestant drops and sprays for more than a few days, though, because prolonged use can cause chronic inflammation of your mucous membranes. And don't give them to children under age 2. There's little evidence that they work in young children, and they may cause side effects.

Self-care for colds

You may not be able to cure your common cold, but you can make yourself as comfortable as possible. These tips may help:

Drink lots of fluids. Avoid alcohol, caffeine and cigarette smoke, which can cause dehydration and aggravate your symptoms.

Get some rest. Consider staying home from work if you have a fever or a bad cough, or are drowsy from medications. This will give you a chance to rest as well as reduce the chances that you'll infect others. Wear a mask when you have a cold if you live or work with someone with a chronic disease or compromised immune system.

Adjust your room's temperature and humidity. Keep your room warm, but not overheated. If the air is dry, a cool-mist humidifier or vaporizer can moisten the air and help ease congestion and coughing. Be sure to keep the humidifier clean to prevent the growth of bacteria and molds.

Soothe your throat. Gargling with warm salt water several times a day or drinking warm lemon water with honey may help soothe a sore throat and relieve a cough.

Use nasal drops. To help relieve nasal congestion, try saline nasal drops. They're available without a prescription and are effective, safe and nonirritating, even for children. To use them, instill several drops into one nostril, then immediately bulb suction that nostril. Repeat in the opposite nostril.

Try chicken soup. Generations of parents have spooned chicken soup into their sick children. Now scientists have put chicken soup to the test, discovering that it does seem to help relieve cold and flu symptoms in two ways. First, it acts as an anti-inflammatory agent by inhibiting the movement of neutrophils — immune system cells that participate in the body's inflammatory response. Second, it temporarily speeds up the movement of mucus through the nose, helping relieve congestion and limiting the amount of time viruses are in contact with the nasal lining. Researchers at the University of Nebraska compared homemade chicken soup with canned versions and found that many, though not all, canned chicken soups worked just as well as soups made from scratch.

Complementary and alternative treatment

Alternative therapies for the common cold are as common as colds. A few may have some value with little risk at typically used doses.

Andrographis. This herb is a popular cold and influenza treatment in Scandinavia and has been used for centuries in Asia. Although independent studies are limited, research suggests that andrographis may reduce the duration and severity of symptoms if taken early, and it might reduce the risk of catching a cold if you take it regularly for a couple of months. It appears safe at standardized commercial doses, but allergic reactions have been noted at higher doses. In addition, it may not be safe in combination with blood sugar lowering drugs, as it might push blood levels too low. Safety for long-term use is unclear.

Vitamin C. There's mixed evidence for using vitamin C to treat a cold. There appear to be no benefits for cold prevention or treatment for most people. However, studies have shown a roughly 50 percent cold-prevention benefit for people in extreme circumstances, such as marathon runners and soldiers in subarctic training. Vitamin C may also reduce the duration of cold symptoms.

Vitamin C supplements are generally considered safe at recommended doses. Higher doses, especially over 2,000 milligrams a day, may be associated with nausea, diarrhea and kidney stones.

Echinacea. Studies of echinacea use for the common cold are mixed, and its effectiveness is unclear. While no studies have shown that taking echinacea can prevent you from getting a cold, there is some evidence that it can modestly relieve symptoms or shorten the duration of a cold, if taken when cold symptoms first appear.

Garlic. Garlic has been used for a long time for the prevention and treatment of colds, but scientific evidence on the subject is slim. Although generally considered safe in quantities found in food, garlic may cause an allergic reaction. It may also increase the risk of bleeding, especially if you're taking a blood-thinning medication.

Nasal irrigation. This therapy is similar to the conventional use of nasal drops (see preceding page), but more aggressive. It's more commonly used for hay fever and is relatively low risk (see page 173).

Probiotics. Taking probiotics during cold and flu season may lower your risk of these illnesses or lessen their severity or duration (see page 92).

When to seek medical advice

A common cold generally goes away in about a week, although it may not disappear as quickly as you'd like. If your signs and symptoms last longer than a week, you may have a more serious illness, such as the flu or pneumonia.

Seek medical attention if you have:

- Fever greater than 102 F
- High fever accompanied by achiness and fatigue
- Fever accompanied by sweating, chills and a cough with colored phlegm
- Symptoms that get worse instead of better

In general, children are more sick with a common cold than are adults and often experience complications such as ear infections. Your child doesn't need to see a doctor for a routine common cold, but you should seek medical attention right away if your child has any of these signs or symptoms:

- Fever of 103 F or higher, chills or sweating
- Fever that lasts more than 72 hours
- Vomiting or abdominal pain
- Unusual sleepiness
- Severe headache
- Difficulty breathing
- Persistent crying
- Ear pain

Coronary artery disease

How healthy are your coronary arteries? If you eat healthy foods, get physical activity every day and don't smoke, you're well on your way to preventing symptoms of coronary artery disease — a leading type of heart disease.

The coronary arteries supply your heart with blood, oxygen and nutrients. When blood flow through the coronary arteries becomes obstructed, it's known as coronary artery disease.

Coronary artery disease is caused by the gradual buildup of fatty deposits in your coronary arteries (atherosclerosis). As the deposits slowly narrow your coronary arteries, your heart receives less blood. Eventually, diminished blood flow may cause chest pain (angina), shortness of breath or other symptoms. A complete blockage can cause a heart attack.

Since coronary artery disease often develops over decades, it can go virtually unnoticed until it produces a heart attack. But there's plenty you can do to prevent coronary artery disease. Start by committing to a healthy lifestyle.

Conventional treatment

Lifestyle changes can promote healthier arteries. If you smoke, quitting is the most important thing you can do. Eat healthy foods, and exercise regularly. Sometimes medication or procedures to improve blood flow are recommended as well.

Medications

Various drugs can be used to treat coronary artery disease, including:

Cholesterol medications. Aggressively lowering your low-density lipoprotein (LDL, or "bad") cholesterol can slow, stop or even reverse the buildup of fatty deposits in your arteries. Boosting your high-density lipoprotein (HDL, or "good") cholesterol may help, too. Your doctor can choose from a range of cholesterol medications, including drugs known as statins and fibrates.

Aspirin. A daily aspirin or other blood thinner can reduce the tendency of your blood to clot, which may help prevent obstruction of your coronary arteries. If you've had a heart attack, aspirin can help prevent future attacks.

Beta blockers. These drugs slow your heart rate and decrease your blood pressure, which decreases your heart's demand for oxygen. If you've had a heart attack, beta blockers reduce the risk of future attacks.

Nitroglycerin. Nitroglycerin tablets, spray and patches can control chest pain by opening up your coronary arteries and reducing your heart's demand for blood.

Angiotensin-converting enzyme (ACE) inhibitors. These drugs decrease blood pressure and may help prevent progression of coronary artery disease. If you've had a heart attack, ACE inhibitors reduce the risk of future attacks.

Calcium channel blockers. These medications relax the muscles that surround your coronary arteries and cause the vessels to open, increasing blood flow to your heart. They also control high blood pressure.

Procedures to restore and improve blood flow

Sometimes more aggressive treatment is needed. On the next page are a few options.

Angioplasty and stent placement (percutaneous coronary revascularization). In this procedure, your doctor inserts a long, thin tube (catheter) into the narrowed part of your artery. A wire with a deflated balloon is passed through the catheter to the narrowed area. The balloon is then inflated, compressing the deposits against your artery walls. A mesh tube (stent) is often left in the artery to help keep the artery open. Some stents slowly release medication that also helps keep the artery open.

Coronary artery bypass surgery. A surgeon creates a graft to bypass blocked coronary arteries using a vessel from another part of your body. This allows blood to flow around the blocked or narrowed coronary artery. Because this requires open-heart surgery, it's most often reserved for cases of multiple narrowed coronary arteries.

Coronary brachytherapy. If the coronary arteries narrow again after stent placement, radiation may be used to help open the artery again.

Laser revascularization. If standard treatments aren't effective, a new surgery known as laser revascularization may be considered. During this procedure, a laser beam is used to make tiny new channels in the wall of the heart muscle. New vessels may grow through these channels and into the heart to provide additional paths for blood flow.

Complementary and alternative treatment

In relation to coronary artery disease, therapies focus primarily on reducing stress and lowering cholesterol (see page 164) or triglycerides.

Omega-3 fatty acids. There appears to be good evidence that omega-3 fatty acids (fish oil), from fish or from supplements, can reduce high triglyceride levels, which are a risk factor for coronary artery disease. Fish oil contains both docosahexaenoic acid (DHA) and eicosapentaenoic acid (EPA). Omega-3 fatty acids are also found in some plant and nut oils.

The American Heart Association recommends 2 to 4 grams (2,000 to 4,000 milligrams) of omega-3 fatty acids daily for people with elevated triglyceride levels. In addition, the association recommends 1 gram (1,000 mg) a day for people with documented coronary artery disease. The supplements should be taken in consultation with a doctor.

Because high doses can cause bleeding, don't take more than 3 grams (3,000 mg) a day unless instructed to do so by your doctor.

Yoga. Yoga, with its emphasis on relaxation, fitness and a healthy lifestyle, may complement standard therapies for coronary artery disease. It may also improve heart disease risk factors such as high blood pressure, high cholesterol and high blood sugar levels. Yoga is generally considered safe, but certain positions may pose a risk if you have spinal problems, atherosclerosis of your neck arteries, glaucoma or other medical problems. Check with your doctor before starting yoga if you have significant medical conditions.

Reducing your risk
Lifestyle changes can help you prevent or slow the progression of coronary artery disease.

- **Stop smoking.** Stopping is the best way to reduce your risk of a heart attack.
- **Control your blood pressure.** Have a blood pressure measurement at least every two years.
- **Check your cholesterol.** Have a baseline cholesterol test when you're in your 20s and then at least every five years.
- **Keep diabetes under control.** Blood sugar control can reduce the risk of heart disease.
- **Get moving.** Exercise helps you achieve and maintain a healthy weight and control diabetes, high cholesterol and high blood pressure — all coronary artery disease risk factors.
- **Eat healthy foods.** Focus on fruits, vegetables and whole grains.
- **Maintain a healthy weight.** Weight loss is especially important for people who have large waist measurements — more than 40 inches for men and more than 35 inches for women.
- **Manage stress.** Practice techniques for managing stress (see page 38).

The cholesterol connection

Cholesterol is found in every cell in your body. This fat-like substance is an important component of cell membranes and is needed to formulate some hormones. Your body makes all the cholesterol it needs. Any cholesterol in your diet is extra — and up to no good.

When there's too much cholesterol in your blood, you may develop fatty deposits in your blood vessels. Eventually, these deposits make it difficult for enough blood to flow through your arteries. Your heart may not get as much oxygen-rich blood as it needs, which increases the risk of a heart attack. Decreased blood flow to your brain can cause a stroke.

But there's good news. High blood cholesterol (hypercholesterolemia) is largely preventable. A healthy diet, regular exercise and other lifestyle changes can go a long way toward reducing high cholesterol. Sometimes medication is needed, too.

Treating high cholesterol

Lifestyle changes play an important role and can help improve your cholesterol level. Eat a healthy diet, get regular physical activity and, if you smoke, stop. If you've made these important lifestyle changes and your total cholesterol — particularly your low-density lipoprotein (LDL) cholesterol — remains high, your doctor may recommend medication.

Medications

The specific choice of medication or combination of medications depends on various factors, including your individual risk factors, age, current health and possible side effects. Common choices include:

- **Statins.** Statins — among the most commonly prescribed medications for lowering cholesterol — block a substance your liver needs to make cholesterol. This depletes cholesterol in your liver cells, which causes your liver to remove cholesterol from your blood. Statins may also help your body reabsorb cholesterol from accumulated deposits on your artery walls, potentially reversing coronary artery disease. Choices include atorvastatin (Lipitor), fluvastatin (Lescol), lovastatin (Altoprev, Mevacor), pravastatin (Pravachol), rosuvastatin (Crestor) and simvastatin (Zocor).

- **Bile-acid-binding resins.** Your liver uses cholesterol to make bile acids, a substance needed for digestion. The medications cholestyramine (Prevalite, Questran), colesevelam (Welchol) and colestipol (Colestid) lower cholesterol indirectly by binding to bile acids. This prompts your liver to use excess cholesterol to make more bile acids, which reduces the level of cholesterol in your blood.

- **Cholesterol absorption inhibitors.** Your small intestine absorbs the cholesterol from your diet and releases it into your bloodstream. The drug ezetimibe (Zetia) helps reduce blood cholesterol by limiting the absorption of dietary cholesterol. Zetia can be used in combination with any of the statin drugs.

- **Combination cholesterol absorption inhibitor and statin.** Ezetimibe-simvastatin (Vytorin) decreases both absorption of dietary cholesterol in your small intestine and production of cholesterol in your liver.

If you also have high triglycerides, your doctor may prescribe:

- **Fibrates.** The medications fenofibrate (Lofibra, TriCor) and gemfibrozil (Lopid) decrease triglycerides by reducing your liver's production of very-low-density lipoprotein (VLDL) cholesterol and by speeding up the removal of triglycerides from your blood. VLDL cholesterol contains mostly triglycerides.

- **Niacin.** Niacin (Niaspan) decreases triglycerides by limiting your liver's ability to produce LDL and VLDL cholesterol. Various prescription and nonprescription preparations are available, but prescription niacin is preferred. Dietary supplements containing niacin aren't effective for lowering triglycerides.

Most of these medications are well tolerated, but effectiveness varies from person to person. The most common side effects are stomach pain, constipation, nausea and diarrhea. If you decide to take cholesterol medication, your doctor may recommend periodic liver function tests to monitor the medication's effect on your liver.

Beyond the basics

In addition to standard medications, some alternative therapies may help lower cholesterol. Research suggests some of these therapies may offer benefits, and the risks appear to be relatively low.

- **Plant sterols or stanols.** These plant components help block the absorption of cholesterol and can lower LDL ("bad") cholesterol. They're now added to some foods, including margarines, orange juice and salad dressings. They're generally considered safe in recommended amounts, but caution should be used if you have certain medical conditions, including asthma or other respiratory conditions, diabetes, or allergies to pine. Talk to your doctor. The American Heart Association recommends plant sterols or stanols only for people who have high levels of LDL cholesterol.

- **Blond psyllium.** Also called ispaghula, this comes from the husks of the seeds of *Plantago ovata* and is high in soluble dietary fiber. It's the main ingredient in many bulk laxatives and has some cholesterol-lowering effects. Blond psyllium can decrease cholesterol by absorbing dietary fats in the gastrointestinal tract. It's generally considered safe, except for people with significant bowel abnormalities or those who have had bowel surgery. In addition, people who frequently handle blond psyllium can be at risk of hypersensitivity reactions.

- **Soy.** Soy supplements have not been shown to be effective in reducing cholesterol. However, studies have shown that substituting soy protein in your diet for other dietary sources of protein, such as red meat, can reduce LDL cholesterol by about 10 percent. Based on this information, the Food and Drug Administration (FDA) allows makers of soy products to claim that consuming 25 grams of soy protein a day reduces the risk of heart disease.

- **Policosanol.** Policosanol contains a mixture of carbon alcohols, which are derived from sugar cane. Clinical research on this supplement is contradictory. Earlier studies, which took place in Cuba, suggested that policosanol reduced total cholesterol and LDL ("bad") cholesterol. Later studies, which took place outside of Cuba, did not find such promising results. Because policosanol has anti-platelet effects, it shouldn't be used by people who take aspirin or other anticoagulant drugs. It may increase risk of bleeding.

- **Garlic.** Research indicates that garlic may be of some benefit, but higher quality studies are less positive. The supplements appear to be of low risk, except in people taking anti-clotting medications.

- **Red yeast rice.** Red yeast rice products are essentially statins in disguise. These products are extracts of rice that have been fermented with a strain of red yeast. The process yields numerous different HMG-CoA reductase inhibitors (statins), one of which is mevinolin, better known as lovastatin (Mevacor). Red yeast rice products are effective, but they can cause the same side effects as statins. Since red yeast rice contains a compound already approved as a drug, the FDA considers red yeast rice products to be unapproved drugs, and, therefore, illegal. However, the products are available on the Internet. Since there's no way to determine the quantity or quality of lovastatin in supplements, you should avoid them.

Depression

In the United States, about 16 percent of adults experience major depression during their lifetime. And, unfortunately, most people don't get adequate treatment.

Depression is a disorder that affects your thoughts, moods, feelings, behavior and even your physical health. People used to think it was "all in your head" and that if you really tried, you could "snap out of it" or just "get over it." But doctors now know that depression is not a weakness, and it's not something you can treat on your own. Depression is a medical disorder with a biological and chemical basis.

Sometimes, a stressful life event triggers depression. Other times, depression seems to occur spontaneously with no identifiable specific cause. Depression is much more than grieving or a bout of the blues.

Depression may occur only once in a person's life. Often, however, it occurs as repeated episodes over a lifetime, with periods free of depression in between. Or it may be a chronic condition, requiring ongoing treatment over a lifetime.

People of all ages and races are affected by depression. Medications are available that are generally safe and effective, even for the most severe depression. With proper treatment, most people with serious depression improve, often within weeks, and can return to normal daily activities.

Conventional treatment

The development of newer antidepressant medications and mood-stabilizing drugs has improved the treatment of depression. Medications can relieve symptoms of depression and have become the first line of treatment for most types of the disorder.

Treatment may also include psychotherapy, which may help you cope with ongoing problems that may trigger or contribute to depression. A combination of medications and a brief course of psychotherapy usually is effective if you have mild to moderate depression. If you're severely depressed, initial treatment usually is with medications or electroconvulsive therapy. Once you improve, psychotherapy can be more effective.

Doctors usually treat depression in two stages. Acute treatment with medications helps relieve symptoms until you feel well. Once your symptoms ease, maintenance treatment typically continues for four to nine months to prevent a relapse. It's important to keep taking your medication even though you feel fine and are back to your usual activities. Episodes of depression recur in the majority of people who have one episode, but continuing treatment greatly reduces your risk of a rapid relapse. If you've had two or more previous episodes of depression, your doctor may suggest long-term treatment with antidepressants.

Medications

Selective serotonin reuptake inhibitors (SSRIs), such as fluoxetine (Prozac, Sarafem), paroxetine (Paxil), sertraline (Zoloft), citalopram (Celexa) and escitalopram (Lexapro), are often first line treatments. Among tricyclic antidepressants are amitriptyline, desipramine (Norpramin), nortriptyline (Pamelor), protriptyline (Vivactil), trimipramine (Surmontil) and a combination of perphenazine and amitriptyline. Tetracyclics include maprotiline and mirtazapine (Remeron).

Other drugs include monoamine oxidase inhibitors (MAOIs), such as phenelzine (Nardil) and tranylcypromine (Parnate), and stimulants such as methylphenidate (Ritalin, Concerta), dextroamphetamine (Dexedrine, Dextrostat) or modafinil (Provigil). Doctors also prescribe lithium (Eskalith, Lithobid) and various mood-stabilizing drugs.

Psychotherapy

There are several types of psychotherapy. Each type involves a short-term, goal-oriented approach aimed at helping you deal with a specific issue. Prolonged psychotherapy is seldom necessary to treat depression.

Electroconvulsive therapy

Despite the images that many people conjure up, electroconvulsive therapy is generally safe and effective. Experts aren't sure how this therapy relieves the signs and symptoms of depression. The procedure may affect levels of neurotransmitters in your brain. The most common side effect is confusion that lasts a few minutes to several hours. This therapy is usually used for people who don't respond to medications and for those at high risk of suicide.

Light therapy

Light therapy may help if you have seasonal affective disorder. This disorder involves periods of depression that recur at the same time each year, usually when days are shorter in the fall and winter. Scientists believe fewer hours of sunlight may increase levels of melatonin, a brain hormone thought to induce sleep and depress mood. Treatment in the morning with a specialized type of bright light, which suppresses production of melatonin, may help if you have this disorder.

Complementary and alternative treatment

Some popular supplements marketed or taken for depression include:

St. John's wort. St. John's wort may work as well as antidepressants in people with mild or moderate depression, and some recent studies indicate it might even be effective for people with severe depression. Adverse reactions may include dry mouth, dizziness, digestive problems, fatigue, headache and sexual problems. In most cases, signs and symptoms are mild. St. John's wort can interfere with the effectiveness of many prescription medications, including antidepressants, drugs to treat human immunodeficiency virus (HIV) infections and AIDS, and drugs to prevent organ rejection in people who've had transplants. If you take *any* prescription medication, talk to your doctor before taking St. John's wort.

SAMe. This is a chemical substance found in all human cells and it plays a role in many body functions. It's thought to work by affecting signaling across nerve cell membranes. Studies have found SAMe to be more effective than a placebo and it may be as effective as some conventional antidepressant medications. SAMe can cause nausea and constipation.

5-HTP. One of the raw materials that your body needs to make serotonin is a chemical called 5-HTP, which is short for 5-hydroxytryptophan. In theory, if you boost your body's level of 5-HTP, you should also elevate your levels of serotonin. But there's not enough evidence to determine if 5-HTP is effective, and there are concerns about its safety.

Omega-3 fatty acids. Found in fish oil and certain nuts and plants, the acids are being studied as a possible mood stabilizer for people with bipolar depression and other psychiatric disorders.

Saffron. Some clinical evidence suggests that saffron extract might improve symptoms of depression. More study is needed.

Some nonsupplement therapies may help

Although supplements are popular for depression, a number of other integrative therapies may help. Work with your doctor to find how these may be used with conventional therapies.

Traditional Chinese medicine. This system, which broadly includes acupuncture, herbal remedies and massage, may provide some help for depression. For example, some studies suggest that acupuncture might be beneficial for depression. Overall, though, the research is inconclusive.

Art therapy. Self-expression through art therapy may help you deal with anxiety, stress, depression, and other mental and emotional issues.

Music therapy. Music therapy can enhance mood, promote relaxation and reduce anxiety.

Spirituality. Prayer may help you develop stronger coping skills and may reduce anxiety.

Electromagnetic therapy. Transcranial electromagnetic stimulation (TMS) is offered at Mayo Clinic as a possible treatment for depression.

Yoga. As an exercise and as a meditative approach, yoga can enhance relaxation and help reduce anxiety.

Diabetes

Type 2 diabetes is a chronic condition that affects the way your body metabolizes sugar (glucose) — your body's main source of fuel. Type 2 diabetes develops when your body becomes resistant to the effects of insulin — a hormone that regulates the absorption of sugar into your cells — or when your body produces some, but not enough, insulin to maintain a normal glucose level.

In contrast, type 1 diabetes results when your pancreas no longer produces insulin.

More than 23 million people in the United States have diabetes, according to the American Diabetes Association. About 90 to 95 percent of people with diabetes have type 2 diabetes. And the condition is on the rise, fueled largely by the growing obesity problem.

The American Diabetes Association estimates that nearly one-third of people who have type 2 diabetes don't even know it. If the condition is left uncontrolled, the consequences can be life-threatening.

There's no cure for type 2 diabetes, but there's plenty you can do to manage — or prevent — the condition. Start by eating healthy foods, getting plenty of exercise and maintaining a healthy weight. If diet and exercise aren't enough, managing your blood sugar with medication can help you continue to live a healthy and active life.

Conventional treatment

Eating a healthy diet, exercising and maintaining a healthy weight may be all that's needed to control your diabetes. When those aren't enough, you may need the help of medication.

Diet

Contrary to popular belief, there's no single diabetes diet. And having diabetes doesn't mean you have to eat only bland, boring foods. Instead, it means you'll eat more fruits, vegetables and whole grains and fewer animal products and sweets. It's the same eating plan that's recommended for everyone. A registered dietitian can help you create a meal plan that fits your health goals, food preferences and lifestyle. To keep your blood sugar consistent, try to eat the same amount of food with the same proportion of carbohydrates, proteins and fats at the same time every day.

Exercise

The same exercises that are good for your heart and lungs also help lower your blood sugar levels. Consult your doctor before beginning an exercise program.

Maintaining a healthy weight

Fat makes your cells more resistant to insulin. But when you lose weight, the process reverses and your cells become more receptive to insulin. For some people with type 2 diabetes, weight loss is all that's needed to restore blood sugar to normal.

Medication

Various drugs may be used to treat type 2 diabetes, including:

Sulfonylurea drugs. These medications stimulate your pancreas to produce and release more insulin, as long as your pancreas already produces some insulin on its own. Second-generation sulfonylureas such as glipizide (Glucotrol, Glucotrol XL), glyburide (DiaBeta, Glynase, Micronase) and glimepiride (Amaryl) are prescribed most often.

Meglitinides. These medications, such as repaglinide (Prandin), have effects similar to sulfonylureas, but they're not as likely to lead to low blood sugar. Meglitinides work quickly, and the results fade rapidly.

Biguanides. Metformin (Glucophage, Glucophage XR) is the only drug in this class available in the United States. It works by inhibiting the production and release of glucose from your liver, which means you need less insulin to transport blood sugar into your cells.

Alpha-glucosidase inhibitors. These drugs block the action of enzymes in your digestive tract that break down carbohydrates. This means sugar is absorbed into your bloodstream more slowly, which helps prevent the rapid rise in blood sugar that usually occurs right after a meal. Drugs in this class include acarbose (Precose) and miglitol (Glyset).

Thiazolidinediones. These drugs, such as rosiglitazone (Avandia) and pioglitazone hydrochloride (Actos), make your body tissues more sensitive to insulin and keep your liver from overproducing glucose.

Insulin. Some people with type 2 diabetes must take insulin every day to replace what their pancreas is unable to produce.

Amylin mimetics. Pramlintide (Symlin), mimics the action of amylin, a protein secreted by the pancreas. This medication slows down the movement of food through your stomach after meals, affecting how rapidly glucose enters your bloodstream.

Incretin mimetics. Exenatide (Byetta) mimics the action of the hormone incretin, which helps regulate fasting glucose levels and glucose levels after meals.

DPP-4 (dipeptidyl-peptidase 4) inhibitors. They stimulate your pancreas to release more insulin when blood sugar levels rise and reduce the amount of blood sugar your liver releases into your bloodstream. They include the drugs sitagliptin (Januvia) and saxagliptin (Onglyza).

Complementary and alternative treatment

Several therapies may have some benefit for diabetes and appear to be low risk. Work with your doctor when considering these, as you will need to monitor your blood sugar carefully, and you may need to modify the dose of your conventional medication to avoid low blood sugar.

Oat bran. It's high in the soluble fiber beta-glucan. Oat bran as part of a healthy diet has been shown to reduce blood sugar levels.

Soy. Preliminary studies suggest it modestly lowers blood sugar. Soy contains soluble and insoluble fibers, but there could be other mechanisms involved in its effect on blood sugar.

Cinnamon. Initial studies suggested that cinnamon could significantly lower blood sugar in people with diabetes. However, more recent studies failed to confirm these promising findings. More research is needed.

Ginseng. This herb is used widely for a number of conditions and research suggests it may also lower blood sugar. More evidence is needed; however, ginseng appears to have little risk of serious side effects when taken in recommended doses.

Other therapies to control blood sugar

Several small studies indicate that **yoga** may help in the treatment of diabetes. Studies conducted in India found a decrease in blood sugar following yoga sessions. One study suggested that the result was due to the effects of yoga on the pancreas. Yoga is considered a relatively low-risk integrative therapy.

Another traditional Indian practice, **ayurveda**, is also used for diabetes, but study results are mixed. Ayurveda involves the use of, among other things, herbs, massage, diet and exercise to cleanse the body and restore energy balance. Some studies have shown modest benefits for diabetes, but the practice has not been well researched. In addition, there are concerns that some ayurvedic medications could be toxic. If you try ayurvedic practices, do so with caution.

Traditional Chinese medicine also may have some benefits for managing diabetes. Acupuncture, which is part of traditional Chinese medicine, has been shown to reduce pain associated with diabetic neuropathy. However, there may be significant risks from unproven Chinese herbs and herb combinations if you ignore conventional therapies, or if you don't continue to monitor your blood sugar closely.

Fibromyalgia

You hurt all over and frequently feel exhausted. Even after numerous tests, your doctor can't seem to find anything specifically wrong with you. If this sounds familiar, you may have fibromyalgia.

Fibromyalgia is a chronic condition characterized by fatigue, widespread pain in your muscles, ligaments and tendons, and multiple tender points — places on your body where slight pressure causes pain. It occurs in about 2 percent of the population in the United States. Women are much more likely to develop the disorder than are men, and the risk of fibromyalgia increases with age.

The cause of fibromyalgia is a bit of a mystery. Current thinking centers around a theory called central sensitization. This theory states that people with fibromyalgia have a lower threshold for pain because of increased sensitivity in the brain to pain signals. Researchers speculate that this oversensitization may be triggered by infections, physical trauma or emotional stress. However, these links have not been proved. Because fibromyalgia tends to run in families, there may be certain genetic mutations that may make you more susceptible to developing the disorder.

Although the intensity of symptoms may vary, they typically never disappear completely. However, fibromyalgia isn't progressive, crippling or life-threatening.

Conventional treatment

In general, treatment for fibromyalgia involves a combination of medication and self-care. The emphasis is on minimizing symptoms and improving general health.

Medications

Medications can help reduce the pain of fibromyalgia and improve sleep. Common choices include:

Analgesics. Acetaminophen (Tylenol, others) may ease the pain and stiffness caused by fibromyalgia. However, its effectiveness varies. Tramadol (Ultram) is a prescription pain reliever that may be taken with or without acetaminophen. Your doctor may recommend nonsteroidal anti-inflammatory drugs (NSAIDs) — such as aspirin, ibuprofen (Advil, Motrin, others) or naproxen sodium (Anaprox, Aleve) — in conjunction with other medications, but NSAIDs haven't proved to be effective in managing the pain of fibromyalgia when taken by themselves.

Antidepressants. Your doctor may prescribe antidepressant medications, such as amitriptyline, nortriptyline (Pamelor) or doxepin to help promote sleep. Fluoxetine (Prozac) in combination with amitriptyline has also been found effective. Sertraline (Zoloft) and paroxetine (Paxil) can help if you're experiencing depression.

Anti-seizure drugs. Medications used to treat epilepsy can be useful in reducing certain types of pain. Gabapentin (Neurontin) is sometimes helpful in reducing fibromyalgia symptoms, while pregabalin (Lyrica) is the first drug approved by the Food and Drug Administration to treat fibromyalgia.

Other medications. Prescription sleeping pills, such as zolpidem (Ambien), may provide short-term benefits for some people with fibromyalgia, but doctors usually advise against long-term use of these drugs. These medications tend to work for only a short time, after which your body becomes resistant to their effects. Ultimately, using sleeping pills tends to create even more sleeping problems in many people.

Benzodiazepines may help relax muscles and promote sleep, but doctors often avoid these drugs in treating fibromyalgia. Benzodiazepines can become habit-forming, and they haven't provided long-term benefits.

Physical therapy

Specific exercises can help restore muscle balance and may reduce pain. Stretching techniques and the application of hot or cold also may help.

Cognitive behavioral therapy

Cognitive behavioral therapy seeks to increase your belief in your own abilities and teaches you methods for dealing with stressful situations.

Therapy can be provided via individual counseling, audiotapes or classes, and may help you manage your fibromyalgia.

Treatment programs

Interdisciplinary treatment programs may be effective in improving your symptoms, including relieving pain. These programs can combine a variety of treatments, such as relaxation techniques, biofeedback, and gentle, graded exercise. Receiving information and learning about chronic pain can be very helpful. There isn't one combination that works best for everybody. Your doctor can create a program based on what works best for you.

Complementary and alternative treatment

Several integrative treatments do appear to safely relieve stress and reduce pain, but many practices remain unproved because they haven't been adequately studied.

Acupuncture. Results of a Mayo Clinic study found that people with fibromyalgia who received acupuncture had a significant reduction in symptoms compared with those who didn't receive the therapy. Acupuncture is generally a low-risk treatment. Make sure to find an experienced practitioner.

Massage. It's a relatively safe way to relax muscles and help ease pain.

Relaxation therapy. A broad range of therapies, from guided imagery to meditation and progressive muscle relaxation, fall under this heading. These are low-risk techniques that may have some benefits.

Capsaicin. This topical cream made from chili peppers is used for a variety of pain syndromes, including fibromyalgia. In one study involving people with fibromyalgia it took four weeks to notice a pain reduction.

SAMe. Two preliminary studies suggest SAMe might be beneficial for some people with fibromyalgia. Larger trials are still needed to determine SAMe's efficacy and safety.

5-HTP. Limited research suggests some benefits, such as reducing the number of tender points, improving sleep and lessening anxiety, from this precursor for the brain chemical serotonin. But safety is uncertain and it should be used only with the supervision of a doctor.

Guaifenesin. Some researchers think that fibromyalgia may result from buildup of phosphate in the muscles. And some suspect that guaifenesin, a derivative of the guaiac tree, might improve phosphate excretion. So far, there's only anecdotal reports that taking guaifenesin helps and no reliable evidence that it works.

Human growth hormone. It is given daily by injection to some people with fibromyalgia. The rationale is that a subset of people with fibromyalgia may have low levels of insulin-like growth factor-1. The therapy is expensive and not recommended.

Self-care for fibromyalgia

Self-care is critical in the management of fibromyalgia.

- **Reduce stress.** Develop a plan to avoid or limit overexertion and emotional stress. Allow yourself time each day to relax. But don't change your routine totally. People who quit work or drop all activity tend to do worse than those who remain active. Try stress management techniques, such as deep-breathing exercises or meditation.

- **Get enough sleep.** Because fatigue is one of the main characteristics of fibromyalgia, getting sufficient sleep is essential. In addition, practice good sleep habits, such as going to bed and getting up at the same time each day and limiting daytime napping.

- **Exercise regularly.** At first, exercise may increase your pain. But doing it regularly often decreases symptoms. Appropriate exercises often include walking, biking, swimming and water aerobics. A physical therapist can help you develop a home exercise program. Stretching, good posture and relaxation exercises also are helpful.

- **Pace yourself.** Keep your activity on an even level. If you do too much on your good days, you may have more bad days.

Hay fever

If spring brings a stuffy nose, scratchy eyes and an extra sneeze tacked on to your usual "achoo!" — you're likely very familiar with hay fever (allergic rhinitis). Hay fever is the common name for an allergic response to specific substances in your environment. It's one of the most common allergic reactions, affecting about 40 million people in the United States.

If you have seasonal hay fever, tree pollen, grasses or weeds may trigger your symptoms. If you're sensitive to indoor allergens such as dust mites, cockroaches, mold or pet dander, you may have year-round symptoms.

People with hay fever are more likely to develop asthma, bronchitis, sinusitis and other respiratory conditions, and other allergic conditions, such as eczema.

Nonprescription medications and self-care measures may be enough to manage your mild hay fever symptoms. But if your signs and symptoms are more severe — or if hay fever is a year-round nuisance — see an allergy specialist for evaluation and treatment.

For some people hay fever symptoms are a minor, temporary nuisance. But if your symptoms are more persistent, they can affect your performance at work, school or leisure activities. Finding the right treatment likely won't eliminate your symptoms — but for most people, it makes a big difference.

Conventional treatment

Typically, the first step in dealing with hay fever is identifying what triggers your symptoms, then helping you develop a plan to avoid these substances. In some cases, avoidance alone can effectively control hay fever problems. Your doctor may also prescribe an oral medication, a nasal spray or eyedrops — alone or in combination — to decrease your signs and symptoms. Conventional treatments for hay fever include:

Medications

Nasal corticosteroids. These are the most effective hay fever medications and are often prescribed first, especially for more troublesome signs and symptoms. Examples include beclomethasone (Beconase) and fluticasone propionate (Flonase). They're generally safe for extended use. Mild side effects can include an unpleasant smell or taste and nasal irritation.

Antihistamines. These oral medications and nasal sprays help relieve itching, sneezing and runny nose but have less effect on congestion. Nonprescription oral antihistamines include diphenhydramine (Benadryl) and chlorpheniramine (Chlor-Trimeton), while prescription drugs include cetirizine (Zyrtec) and fexofenadine (Allegra). Some can cause drowsiness.

Decongestants. Often used in combination with antihistamines, these are available in nonprescription and prescription liquids, tablets and nasal sprays. Oral decongestants include pseudoephedrine (Sudafed, Actifed, others). Nasal decongestants include phenylephrine (Neo-Synephrine) and oxymetazoline (Afrin). Avoid them if you have high blood pressure (hypertension). Oral decongestants can worsen the symptoms of prostate enlargement, making urination more difficult.

Cromolyn sodium. This nonprescription nasal spray (NasalCrom, others) helps relieve hay fever symptoms by preventing the release of histamine. It's not associated with any serious side effects.

Leukotriene modifier. Montelukast (Singulair) is a prescription tablet that blocks leukotrienes — immune system chemicals that cause allergy symptoms such as excess mucus production. Possible side effects include headache and, less commonly, abdominal pain, cough and dental pain.

Nasal atropine. Available in a prescription nasal spray, ipratropium bromide (Atrovent) helps relieve a severe runny nose by preventing the glands in your nose from producing excess fluid. Mild side effects include nasal dryness, nosebleeds and sore throat. Rarely, it can cause more severe side effects such as blurred vision, dizziness and difficult urination. It's not recommended if you have glaucoma or an enlarged prostate.

If you're taking any other medications or have a chronic health condition, talk to your doctor or pharmacist before starting any treatment for hay fever, to be sure you're not at risk of a drug interaction or other adverse effect.

Allergy shots

If medications don't relieve your symptoms, your doctor may recommend allergy shots (immunotherapy or desensitization therapy). For three to five years, you receive injections containing purified allergen extracts. The goal is to desensitize you to specific allergens.

Self-care

For pollen and molds. Close doors and windows during pollen season. Use air conditioning in your house and car. Stay indoors on dry, windy days. Use a high-efficiency particulate air (HEPA) filter in your bedroom.

For dust mites. Use allergy-proof covers on mattresses and pillows. Wash sheets and blankets in at least 130 F water. Vacuum carpets weekly with a small-particle or HEPA filter. Consider removing carpet.

For pet dander. Remove pets from the house and bathe pets weekly. If pets are in the house, keep them out of your bedroom.

Complementary and alternative treatment

Nasal irrigation is a commonly used alternative therapy for hay fever. It provides symptom relief with little risk.

Common therapies

Nasal irrigation. This therapy is often associated with yoga. There are several variations, but one common technique uses a small container, called a neti pot, that you fill with a mild solution of warm salt water. You tip your head forward and slightly sideways over a sink and place the tip of the pot's spout in one nostril. The solution runs in that nostril, through your sinuses and out the other nostril. Repeat on the other side.

The therapy appears to have little risk and is recommended by the International Consensus Report on the Diagnosis and Management of Rhinitis. If you have frequent nosebleeds, have had recent nose surgery or your gag reflex is impaired, talk with your doctor before trying this.

Butterbur. It is the best studied dietary supplement for treatment of hay fever. Extracts of this shrub may have some effectiveness in preventing hay fever symptoms. Because raw butterbur contains potentially toxic substances, use only a commercially prepared product labeled UPA-free. Look for products standardized to contain 8 milligrams petasin and isopetasin. Don't take it with other medications without your doctor's supervision.

Stinging nettle. It's commonly promoted for allergic rhinitis and there's preliminary evidence that it modestly reduces symptoms. More research is still needed to determine its effectiveness and safety.

Tinospora cordifolia. This ayurvedic medicine seems to have immuno-stimulatory effects. Some evidence suggests taking a specific extract (Tinofend) daily can decrease symptoms, but more study is needed.

Headache

Although headache pain sometimes can be severe, in most cases it's not the result of an underlying disease. The vast majority of headaches are so-called primary headaches. These include migraine and tension headache.

A tension headache is the most common headache, and yet it's not well understood. A tension headache generally produces a diffuse, usually mild to moderate pain over your head. Many people liken the feeling to having a tight band around their head. In many cases, there's no clear cause for a tension headache.

Migraines affect more than 28 million Americans — three times more women than men. A migraine is often disabling. In some cases, these painful headaches are preceded or accompanied by a sensory warning sign (aura), such as flashes of light, blind spots, or tingling in your arm or leg. A migraine can also often be accompanied by other signs and symptoms, such as nausea, vomiting, and extreme sensitivity to light and sound.

Managing headaches is often a balance between fostering healthy habits, finding effective nondrug treatments and using medications appropriately. In addition, a number of preventive, self-care and alternative treatments may help you deal with headache pain.

Conventional treatment

Treatment for headaches depends on the type. Here's an overview of treatment options for two main types of headaches:

Tension headaches

A variety of medications, both nonprescription and prescription, are available for treating tension headaches. You may find fast, effective relief by taking pain relievers such as aspirin, ibuprofen (Advil, Motrin, others) or acetaminophen (Tylenol, others). These medications are inexpensive and readily available and don't require a prescription from your doctor. People with severe or chronic tension headache may require stronger painkillers or preventive medications. Which drug works best varies from one person to another.

Whether you have episodic or chronic headaches, don't overuse nonprescription medications. Limit your use of painkillers to two days a week. Try to take the medications only when necessary, and use the smallest dose needed to relieve your pain. Overusing pain medications can cause rebound headaches or the development of chronic daily headache, triggering the very symptoms you're trying to stop. In addition, all medications used to treat headache have side effects, some of which may be serious. For prescription medications, follow the recommended dosage.

Medications don't cure headaches, and over time painkillers and other medications may lose their effectiveness. If you take medications regularly, discuss the risks and benefits with your doctor. Also, remember that pain medications aren't a substitute for recognizing and dealing with the stressors that may be causing your headaches.

Migraines

Pain-relieving medications. These drugs are taken to stop pain once it has started. For best results, take pain-relieving drugs as soon as you experience signs or symptoms of a migraine. It may help if you rest or sleep in a dark room after taking them.

Examples include nonsteroidal anti-inflammatory drugs (NSAIDs), such as ibuprofen (Advil, Motrin, others) or aspirin; triptans, such as sumatriptan (Imitrex), rizatriptan (Maxalt) and naratriptan (Amerge); and ergots, such as ergotamine (Ergomar) and dihydroergotamine (D.H.E. 45).

Preventive medications. These drugs help reduce or prevent migraines. Choosing a preventive strategy depends on the frequency and severity of your headaches, the degree of disability your headaches cause and other medical conditions you may have. You may be a candidate for preventive therapy if you have two or more debilitating attacks a month, if you use pain-relieving medications more than twice a week, if pain-relieving medications aren't helping or if you have uncommon migraines.

Preventive medications include cardiovascular drugs such as beta blockers, calcium channel blockers — especially verapamil (Calan, Isoptin) — and the high blood pressure drugs lisinopril (Prinivil, Zestril) and candesartan (Atacand). Antidepressants — especially tricyclic antidepressants, such as amitriptyline, nortriptyline (Pamelor) and protriptyline (Vivactil) — also are used, as are NSAIDs and anti-seizure drugs such as divalproex sodium (Depakote), valproic acid (Depakene) and topiramate (Topamax).

Also on the list of preventive medications are cyproheptadine, an antihistamine that affects serotonin activity, and botulinum toxin type A (Botox), which is injected into the muscles of the face and head.

Complementary and alternative treatment

Nontraditional therapies used for headache pain include:

Acupuncture. Among other benefits, acupuncture may be helpful for headache pain. This treatment uses thin, disposable needles that generally cause little or no pain or discomfort. Find an experienced practitioner.

Biofeedback. Biofeedback appears to be effective in relieving migraines and tension headaches. This relaxation technique uses special equipment to teach you how to monitor and control certain physical responses, such as muscle tension.

Massage. Although massage is a wonderful way to reduce stress and relieve tension, its value in treating headaches hasn't been fully determined. For people who have tight, tender muscles in the back of the head, neck and shoulders, massage may help relieve headache pain.

Herbs, vitamins and minerals. There is some evidence that the herbs feverfew and butterbur may prevent migraines or reduce their severity. A high dose of riboflavin (vitamin B-2) also may prevent migraines by correcting tiny deficiencies in the brain cells. Magnesium supplements seem to be of help for some people with migraines. Most people who benefit have low levels of magnesium. Coenzyme Q10 is being studied as a potential preventive agent for migraines. Research suggests it can decrease migraine frequency by about 30 percent. It may take up to three months to notice benefits.

Rubbing peppermint oil on the forehead and temples might reduce the intensity of tension headaches. Most peppermint oil contains menthol, which probably works more to relieve headache pain.

Ask your doctor if any of these treatments are right for you.

High blood pressure

You can have high blood pressure (hypertension) for years without experiencing a single symptom. But silence isn't golden in this case. Uncontrolled high blood pressure increases your risk of serious health problems, including heart attack and stroke.

Blood pressure is determined by the amount of blood your heart pumps and the amount of resistance to blood flow in your arteries. The more blood your heart pumps and the narrower your arteries, the higher your blood pressure.

High blood pressure affects nearly a third of American adults, and about half of Americans age 60 and older, according to the National Heart, Lung, and Blood Institute. Fortunately, high blood pressure can be easily detected. And once you know you have high blood pressure, you can work with your doctor to control it.

Conventional treatment

Changing your lifestyle can go a long way toward controlling high blood pressure. But sometimes lifestyle changes aren't enough. In addition to diet and exercise, your doctor may recommend medication.

Which category of medication your doctor prescribes depends on your stage of high blood pressure and whether you also have other medical conditions. To reduce the number of doses you need a day, which can reduce side effects, your doctor may prescribe a combination of low-dose medications rather than larger doses of one single drug. In fact, two or more blood pressure drugs often work better than one.

The major types of medication used for high blood pressure include:

Thiazide diuretics. These medications act on your kidneys to help your body eliminate sodium and water, reducing blood volume. Thiazide diuretics are often the first — but not the only — choice in high blood pressure medications. In a 2006 study, diuretics were a key factor in preventing heart failure associated with high blood pressure.

Beta blockers. These medications reduce the workload on your heart, causing your heart to beat slower and with less force. When prescribed alone, beta blockers don't work as well in blacks — but they're effective when combined with a thiazide diuretic.

Angiotensin-converting enzyme (ACE) inhibitors. These medications help relax blood vessels by blocking the formation of a natural chemical that narrows blood vessels. ACE inhibitors may be especially important in treating high blood pressure in people with coronary artery disease, heart failure or kidney failure. Like beta blockers, ACE inhibitors don't work as well in blacks when prescribed alone, but they're effective when combined with a thiazide diuretic.

Angiotensin II receptor blockers. These medications help relax blood vessels by blocking the action — not the formation — of a natural chemical that narrows blood vessels. Like ACE inhibitors, angiotensin II receptor blockers often are useful for people with coronary artery disease, heart failure and kidney failure.

Calcium channel blockers. These medications help relax the muscles of your blood vessels. Some slow your heart rate. A word of caution for grapefruit lovers. Grapefruit juice interacts with some calcium channel blockers, increasing blood levels of the medication and putting you at higher risk of side effects. Researchers have identified the substance in grapefruit juice that causes the interaction, which may one day lead to commercial grapefruit juices that don't pose such a risk.

If you're having trouble reaching your blood pressure goal with combinations of the above medications, your doctor may prescribe:

Alpha blockers. These medications reduce nerve impulses to blood vessels, reducing the effects of natural chemicals that narrow vessels.

Alpha-beta blockers. In addition to reducing nerve impulses to blood vessels, alpha-beta blockers slow the heartbeat to reduce the amount of blood that must be pumped through the vessels.

Central-acting agents. These prevent your brain from telling your nervous system to increase your heart rate and narrow your blood vessels.

Vasodilators. These medications work directly on the muscles in the walls of your arteries, preventing your arteries from narrowing.

Complementary and alternative treatment

Several integrative therapies appear to have value for high blood pressure.

Omega-3 fatty acids. Omega-3s can be found in fish oil and in some plant and nut oils. There's little evidence that omega-3 fatty acids lower blood pressure. However, they are beneficial in reducing heart disease risk and mortality. Therefore, consuming omega-3 fatty acids or taking a fish oil supplement makes sense.

Calcium and magnesium. These supplements may modestly reduce blood pressure.

Dark chocolate. The cocoa polyphenols in dark chocolate can lower systolic blood pressure about 5 mm Hg and diastolic by about 3 mm Hg. Milk chocolate contains less polyphenols than does dark chocolate and white chocolate doesn't contain any.

Blond psyllium. Preliminary research suggests it may modestly lower blood pressure due to its high fiber content.

Wheat bran. Like psyllium, it may have a modest effect on blood pressure.

Paced respiration. Paced respiration refers to slow, deep breathing. In various clinical trials, regular use of an over-the-counter device (Resperate) that analyzes breathing patterns and helps guide inhalation and exhalation was found to help lower blood pressure. You can also practice such breathing on your own, without the use of a device.

Yoga. Yoga may improve high blood pressure, as well as high cholesterol and high blood sugar levels. It's generally considered safe, but certain positions may pose a risk if you have spine problems, atherosclerosis of neck arteries, glaucoma or other medical problems. Check with your doctor before starting yoga if you have serious or unstable medical conditions.

Qi gong. In combination with conventional therapies, this traditional Chinese practice may help lower blood pressure. There are many different forms of qi gong, ranging from a practitioner who uses his or her hands on an individual to forms that use meditation and exercise.

Acupuncture. This traditional Chinese therapy involves the insertion of fine needles into the skin at certain points to restore proper energy flow. There's mixed evidence on its effectiveness for high blood pressure, but it's generally a low-risk treatment. Find an experienced practitioner.

Insomnia

Almost everyone has occasional sleepless nights, perhaps due to stress, heartburn, or drinking too much caffeine or alcohol. Insomnia is a lack of sleep that occurs on a regular or frequent basis, and often for no apparent reason.

How much sleep is enough varies from person to person. Although 7 ½ hours of sleep is about average, some people do well on four to five hours of sleep. Other people need nine to 10 hours of sleep each night.

Insomnia can affect not only your energy level and mood, but also your health because sleep helps bolster your immune system. Fatigue, at any age, leads to diminished mental alertness and concentration. Lack of sleep caused by insomnia is linked to accidents both on the road and on the job.

Insomnia may be either temporary or chronic. You don't necessarily have to live with the sleepless nights of insomnia. Some simple changes in your daily routine and habits may result in better sleep.

Conventional treatment

No matter what your age, insomnia usually is treatable. The key often lies in changes to your routine during the day and when you go to bed.

Coping skills

Key coping skills that can help overcome sleep problems include:
- Sticking to a sleep schedule
- Limiting your time in bed
- Avoiding "trying" to sleep
- Hiding the bedroom clocks
- Exercising and staying active
- Avoiding or limiting caffeine, alcohol and nicotine
- Checking your medications for drugs that may affect sleep
- Dealing with painful health conditions
- Finding ways to relax
- Avoiding or limiting naps
- Minimizing sleep interruptions

Medication

If self-help measures don't work or you believe that another condition, such as depression, restless legs syndrome or anxiety, is causing your insomnia, talk to your doctor. He or she may recommend that you take medications to promote relaxation or sleep.

Prescription medications. Taking prescription sleeping pills, such as zolpidem (Ambien), eszopiclone (Lunesta), zaleplon (Sonata) or ramelteon (Rozerem), for a couple of weeks until there's less stress in your life may help you get to sleep until you notice benefits from behavioral self-help measures. The antidepressant trazodone also may help with insomnia.

Doctors generally don't recommend prescription sleeping pills for the long term because they may cause side effects. Plus, your goal is to develop the ability to sleep without the help of medication. In addition, sleeping pills can become less effective after a while.

Nonprescription medications. Nonprescription sleep aids contain antihistamines to induce drowsiness. They're OK for occasional sleepless nights, but they, too, often lose their effectiveness the more you take them. Many sleeping pills contain diphenhydramine, which can cause difficulty urinating and a drowsy feeling in the daytime.

Complementary and alternative treatment

There are many nonconventional treatments used for insomnia, and several may offer some benefit.

Melatonin. Melatonin is a hormone produced naturally in the brain. Supplements contain synthetic melatonin. Although widely used for prevention of jet lag, it's also used for sleep problems, where it seems most effective in older people. Melatonin is generally considered safe at recommended levels but may cause clotting abnormalities in people taking the blood thinner warfarin (Coumadin). It shouldn't be taken if you're pregnant or trying to become pregnant.

Valerian. Research suggests that valerian, a perennial plant, may help you get to sleep faster and improve sleep quality. It's generally considered safe at recommended doses. It's also used for anxiety. Research from a multicenter study also suggests that the combination of valerian and hops may help insomnia.

Guided imagery. This can refer to a number of therapies, including visualization. The goal is to help you relax and visualize a positive outcome, in the case of insomnia, sleep. Guided imagery has been shown to alter breathing, heart rate and blood pressure. It's generally considered safe.

May help and likely won't hurt

Although research is unclear about the value of these therapies for insomnia, the risk of trying them is relatively low:

Acupuncture. A small Korean study of people 65 and older found acupuncture to be effective for insomnia, and another study found acupuncture helped insomnia during pregnancy.

Hypnosis. One study of school-age children found hypnosis beneficial in overcoming insomnia.

Lavender. A study of female college students found that lavender fragrance was effective for both insomnia and depression.

Music therapy. A small study of women in two domestic abuse centers found that music therapy improved sleep quality and also reduced anxiety.

Don't ignore sleep problems

Sleep is as important to your health as a healthy diet and regular exercise. Whatever your reason for sleep loss, insomnia can impact you both mentally and physically.

The impact can be cumulative. People with chronic insomnia are more likely than others to develop psychiatric problems such as depression and anxiety disorders. Long-term sleep deprivation can also increase the severity of chronic diseases, such as high blood pressure and diabetes.

And it's clear that insufficient sleep can lead to serious or even fatal accidents. According to the National Highway Traffic Safety Administration, more than 100,000 crashes each year are due to drivers falling asleep at the wheel.

Irritable bowel syndrome

Irritable bowel syndrome (IBS) is one of the most common disorders that doctors see. Yet it's also one that many people aren't comfortable talking about.

Irritable bowel syndrome is characterized by abdominal pain or cramping and changes in bowel function — including bloating, gas, diarrhea and constipation — problems most people don't like to discuss. What's more, for many years irritable bowel syndrome was considered a psychological rather than a physical problem.

Up to 1 in 5 American adults has irritable bowel syndrome. The disorder accounts for more than 1 out of every 10 doctor visits. For most people, signs and symptoms of irritable bowel disease are mild. Only a small percentage of people have severe signs and symptoms.

Fortunately, unlike more serious intestinal diseases such as ulcerative colitis and Crohn's disease, irritable bowel syndrome doesn't cause inflammation or changes in bowel tissue or increase your risk of colorectal cancer. In many cases, you can control irritable bowel syndrome by managing your diet, lifestyle and stress.

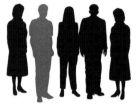

Up to 1 in 5 American adults has irritable bowel syndrome.

Conventional treatment

Because it's still not clear what causes irritable bowel syndrome, treatment focuses on the relief of symptoms so that you can live your life as fully and normally as possible.

In most cases, you can successfully control mild symptoms of irritable bowel syndrome by learning to manage stress and making changes in your diet and lifestyle. But if your problems are moderate or severe, you may need more help than lifestyle changes alone can offer. Your doctor may suggest:

Fiber supplements. Taking fiber supplements such as psyllium (Metamucil) or methylcellulose (Citrucel) with fluids may help control constipation.

Anti-diarrheal medications. Over-the-counter medications such as loperamide (Imodium) can help control diarrhea.

Eliminating high-gas foods. If you have significant bloating or are passing significant amounts of gas, your doctor may also ask you to cut out such items as carbonated beverages, salads, raw fruits and vegetables, cabbage, broccoli and cauliflower.

Anticholinergic medications. Some people need drugs that affect certain activities of the nervous system (anticholinergics) to relieve painful bowel spasms.

Antidepressant medications. If your symptoms include pain and depression, your doctor may recommend a tricyclic antidepressant or a selective serotonin reuptake inhibitor (SSRI). These medications help relieve depression as well as inhibit the activity of neurons that control the intestines. For diarrhea and abdominal pain, your doctor may suggest tricyclic antidepressants, such as imipramine (Tofranil) and amitriptyline. Side effects of these drugs include drowsiness and constipation. SSRIs such as fluoxetine (Prozac, Sarafem) or paroxetine (Paxil) may be helpful if you're depressed and have pain and constipation.

Counseling. If antidepressant medications don't work, you may have better results from counseling if stress tends to exacerbate your symptoms.

Medications specifically for IBS

There are currently two drugs available to treat IBS: alosetron (Lotronex) and tegaserod (Zelnorm).

Alosetron. This drug is a nerve receptor antagonist that's supposed to relax the colon and slow the movement of waste through the lower bowel. But the drug was removed from the market just nine months after its approval when it was linked to at least four deaths and severe side effects in 197 people. In June 2002, the Food and Drug Administration (FDA) decided to allow alosetron to be sold again —

with restrictions. The drug can be prescribed only by doctors enrolled in a special program and is intended for severe cases of diarrhea-predominant IBS in women who don't respond to other treatments. It isn't approved for men.

Tegaserod. For women who have IBS with constipation, the FDA has approved the medication tegaserod (Zelnorm). It's approved for short-term use in women and hasn't been shown to be effective for treating men with IBS. Tegaserod imitates the action of the neurotransmitter serotonin and helps to coordinate the nerves and muscles in the intestine. Some reports have suggested a risk of rare, dangerous side effects similar to those of alosetron, but the drug is still available.

Complementary and alternative treatment

The following nontraditional therapies may help relieve symptoms of irritable bowel syndrome:

Probiotics. Probiotics are "good" bacteria that normally live in your intestines and are found in certain foods, such as yogurt, and in dietary supplements. It's been suggested that people with irritable bowel syndrome may not have enough good bacteria, and that consuming foods with probiotics may help ease symptoms. Some studies have shown that probiotics can help IBS. Not all studies on probiotics have had positive results, however. Use of probiotics is generally considered safe at recommended doses.

Peppermint oil. Peppermint is a natural antispasmodic that relaxes smooth muscles in the intestines. Study results haven't been consistently encouraging, but there's some evidence that peppermint oil can reduce abdominal pain, flatulence and diarrhea. Because peppermint may aggravate heartburn, it's best to take enteric-coated preparations of peppermint oil.

Artichoke leaf extract. Some research suggests it can help relieve cramping, flatulence and constipation.

Blond psyllium. For constipation-predominant IBS, the fiber in psyllium may improve symptoms. Fiber tends to normalize bowel movements; however, it may take up to four weeks before the effects become noticeable.

Acupuncture. Researchers at the National Institutes of Health (NIH) have found that acupuncture can provide relief from chronic pain. Although study results on the effects of acupuncture on symptoms of irritable bowel syndrome have been mixed, some people use acupuncture to help relax muscle spasms and improve bowel function.

Dealing with stress may prevent IBS

Finding ways to deal with stress can be extremely helpful in preventing or alleviating symptoms of IBS. These include:

Counseling. Sometimes, a health care professional such as a psychologist or psychiatrist can help you learn how to reduce stress.

Biofeedback. This stress-reduction technique helps you reduce muscle tension and slow your heart rate with the feedback of a machine.

Regular exercise, yoga, massage or meditation. You can take classes in yoga and meditation or practice the therapies at home using books or tapes.

Progressive relaxation exercises. Start by tightening the muscles in your feet, then concentrate on slowly letting all of the tension go. Next, tighten and relax your calves. Continue until the muscles in your body, including those in your eyes and scalp, are completely relaxed.

Deep breathing. Most adults breathe from their chests. But you become calmer when you breathe from your diaphragm, the muscle that separates your chest from your abdomen. When you inhale, allow your belly to expand with air; when you exhale, your belly contracts.

Hypnosis. A trained professional teaches you how to relax and then guides you as you imagine your intestinal muscles becoming smooth and calm.

Memory problems

Increasing evidence suggests that the phrase "Use it or lose it" may indeed apply to your body's most powerful organ — your brain. And that intellectual stimulation — especially, perhaps, in your later years — is key to keeping your brain alive and well.

Will your mental ability change as you age? Research indicates that the answer is yes, it probably will. Like physical performance, mental performance generally tends to decline with age.

It's important to remember, too, that many factors besides age affect mental ability. Depression and chronic stress are the most common. Both can cause difficulty with short-term memory, decreased focus and concentration, and impaired decision-making ability. Both are also treatable.

Memory does depend on the individual, but most people generally can develop valuable habits to help offset age-related memory changes. Mentally stimulating activities such as reading regularly, taking classes, learning new skills and engaging in active conversations with friends may lead to preservation of mental abilities with age.

Conventional treatment

Are there things that you can do later in life to preserve your mental capacities? Research says, absolutely, yes. Older adults can learn just as well as can younger adults, and it's possible to increase brain cell connections, regardless of your age. Other lifestyle measures also have been shown to benefit mental functioning, such as physical activity, limiting alcohol use and managing stress.

And even if research hasn't outlined all of the ins and outs of the human intellect, keeping your brain active and engaged in the world around you makes for an interesting life — and who can resist that possibility? Being engaged with life pays.

Here are practical strategies to help you keep your brain in shape:

Use reminders and keep organized
In today's world, information comes at you constantly from multiple sources. You need to find a way to get beyond the information overload. To get organized, create a way to track each type of information. List appointments in a personal calendar. Create to-do lists for unscheduled tasks. Maintain a personal file with names, addresses and phone numbers. Even a simple list above the phone will do. A wide variety of tools are available to help you organize, maintain and remember data — ranging from simple paper records to sophisticated computer software.

Create routines, rituals and cues
Keep frequently used items in the same place, whether at work or at home. Have a designated spot to put your car or house keys after each time you use them. Keep the kitchen utensils that you use every day in the same location.

Rituals also can help. Complete common tasks in the same order or at the same time. Also set up cues. For example, place packages to mail close to the front door so that you don't forget them.

Experiment with memory techniques
Experiment with the following to see what works for you:

Make associations. One way to remember something new is to associate it with something else that you already know. You did this as a child when you learned to recognize Italy on a world map by remembering that the country is shaped like a boot.

Choose your memories. Sometimes it's necessary to remind yourself of what's truly important. When meeting many new people at the same time, for example, focus on remembering just a handful of key names. When reading a book or article, give it a quick skim to decide what facts or ideas are important to remember, then let go of the rest.

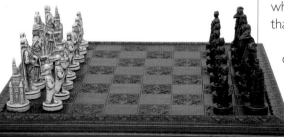

Repeat, rehash and revisit. Exercise your memory by retrieving key information. Repeat essential facts — names, dates, numbers — several times when you first try to learn them.

Don't be afraid of challenges

Test your limits. Take classes — learn yoga or Pilates or take a philosophy course. Switch careers or start a new one. Take up a new hobby.

Take care of yourself

Caring for your body will help your mind. Staying physically active, getting enough sleep, limiting your alcohol intake and managing your stress levels all contribute to keeping your brain at its optimum functioning level.

Complementary and alternative treatment

There are a variety of nonconventional approaches to memory preservation, many of which need further study. Among them are:

Ginkgo. Ginkgo was thought to enhance cognitive function, but recent studies suggest it's not effective. Ginkgo appears safe when consumed in recommended quantities, but it can increase the risk of bleeding. Talk to your doctor before using ginkgo if you're on a blood-thinning medication.

Omega-3 fatty acids. Limited evidence suggests that consuming higher amounts of omega-3 fatty acids (fish oil) may be associated with improved cognitive function and reduced risk of dementia later in life.

Vitamin E. It might help slow the progression of moderately severe Alzheimer's disease. Often times it is combined with the medication selegiline. There is concern, however, that unhealthy people who take high doses of vitamin E may increase their risk of cardiovascular death. Therefore, it's important to discuss use of vitamin E with your doctor beforehand.

Huperzine A. A couple of studies suggest this supplement made from Chinese club moss may improve memory and cognitive function. It appears to work similar to the prescription medications cholinesterase inhibitors. More study is needed to determine safety and effectiveness.

Vinpocetine. This derivative of the periwinkle plant appears to modestly improve cognitive function in some individuals who take it. It helps dilate blood vessels. In people who use anti-platelet or anticoagulant drugs, it may increase bruising and bleeding.

Acetyl-L-carnitine. Some studies suggest it provides some memory benefit, but there have been negative findings as well. Younger individuals with early-onset symptoms are more likely to experience some benefit. Although generally well tolerated, it can cause nausea and vomiting.

Phosphatidylserine. This lecithin derivative may improve attention and memory in people with cognitive deterioration.

Medications can affect your memory

If you're concerned about your ability to remember, ask your doctor about the side effects of medications you're taking.

Some medications have side effects that can interfere with memory. When you talk to your doctor, mention everything you're taking, including vitamins, minerals, over-the-counter drugs and herbal supplements.

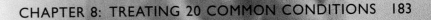

Menopause symptoms

Although your mother or grandmother may have used "the change" to refer to menopause, it isn't a single event. Instead, it's a transition that can start in your 30s or 40s and last into your 50s or even 60s. You may begin to experience signs and symptoms of menopause well before your periods stop permanently. Once you haven't had a period for 12 consecutive months, you've reached menopause.

Menopause is a natural biological process. Although it's associated with hormonal, physical and psychosocial changes in your life, menopause isn't the end of your youth or of your sexuality. Several generations ago, few women lived beyond menopause. Today, you may spend as much as half of your life after menopause.

In recent decades, hormone therapy (HT) has been widely used to relieve the signs and symptoms of menopause and — doctors thought — to prevent diseases associated with aging. However, long-term evidence demonstrated that HT may actually increase your risk of serious health conditions, such as heart disease, breast cancer and stroke.

Hormone therapy is still a safe, short-term option for some women, but numerous other therapies also are available to help you manage menopausal symptoms and stay healthy during this important phase of your life.

Conventional treatment

Treatments for menopause focus on relieving bothersome signs and symptoms and on preventing or lessening chronic conditions that may occur with aging. Conventional treatments include:

Medications

Hormone therapy. Hormone therapy — estrogen or a combination of estrogen and progestin — remains the most effective treatment option for menopausal symptoms such as hot flashes and vaginal discomfort. However, certain risks exist with long-term hormone therapy, including a slightly increased risk of heart disease, stroke and breast cancer. Depending on your personal and family medical history, your doctor may recommend hormone therapy in the lowest dose needed to provide symptom relief.

Low-dose antidepressants. Venlafaxine (Effexor), an antidepressant related to a class of drugs called selective serotonin reuptake inhibitors (SSRIs), may decrease hot flashes by up to 60 percent. Other SSRIs may also be helpful. Side effects may include nausea, dizziness or sexual dysfunction.

Gabapentin (Neurontin). This drug is commonly used to treat seizures and chronic pain, but it has also been shown to significantly reduce hot flashes. Side effects may include drowsiness, dizziness, nausea and swelling.

Clonidine (Catapres, others). Clonidine, a pill or patch typically used to treat high blood pressure, may reduce the frequency of hot flashes, but side effects such as dizziness, drowsiness, dry mouth and constipation are common.

Bisphosphonates. Doctors may recommend these nonhormonal medications, such as alendronate (Fosamax) and risedronate (Actonel), to reduce bone loss and risk of fractures. In women, these medications have replaced estrogen as the main treatment for osteoporosis. Side effects may include nausea, abdominal pain and irritation of the esophagus.

Selective estrogen receptor modulators (SERMs). SERMs are a group of drugs that includes raloxifene (Evista). Raloxifene mimics estrogen's beneficial effects on bone density in postmenopausal women, without some of the risks associated with estrogen. Hot flashes are a common side effect of raloxifene. You shouldn't use this drug if you have a history of blood clots.

Vaginal estrogen. To relieve vaginal dryness, estrogen can be used in vaginal tablet, ring or cream form. This treatment releases a small amount of estrogen locally to vaginal tissue, and can help relieve vaginal dryness, discomfort with intercourse and some urinary symptoms. Before deciding on any form of treatment, talk with your doctor about your options and the risks and benefits involved with each.

Self-care

Cool hot flashes. If you're experiencing hot flashes, get regular exercise and try to pinpoint what triggers your hot flashes. Triggers may include hot beverages, spicy foods, alcohol, hot weather and even a warm room.

Decrease vaginal discomfort. For vaginal dryness or discomfort with intercourse, use over-the-counter water-based vaginal lubricants (Astroglide, K-Y Jelly), moisturizers (Replens, Vagisil) or vaginal estrogen. Staying sexually active also helps.

Optimize your sleep. If you have trouble sleeping, avoid caffeinated beverages and don't exercise right before bedtime.

Complementary and alternative treatment

Many therapies have been promoted as aids in managing the symptoms of menopause. Some complementary and alternative approaches include:

Isoflavones. Soy is a common source of isoflavone phytoestrogens — plant-derived compounds that have weak estrogen-like effects. These compounds may help with hot flashes. Study results regarding their safety and effectiveness are mixed — some indicate that isoflavones may increase breast cancer growth, others that they may inhibit it. If you've had breast cancer, talk to your doctor before taking isoflavone pills, such as soy.

Flaxseed. Flaxseed is a rich source of lignan phytoestrogens, as well as omega-3 fatty acids and alpha-linolenic acid. Some research suggests daily consumption of flaxseed improves mild menopause symptoms, such as hot flashes. Flaxseed is a healthy alternative to other fats and it's safe. However, it shouldn't be consumed in high amounts by people who take warfarin (Coumadin).

Black cohosh. This herb is used for treating hot flashes and other menopausal symptoms. The North American Menopause Society supports short-term use of black cohosh for relieving menopausal symptoms because it seems to have a low risk of side effects when taken for a short period. However, some women taking black cohosh have experienced liver damage. How it works and the effects of long-term use are uncertain.

Ginseng. Ginseng may help improve fatigue and mood and sleep problems, but it doesn't help with hot flashes.

Other therapies. Techniques that focus on relaxation (deep breathing, guided imagery, yoga) don't directly target the hormonal fluctuations of menopause, but they may help you cope with mood swings, stress and sleep disturbances.

Conflicting or unclear evidence

A number of other alternative therapies are used for menopausal symptoms, including vitamin E, red clover, chasteberry and evening primrose oil. Scientific evidence as to their effectiveness and long-term safety is lacking.

Overweight

Do you weigh more than you should? If so, you're like the two-thirds of American adults who are overweight. About 1 in 3 American adults is considered to be obese. And childhood obesity is at an all-time high.

Obesity is more than a cosmetic concern. Being seriously overweight puts you at greater risk of developing high blood pressure and many other serious health risks that may ultimately be life-threatening.

The good news is that even a modest weight loss — reducing your weight by about 5 to 10 percent — can bring health improvements. This can often be done through diet and exercise modifications. If that isn't enough, other forms of treatment, including medications and surgery may help.

Talking to your doctor openly and honestly about your weight is one of the best things you can do for your health. The more your weight increases, the more health problems you may face. In addition to high blood pressure, added weight puts you at risk of high blood cholesterol, diabetes and arthritis. All of these conditions may improve if you're able to lose weight.

When it comes to weight loss, there's no shortage of advice. But what you should be looking for is something that works for a lifetime — that can help you stay at a healthy weight — not a "quick fix."

Conventional treatment

The safest and most effective way to lose weight is to eat a healthier diet, exercise and change unhealthy behaviors. But this requires a lifelong commitment. In some cases, you may need additional help, perhaps in the form of prescription medications or surgery.

Lifestyle changes

Diet. Calories you eat but don't use up are stored as fat on your body. Consuming fewer calories is an important factor for successful weight loss. The number of calories you need to maintain weight each day depends on several factors, including your age and activity level. Ask your doctor to help you determine your calorie goals to lose weight. He or she may recommend that you also work with a dietitian or a reputable weight-loss program.

Exercise. Changing your diet will help you consume fewer calories, but increasing your physical activity will help you burn calories you've stored up. In the long run, regular exercise is a key component to maintaining weight loss. Use aerobic exercise to burn body fat and strength training to build lean muscle tissue.

Behavior. Last but not least, it's important to change your approach to eating and activity. Long-term weight control relies on lifestyle changes that last. To be successful, you may need to change entrenched habits and beliefs that have hindered weight loss for you in the past. A therapist or a professionally led support group can often be helpful.

Medications

Sibutramine (Meridia). This medication changes your brain chemistry, making you feel full more quickly. Studies have shown that after a year, Meridia users lost an average of about 10 pounds more than did people simply following a low-calorie diet and taking an inactive pill (placebo). Side effects can include increased blood pressure, headache, dry mouth, constipation and insomnia.

Orlistat (Xenical). Orlistat inhibits the absorption of fat in your intestines. Unabsorbed fat is eliminated in the stool. Side effects include oily and frequent bowel movements, but these improve with decreased fat intake. Average weight loss with Xenical is modest, similar to Meridia. Because Xenical blocks absorption of some nutrients, your doctor may recommend that you also take a multivitamin. Alli is a reduced-strength version of orlistat sold without a prescription.

Surgery

When appropriate, weight-loss surgery can result in dramatic improvements in weight and health. In the first year or two, most people lose up to 50 percent of their excess weight. Generally, those who follow dietary and exercise recommendations keep most of that weight off long term.

Most procedures create a small pouch at the top of your stomach that can hold only about an ounce or two of food, though this can later expand to several ounces. After the operation, you can eat only small portions of food at a time without feeling nausea or discomfort. A variation on this procedure adds a bypass around part of your small intestine, where most of the calories from foods that you eat are absorbed. It reduces what you can eat, and it reduces the calories your body absorbs.

Complementary and alternative treatment

Many herbal supplements have been touted as weight-loss aids. Unfortunately, there doesn't seem to be any specific supplement that works well, and some may have potentially dangerous side effects.

Small, preliminary studies suggest the following supplements may have weight-loss potential, but the evidence is still far from conclusive.

Conjugated linoleic acid (CLA). Preliminary studies suggest that this compound may reduce body fat and increase muscle. Occasional side effects may include nausea and indigestion.

Calcium. There's some evidence that increasing calcium consumption from dairy products such as yogurt may increase weight reduction. Calcium supplements don't appear to produce the same effect.

Chromium. Taking chromium supplements might produce modest weight loss, but not all studies have produced positive benefits.

Omega-3 fatty acids. There's some evidence that the fatty acids in fish oil can improve weight loss.

Vitamin D. A few studies suggest it also may play a role in weight loss.

Products to avoid

Some weight-loss supplements are best left on the shelf, including ephedra, bitter orange and country mallow (heartleaf). These supplements can cause potentially dangerous cardiovascular problems. Ephedra supplements have been banned from the marketplace. The ban has been challenged but to date it's still in place. Ephedra may still be sold legally as a tea. Ephedra products also can be found on the Internet.

For more information on herbal weight-loss products, see page 55.

Are you a fidgeter?

Some people have a built-in mechanism for keeping weight off through their everyday movements. Studies show that people who fidget burn extra calories. Fidgeting appears to help them control their weight, even when they overeat.

In one of the most detailed and data-rich studies on obesity ever performed, Mayo Clinic researchers found that people who move more during the day — including fidgeting, tapping their toes, wiggling and changing posture — are less likely to gain weight than are people who move less. Researchers labeled this factor non-exercise activity thermogenesis, or NEAT.

The study provides an optimistic message, even if you're not a fidgeter. Every calorie you burn by moving counts. Even browsing in a store takes twice as much energy as sitting in a chair. If you move more each day, you'll tend to stay leaner than if you sit still.

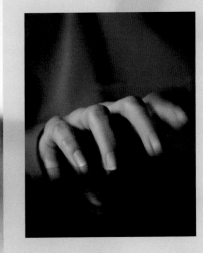

Premenstrual syndrome (PMS)

Mood swings, tender breasts, a swollen abdomen, food cravings, fatigue, irritability and depression. If you experience some or all of these symptoms in the days before your monthly period, you may have premenstrual syndrome (PMS).

An estimated 3 of every 4 menstruating women experience some form of premenstrual syndrome. These problems are more likely to trouble women between their late 20s and early 40s, and they tend to recur in a predictable pattern. Yet the physical and emotional changes you experience with premenstrual syndrome may be more or less intense with each menstrual cycle.

Still, you don't have to let such problems control your life. In recent years, much has been learned about premenstrual syndrome. Treatments and lifestyle adjustments can help you reduce or manage the signs and symptoms of premenstrual syndrome.

If you've tried managing your premenstrual syndrome with lifestyle changes, but with little or no success, and signs and symptoms of PMS are seriously affecting your health and daily activities, see your doctor.

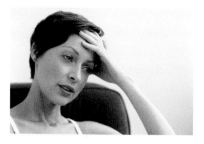

Conventional treatment

Your doctor may prescribe one or more medications for premenstrual syndrome. The success of medications in relieving symptoms varies from one woman to the next. There are also self-care measures that you can try to ease your symptoms.

Medications

Nonsteroidal anti-inflammatory drugs (NSAIDs). Taken before or at the onset of your period, NSAIDs such as ibuprofen (Advil, Motrin, others) or naproxen sodium (Aleve) can ease cramping and breast discomfort common to PMS.

Oral contraceptives. Oral contraceptives stop ovulation and stabilize hormonal swings, thereby helping to relieve PMS symptoms.

Antidepressants. Selective serotonin reuptake inhibitors (SSRIs), which include fluoxetine (Prozac, Sarafem), paroxetine (Paxil) and sertraline (Zoloft), have been successful in reducing symptoms such as fatigue, food cravings and sleep problems. These drugs are generally taken daily. But for some women with PMS, use of antidepressants may be limited to the two weeks before menstruation begins.

Medroxyprogesterone acetate (Depo-Provera). For severe PMS, this injection can be used to temporarily stop ovulation. However, Depo-Provera may cause an increase in some signs and symptoms of PMS, such as increased appetite, weight gain, headache and depressed mood.

Self-care

Modify your diet. The following may reduce symptoms:
- Eat smaller, more frequent meals each day to reduce bloating and the sensation of fullness.
- Limit salt and salty foods to reduce bloating and fluid retention.
- Choose foods high in complex carbohydrates, such as fruits, vegetables and whole grains.
- Choose foods rich in calcium. If you can't tolerate dairy products or aren't getting adequate calcium in your diet, you may need a daily calcium supplement.
- Take a daily multivitamin supplement.
- Avoid caffeine and alcohol.

Incorporate exercise into your regular routine. Go for a brisk walk, cycle, swim or do another aerobic activity most days of the week. Regular exercise can alleviate symptoms such as fatigue and a depressed mood.

Reduce stress. Get plenty of sleep. For those days when you don't feel well, keep your schedule simple.

Record your symptoms for a few months. Identify the triggers and timing of your symptoms so that you can intervene to help lessen them.

Complementary and alternative treatment

Here are some of the more common complementary products and remedies used to soothe the symptoms of premenstrual syndrome:

Calcium. Consuming 1,000 to 1,200 milligrams (mg) of dietary and supplemental calcium daily, such as chewable calcium carbonate (Tums, Rolaids, others), may reduce physical and psychological symptoms of PMS. Regular use of calcium carbonate also reduces your risk of osteoporosis.

Research also suggests that a high intake of calcium and vitamin D may reduce a woman's risk of PMS.

Magnesium. Taking 400 mg of supplemental magnesium daily may help to reduce fluid retention, breast tenderness and bloating in women with premenstrual syndrome.

Vitamin B-6. A daily dose of 50 to 100 mg of vitamin B-6 (pyridoxine) may help some women with troublesome PMS symptoms.

Vitamin E. This vitamin, taken in 400 international units (IU) daily, may ease PMS symptoms, including cramps and breast tenderness. However, reports have questioned its safety when taken in higher doses over a long term. Talk with your doctor about the amount you should take.

Chasteberry. The fruit of the chaste tree, called the chasteberry, has been used for centuries to treat women's hormone-related problems. Research suggests that chasteberry may reduce breast pain, swelling, constipation, irritability, depressed mood, anger and headache. In general, it seems to be well tolerated with only mild side effects. However, chasteberry isn't considered safe if you're pregnant or breast-feeding.

Ginkgo. There's some evidence that ginkgo may decrease fluid retention associated with PMS.

Natural progesterone creams. These are derived from wild yams and soybeans. Some women report that these creams relieve symptoms; however, no scientific studies have proved their effectiveness.

Relaxation therapy. Practicing progressive muscle relaxation or deep-breathing exercises can help reduce headaches, anxiety or insomnia.

Lacking evidence

There are other supplements that are sometimes used to manage symptoms of PMS. These include products such as manganese, SAMe, soy, St. John's wort, evening primrose oil and the Chinese herb dong quai. At this point, studies have not found sufficient evidence that the products work or that they are safe to use on a regular basis. Research into the effectiveness of these and other potential PMS therapies is ongoing.

Premenstrual dysphoric disorder: A severe form of PMS

Up to 8 percent of menstruating women have PMDD — a severe, sometimes disabling form of premenstrual syndrome.

PMDD is distinguished from PMS by the severity of its symptoms and its impact on relationships and daily activities. Symptoms may include persistent sadness, anxiety, fatigue, feelings of being overwhelmed, flu-like symptoms, and changes in sleeping and appetite patterns.

What causes PMDD isn't clear. Frequently, women with PMDD also have major depression, but not always.

A doctor may diagnose premenstrual dysphoric disorder based on its pattern of symptoms. Your doctor may recommend that you keep a diary to record the type, severity, duration and timing of your symptoms. This information may help your doctor diagnose PMDD and determine the most appropriate treatment for you.

Antidepressants known as selective serotonin reuptake inhibitors (SSRIs) are often the first line of therapy for PMDD. Other therapies used to treat premenstrual syndrome, including chasteberry, may also be helpful for PMDD.

Sexual problems

Although you may feel as if you're the only one who experiences difficulties with your sexual life, you're far from being alone. Many people — both men and women — experience sexual problems at some point in their lives. However, such concerns tend to become more common with age.

For men, erectile dysfunction (impotence) is a common problem. Patterns of erectile dysfunction may range from an occasional inability to obtain a full erection to an inability to maintain an erection throughout intercourse to an inability to achieve an erection at all.

For women, sexual dysfunction implies persistent or recurrent problems encountered in one or more of the stages of sexual response. This may include low or absent desire for sex, difficulty in achieving or maintaining sexual arousal, inability to achieve orgasm and painful sexual intercourse.

When sexual problems prove to be persistent and distressing, they can interfere with a person's self-image and his or her relationships. Although sexual problems are often multifaceted, they are treatable. And whereas sexual concerns were once considered a taboo subject, doctors and their patients are realizing that frank communication and better understanding of the nature of the problems are important steps toward sexual health.

Conventional treatment

For both men and women, treatment often requires first addressing an underlying medical condition or adjusting medications that have sexual side effects. Counseling or psychotherapy can be useful not only for the person experiencing difficulties but also for his or her partner.

For men

Oral medications. These include sildenafil (Viagra), tadalafil (Cialis) and vardenafil (Levitra). They work by enhancing the effects of nitric oxide, a chemical messenger that relaxes smooth muscles in the penis. This increases blood flow and allows an erection to occur in response to sexual stimulation. Don't combine these medications with nitrate drugs, such as nitroglycerin. Together, they can cause dizziness, low blood pressure and loss of consciousness.

Prostaglandin E (alprostadil). Alprostadil is a synthetic version of the hormone prostaglandin E, which helps enhance blood flow needed for an erection. The medication can be injected with a fine needle at the base of the penis or as a tiny suppository inserted into the tip of the penis.

Hormone therapy. For the small number of men who have testosterone deficiency, testosterone replacement therapy may be an option.

Vacuum devices. This treatment involves using a hand pump to pull blood into the penis and create an erection. A tension ring placed around the base of the penis maintains the erection during intercourse.

Vascular surgery. Surgery is usually reserved to correct blood flow in men who've experienced an injury to the penis or pelvic area.

Penile implants. This treatment involves surgically placing an inflatable or semirigid device into the two sides of the penis, which you manipulate at will. This treatment isn't usually recommended until other methods have been considered.

For women

Pelvic floor exercises (Kegels). These exercises strengthen the muscles involved in pleasurable sexual sensations and may help with arousal and orgasm difficulties. To do the exercises, tighten your pelvic muscles as if you're stopping your stream of urine. Hold for a count of five, relax and repeat several times a day.

Estrogen therapy. Localized estrogen therapy in the form of a vaginal cream, gel or tablet can help with sexual changes due to menopause. Estrogen may help improve the tone and elasticity of vaginal tissues, increase vaginal blood flow and enhance lubrication.

Progestin therapy. Some studies suggest that progestin hormonal therapy, in combination with estrogen, may lead to improvements in desire and arousal. More research is needed.

Testosterone therapy. Testosterone is important for sexual function in women as well as men, although at a much lower level. But its use for sexual dysfunction is controversial.

Complementary and alternative treatment

Although there are a number of proposed alternative remedies for sexual dysfunction, scientific evidence as to their safety and effectiveness is limited. These remedies include:

Acupuncture. A few small, preliminary studies suggest that acupuncture may possibly help improve erectile dysfunction. Acupuncture uses ultrafine needles inserted at strategic points on your body to improve your body's flow of vital energy. Acupuncture risks are generally low.

DHEA. In its natural form, dehydroepiandrosterone (DHEA) is the raw material from which male and female sex hormones are generated. DHEA levels in the body begin to decline after age 30. A few clinical trials suggest that, in its synthetic form, DHEA may possibly increase libido in premenopausal women and improve erectile dysfunction in men, but more study is needed. Acne is a common side effect.

Ginkgo. This herbal extract may help erectile dysfunction by improving blood flow to the penis. It may also improve sexual side effects of antidepressants in both men and women. Ginkgo may increase your risk of bleeding, so talk to your doctor before taking it if you're also on blood-thinning medications.

L-arginine. L-arginine is a protein that occurs naturally in the body. In its supplement form, it may help erectile dysfunction by enhancing the effects of nitric oxide, not unlike the action of Viagra and similar medications. Side effects may include nausea, abdominal cramps and diarrhea, especially at higher doses. Don't take L-arginine with Viagra.

Be cautious

Yohimbe bark extract. Derived from the yohimbe tree of western Africa, this bark extract has been traditionally used as an aphrodisiac and mild hallucinogen, but little research has been done on it. Its close cousin, yohimbine hydrochloride (Yocon) — a standardized prescription drug — is used for treating sexual side effects of antidepressants, female sexual dysfunction and erectile dysfunction. Yohimbe bark extract may contain yohimbine but levels vary, so it's difficult to know what you're getting. High doses can be dangerous. All forms may increase heart rate and raise blood pressure. Therefore, it's best to avoid this product.

'Herbal viagras.' Sildenafil (Viagra) is a prescription medication used to treat erectile dysfunction. Many herbal products are touted as "herbal viagras," but they're not the same as Viagra. For more information on these products, see page 72.

Coping with ED

Whether the cause is physical or psychological, or a combination of both, erectile dysfunction (ED) can become a source of mental and emotional stress for a man — and his partner.

If you experience erectile dysfunction only on occasion, try not to assume that you have a permanent problem or to expect it to happen again during your next sexual encounter. Don't view one episode as a lasting comment on your health, virility or masculinity.

In addition, if you experience occasional or persistent erectile dysfunction, remember your sexual partner. Your partner may see your inability to have an erection as a sign of diminished sexual desire. Your reassurance that this is not the case can be helpful.

To appropriately treat erectile dysfunction and strengthen your relationship with your partner, try to communicate openly and honestly about your condition. Couples may also want to seek counseling to confront any concerns they may have about erectile dysfunction and to learn how to discuss their feelings. Try to maintain this communication throughout the diagnosis and treatment process.

Treatment is often more successful if couples work together as a team.

Stress and anxiety

Modern life is full of pressures, fears and frustration. In other words, it's stressful. Racing against deadlines, sitting in traffic, arguing with your spouse — all of these situations make your body react as if you were facing a physical threat.

This reaction — called the "fight-or-flight response" — gave early humans the energy to fight aggressors or run from predators. It helped the species survive. Today, instead of protecting you, stress may — if constantly activated — make you more vulnerable to health problems.

It's normal to feel anxious or worried at times — everyone does. But if you often feel anxious without reason and your worries disrupt your daily life, you may have what's called generalized anxiety disorder (GAD). This condition causes excessive or unrealistic anxiety and worry about life circumstances, usually without a readily identifiable cause.

Fortunately, there's help for chronic stress and anxiety. Treatment ranges from learning new coping skills to medications to professional counseling or therapy. Several complementary and alternative therapies may also prove helpful in easing your emotional and physical burden.

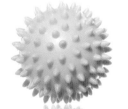

Conventional treatment

If you're under continuous stress that appears to have no endpoint in sight, you may be able to help yourself by implementing some key changes in your life. Professional counseling also can help. A buildup of stress can lead to generalized anxiety disorder, in which case a combination of medications and psychotherapy is often recommended.

Self-care

There are three fundamental ways in which to manage stress: By changing your environment so that daily demands aren't so high, by learning how to better cope with the demands in your environment, or by doing both.

Techniques that can help you manage stress include identifying and addressing those problems you can change, letting go of stressors beyond your control, taking good care of yourself, maintaining a healthy diet, exercising and finding time for relaxation, and relying on certain people to help you through the rough spots.

Medications

Anti-anxiety drugs. Benzodiazepines are sedatives that often ease anxiety within 30 to 90 minutes. Because they can be habit-forming, your doctor may prescribe them for only a short time to help you get through a particularly anxious period. Side effects include unsteadiness, drowsiness, reduced muscle coordination and problems with balance. Higher doses and long-term use can cause memory problems.

Antidepressants. These drugs influence the activity of certain brain chemicals (neurotransmitters) to help nerve cells (neurons) in your brain send and receive messages. Antidepressants usually begin to work within two weeks, but it may take up to eight weeks before you notice their full effects. You may need to try more than one to find which drug works best for you.

Psychotherapy

A common form of psychotherapy used to treat anxiety is cognitive behavioral therapy. During treatment sessions, a therapist helps you identify distorted thoughts and beliefs that trigger psychological stress, fear or depression. You learn to replace negative thoughts with more positive, realistic perceptions, and you learn ways to view and cope with life events differently.

Complementary and alternative treatment

Various forms of complementary and alternative therapies are used to treat stress and anxiety. The success of these treatments often depends on each individual's response. With the exception of some herbal thera- pies, most are relatively safe and have few side effects.

Herbal therapy. Kava, St. John's wort, passionflower and valerian are some of the most common herbal extracts used for anxiety. Research shows kava to be effective in soothing tension and agitation, but reports of severe liver damage have been associated with its use, therefore it's not recommended. Kava has been banned from sale in some countries, and other countries are considering similar action.

St. John's wort has mostly been studied for treatment of depression, but there's some evidence that it may also help relieve anxiety. St. John's wort can interact with many different medications and supplements, so be sure to talk with your doctor before taking this supplement.

Passionflower and valerian — often taken in the form of bedtime tea — appear to have mild sedative and tranquilizing properties with few side effects.

Biofeedback. For this technique, a practitioner measures your body's physiological response to stress or anxiety, which is displayed to you as auditory or visual signals. By increasing your awareness of your body's responses, you attempt to counter the signals with relaxation methods.

Relaxation therapy. Relaxation therapy encompasses numerous tech- niques ranging from paced respiration and deep breathing to meditation and progressive muscle relaxation. Most involve repetition of a single word, phrase or muscular activity and promote "emptying" your mind of external thoughts and stressors.

Massage. A number of studies indicate that massage can help reduce stress and anxiety symptoms.

Aromatherapy. Aromatherapy is the science of using oils from various plants to treat illness and promote health. The oils are often vaporized and inhaled or used as massage oils. It's believed that compounds in the oils activate certain parts of your brain, releasing different brain chemicals that may have a relaxing effect.

Art and music therapy. Art therapy involves the use of drawing, paint- ing, clay or sculpture to allow expression and organization of your inner thoughts and emotions when talking about them is difficult. The creation of art itself, or interpretation of an art piece, is thought to be therapeutic. Playing of music — even during medical procedures — has also been shown to produce relaxing and calming effects.

Yoga. When practiced regularly, yoga may help reduce daily stress and anxiety. Kundalini yoga, a type of yoga that's been studied specifically for anxiety disorder, combines poses and breathing techniques with chanting and meditation.

Acupuncture. A study conducted at Mayo Clinic found that acupunc- ture helped reduce anxiety symptoms associated with fibromyalgia.

Vaginal yeast infections

For many women, the itching, burning vaginal sensations and white, lumpy discharge that accompany vaginal yeast infections are all too familiar. And they usually produce the feeling of "Oh, no, not again."

Yeast infections are common — an estimated 3 out of 4 women will have a yeast infection in their lifetimes, and about half of women have two or more infections.

Yeast infections occur when certain internal or external factors change the normal environment of your vagina and trigger an overgrowth of a microscopic fungus — the most common being a fungus called *Candida albicans* (*C. albicans*). A yeast infection isn't considered a sexually transmitted disease.

Certain medications (antibiotics, steroids), uncontrolled diabetes, and hormonal changes caused by pregnancy or birth control pills can make you more prone to yeast infections. Bubble baths, vaginal contraceptives, damp or tightfitting clothing, and feminine hygiene sprays and deodorants also may increase your susceptibility to infection.

Fortunately, treatment is readily available. Once you've learned to recognize a yeast infection, you can usually treat it with over-the-counter products, with the approval of your doctor.

Conventional treatment

Yeast infections generally are treated with an antifungal cream or suppository. You should see your doctor if this is your first vaginal infection, you've had more than one kind of vaginal infection, you've had multiple sex partners or a recent new partner, or your symptoms persist despite treatment. Also see your doctor if you experience a fever or develop a particularly unpleasant vaginal odor. It's possible you have something other than a yeast infection.

Self-care

If you've talked to your doctor and you know that you have a yeast infection, your doctor may recommend going ahead with treatment on your own, taking these steps:

- Use an over-the-counter medication specifically for yeast infections. Options include one-day, three-day or seven-day courses of cream or vaginal suppositories. The active ingredient in these products is clotrimazole (Gyne-Lotrimin), miconazole (Monistat) or tioconazole (Vagistat). Some products also come with an external cream to apply to the labia and opening of the vagina to soothe itching. Follow package directions and complete the entire course of treatment even if you're feeling better right away.
- To ease discomfort until the antifungal medication takes full effect, apply a cold compress, such as a washcloth, to the labial area.

If you experience persistent infections, your doctor may also prescribe for you a single dose of the oral medication fluconazole (Diflucan).

Preventive care

To help prevent vaginal yeast infections, consider the following:

- Don't douche. The vagina doesn't require cleansing other than normal bathing. Repetitive douching disrupts the normal organisms that live in the vagina and can actually increase the risk of vaginal infection. Douching won't clear up a vaginal infection.
- Avoid potential irritants, such as scented tampons or pads.
- Wear cotton underwear and pantyhose with a cotton crotch. Don't wear underwear to bed. Yeast thrives in moist environments.
- Change out of wet swimsuits and damp clothing as soon as possible.

Complementary and alternative treatment

Some popular home remedies for treating or preventing vaginal yeast infections include a cream made from tea tree oil, vaginal suppositories made with garlic or boric acid, and douching with vinegar. Anecdotally, some women report success with these home remedies. However, well-designed controlled trials are needed to investigate their safety and effectiveness before any reliable recommendations can be made.

Probiotics. Probiotics refers to dietary supplements or foods that contain beneficial ("good") bacteria normally found in the body. *Lactobacillus acidophilus* (*L. acidophilus*) is a type of beneficial bacteria normally found in the vagina. One study found that vaginal suppositories containing *L. acidophilus* improved symptoms of vaginal yeast infections. However, other studies of oral preparations of *L. acidophilus* found little benefit. Another option is to eat yogurt that contains active lactobacillus cultures. This is a healthy habit that may have the added bonus of reducing recurrent vaginal yeast infections. Evidence as to the effectiveness of eating yogurt to fend off such infections is inconclusive, but there's no risk in giving it a try.

Echinacea. One study found taking echinacea supplements in combination with a topical antifungal cream was effective in preventing recurrent vaginal yeast infections.

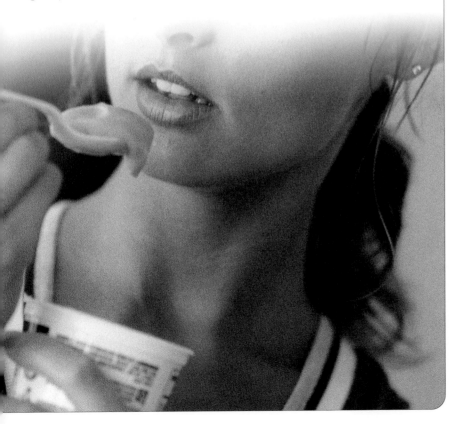

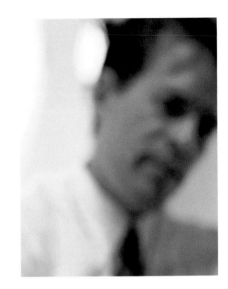

Can men get yeast infections?

A man can get a yeast infection from sexual contact with a woman who has a yeast infection. However, not every man exposed to a yeast infection will get one. Men are at increased risk of such an infection if they have diabetes or are uncircumcised.

Signs and symptoms of male yeast infection include:

- Itching or burning at the head of the penis
- Red rash on the penis

A male yeast infection is usually a relatively minor problem that can be easily treated with the same antifungal creams or ointments used to treat female yeast infections.

If the rash doesn't go away after about a week or it recurs frequently, see your doctor.

Chapter 9

Be Smart, Be Safe

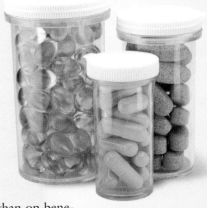

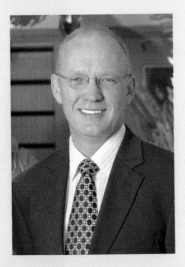

Larry Bergstrom, M.D.
Complementary and
Integrative Medicine Program

" Unfortunately, when it comes to alternative therapies, the information available about many products is based on benefits to the company advertising the product rather than on benefits to the user. "

"It's natural!" That's the answer I get frequently from my patients when I inquire why they're taking a dietary supplement.

More than ever before, people are involved and interested in their health care. The Internet makes it easy to seek out information about the latest in treatments and practices reported to be beneficial to a person's health and happiness. Unfortunately, when it comes to alternative therapies, the information available about many products is based on benefits to the company advertising the product rather than on benefits to the user. Your doctor can help direct you to reliable information about the supplements you're interested in taking.

I'm also finding that a number of my patients use multiple products, in the belief that they're helping themselves. When it comes to dietary supplements, I remind them that supplements are just that — supplements to their diet! Their efforts should first and foremost be to eat a healthy diet. Taking lots of supplements doesn't substitute for a good diet. A good diet has long-lasting health benefits. The same cannot be said for nutrients from a pill.

People also trust that the products they purchase or therapies they practice are safe. Alternative products and practices may offer benefits when it comes to your health, but some of them also pose risks — serious risks. Some supplements come from plants whose ingredients are powerful agents. St. John's wort, for example, interacts with many prescription medications and can lead to serious health risks for individuals who combine the supplement with a medication.

The option to pick and choose among treatments — alternative and conventional — provides opportunities to maintain health and happiness. But it also makes the complicated world of health care even more so. Take a careful look at your options. Make sure the therapy you're considering will do you more good than harm — consider its safety as well as its effectiveness. A safe practice is one that does no harm when it's used as intended.

Finally, to reduce potential risks, you need to be upfront with your doctor. Your health is your doctor's No. 1 priority, but he or she can't help protect you if you don't provide honest answers. Many people neglect to report all of the products and practices they're using, either because they don't consider them to be relevant or because they're uncertain how their doctor may react. Your doctor needs to know about everything you're taking or using.

Remember, your doctor has the same goal that you do — to help you live a healthy and long life.

Protecting yourself

It's becoming increasingly evident that alternative medicine can play a role in better health. But it's important to remember that there are some important differences between conventional treatments and alternative therapies.

If you decide to use alternative treatments, learn about the treatments. And before choosing a treatment, evaluate the benefits and risks.

5 steps to follow

When considering any product or practice, do your homework.

1. **Gather information.** The Internet offers an ideal way to keep up with the latest on alternative treatments. But beware — the Internet is also a great source of misinformation.
2. **Evaluate the providers.** After gathering information about a treatment, you may decide to find a practitioner who offers it. Choosing a name from the classified section of the phone book is risky if you have no other information about the provider.
   - Check your state government listings for agencies that regulate and license health providers.
   - Talk with your doctor or another trusted health care professional to get advice.
   - Talk to people who've received the treatment you're considering and ask about their experience with specific providers.
3. **Consider the cost.** Many alternative approaches aren't covered by health insurance. Find out exactly how much the treatment will cost you. When possible, get the amount in writing before you begin treatment.
4. **Check your attitude.** When it comes to alternative medicine, steer a middle course between uncritical acceptance and outright rejection. Stay open to various treatments, but evaluate them carefully.
5. **Opt for therapies that are complementary.** The best use of alternative therapies is to complement rather than replace conventional medical care.

You can use alternative treatments to maintain good health and to relieve some symptoms. But continue to rely on conventional medicine to diagnose a problem and treat the sources of disease.

Also, remember that lifestyle choices make an enormous difference. Most medical practitioners — conventional and alternative — will tell you that good nutrition, exercise, not smoking, stress management and basic safety practices are keys to a long life and good health.

Is it helping?

Once you begin using a particular therapy, make sure to periodically assess if the product or practice is working. You likely won't see changes overnight, but after a period of four to six weeks you should be able to determine if it's helping you.

Ask yourself the following questions:

- **Am I noticing a difference?** Has the pain lessened, or your stress level eased? Do you feel better? Are you getting fewer colds?
- **Am I bothered by side effects?** Are you experiencing unwanted effects from the therapy, such as headache, nausea or muscle pain? Do the benefits outweigh the side effects?
- **What's my goal?** Is the product or therapy working well enough to help you achieve your goal?

If you're not seeing the results that you'd hoped for, talk with your doctor. It may be that you're not using the therapy correctly, or that you're not taking the right amount. Or it could be that the product or practice simply doesn't work for you. You and your doctor may want to consider try a different approach.

Dietary supplements: Not your typical pills

Dietary supplements aren't subject to the same regulations as are drugs.

Limited regulation

The Dietary Supplement Health and Education Act (DSHEA) limits the Food and Drug Administration's (FDA) control over dietary supplements. It states that manufacturers don't have to prove to the FDA that a product is safe or effective before it goes on the market. As a result, in the United States dietary supplements can be marketed with limited regulation.

Recent legislation passed in 2007 — current good manufacturing practices (cGMPs) for dietary supplements — mandates supplement manufacturers to follow high standards. When fully enacted in 2010, this will make the quality of dietary supplements manufactured in the United States more consistent. The legislation, however, does not address if a supplement is effective.

Safe use

If you use dietary supplements:

- **Follow directions.** Herbal products have active ingredients that can affect how your body functions. Don't exceed the recommended dosages.

- **Tell your doctor what you're taking.** Some herbs may interfere with the effectiveness of prescription or over-the-counter drugs or have other harmful effects.

- **Read the label and look for a seal of approval.** An example is the U.S. Pharmacopeia's "USP Dietary Supplement Verified" mark, indicating that the supplements meet certain standards of quality.

- **Avoid supplements if you're pregnant or breast-feeding, unless your doctor approves.** They could harm the baby.

- **Be cautious about products manufactured or purchased outside the United States.** Some European herbs, such as German herbs, are well regulated and standardized. But toxic ingredients (including lead and mercury) and prescription drugs (such as prednisone) have been found in herbal supplements manufactured elsewhere, particularly China, India and Mexico.

- **Avoid potentially dangerous herbs altogether.** These include chaparral, ephedra (mahuang) and kava. Overdoses can be fatal. Though some of these are "banned," they're still available on the Internet.

When medicines and herbs don't mix

What happens when herbs are mixed with prescription or nonprescription medications? Researchers are studying this question. For the time being, think twice before mixing any herb with a prescription or nonprescription drug. Certain herbs have been recognized as having a high risk of interactions.

Herbs of concern
Don't mix medications with these popular herbs without your doctor's approval because of possible risk of harmful interactions:

- Echinacea
- Feverfew
- Garlic
- Ginger
- Ginkgo
- Ginseng
- Kava
- St. John's wort

Medications of concern
Some medications have a narrow therapeutic window. That is, problems can develop if the level is too low or too high. An example is the anticoagulant medication warfarin (Coumadin). If the level is too low, dangerous blood clotting can occur. If the level is too high, dangerous bleeding can occur. Other medications with narrow therapeutic windows include those that control heart arrhythmias, prevent organ rejection and control seizures.

To find a qualified practitioner, you might try checking with:

State regulators

Check your state government listings for agencies that regulate and license health care providers. These agencies may list practitioners in your area and offer a way to check credentials.

National associations

National associations and their local affiliates can usually provide you with the names of certified practitioners in your area.

Friends and family

If you know someone who's received the same treatment you're considering, ask about his or her experiences with a specific provider.

Points to keep in mind

When deciding on a practitioner:

- Gather information about each. Ask questions about their credentials and practice. What licenses or certifications do they have?

- After you select a practitioner, make a list of questions to ask at your first visit. Decide if the potential benefits outweigh the risks.

- Assess your first visit and decide if the practitioner is right for you and the treatment plan is reasonable.

Sounds too good to be true? Maybe it is

The Food and Drug Administration and the National Council Against Health Fraud recommend that you watch for the following claims or practices. These are often warning signs of potentially fraudulent dietary supplements or other so-called "natural" treatments:

- The advertisements or promotional materials include words such as *breakthrough, magical* or *new discovery*. If the product were in fact a cure, your doctor would recommend it.

- Promotional materials include pseudo-medical jargon such as *detoxify, purify* or *energize*. Such claims are difficult to define and measure.

- The manufacturer claims that the product can treat a wide range of symptoms, or cure or prevent a number of diseases. No single product can do this.

- The product is supposedly backed by scientific studies, but references aren't provided, are limited or are out of date.

- The product's promotional materials mention no negative side effects, only benefits.

- The manufacturer of the product accuses the government or medical profession of suppressing important information about the product's benefits. There is no reason for the government or medical profession to withhold information that could help people.

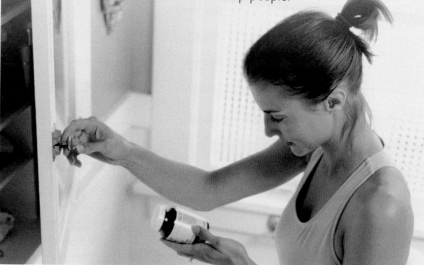

Working with your doctor

You may be a little gun-shy when it comes to talking with your doctor about alternative therapies that you're using, or are considering using.

Perhaps you're worried that your doctor will criticize you or tell you to stop using the treatment. If the therapy isn't dangerous, this shouldn't be the case. Most doctors are well aware that unconventional products and practices are highly popular, and they want to help their patients use the therapies safely.

Surveys also show that because people often consider therapies such as herbs to be "natural," they don't feel they're worth discussing with their doctor. Natural doesn't mean safe. Tell your doctor about everything you take.

Act sooner, rather than later

It's best to talk with your doctor before taking any dietary supplement. Also inform your doctor about other therapies you may be considering, such as meditation or acupuncture.

Why? Your doctor is there to help you. He or she can:

- Determine if the treatment has any potentially dangerous side effects

- Help you determine the appropriate dosage

- Provide advice on which therapies are most appropriate for you

- Inform you if a product you're considering taking may interact with a medication you currently use

- Put you in touch with someone who can perform a particular therapy or who can teach you how to do it

It's important that you answer your doctor's questions accurately. Honest communication between you and your doctor helps your doctor to better monitor your health and assess potential health risks.

Understand the unease

When it comes to dietary supplements, don't be surprised if your doctor may be cautious about endorsing or embracing some of them. This is often because relatively few good studies have been done on dietary supplements.

Understandably, the more evidence there is to support a particular product or practice, the more comfortable doctors feel in recommending it.

However, a growing number of doctors are working to better understand herbal and other supplemental therapies so that they can help you make informed decisions about your health care.

If your doctor isn't comfortable discussing dietary supplements with you, ask for a referral to a pharmacist or specialist who is knowledgeable in this area.

Where to go from here

We hope you've found this book to be thought provoking and informative. We also hope you've been challenged to take some positive steps toward improving your health by incorporating what you've learned into your daily lifestyle. Whether it be paying more attention to what you eat or adding massage to your weekly routine, the therapies discussed in this book can play a critical role in your personal health — mind, body and spirit.

But at the same time, making healthier changes may seem a bit daunting. How do you know where to start? We posed this question to hundreds of readers from the first edition of this book, and their responses were remarkably uniform.

5 key strategies for moving forward

1. **Make a commitment.** Whether you're a seasoned yoga practitioner or someone who is taking a first step into this realm of wellness, you can improve your current health status. Make improvement a priority. Many readers told us that writing down their health goals helped them make — and keep — healthy habits.

2. **Start small.** Pick one or two therapies from this book that resonate with you — or have been shown to target an area of concern for you. For example, if you have fibromyalgia, adding in a weekly massage may be a great first step. If you start off trying to do too much, you probably won't succeed.

3. **Stick with it.** Tai chi, yoga, meditation — none of these health-enhancing approaches can be picked up overnight. In some cases, it may take a few weeks before you begin to see significant benefits from a new practice. Try to give any new therapy at least four to six weeks.

4. **Reassess.** Once you've made a change, ask yourself if the change is helping you as much as you'd hoped that it would. If the answer is yes, keep going! On the other hand, if you're not seeing hoped for improvements, don't despair. Talk with your doctor or an instructor and see if there are things you can do that might yield better results. If you still don't see benefits, then it's probably time to try something else. Not everything works for everybody. Keep exploring until you find practices that fit you and your needs.

5. **Grow.** Even the most advanced meditator won't live long on meditation alone. It's important to nurture all aspects of your life — mind, body and spirit. If you've started out small, you have stuck with it, and you're finding that the practice is meeting your needs, it's probably time to expand. Select another area of your personal wellness that might benefit from greater attention and follow the same steps — make a commitment, start small, stick with it and then reassess.

Our hope is that this book can start you on a path to better health, but we also recognize that the information provided here is really just a starting point. Hopefully, we've been able to show you why therapies such as massage, meditation and acupuncture are valuable. Now you have to do some homework to find out what meets your needs and fits your individual lifestyle. We've included a number of resources where you can obtain more detailed information from trusted and reliable sources.

Remember, too, that this should be a team effort. Talk with your doctor about what you've found. Then work with him or her to make sure any changes you're contemplating won't interfere with the good care you're already receiving.

Your goal is to integrate the best alternative practices with the best of conventional medicine to achieve a lifetime of health and wellness.

Visiting Mayo Clinic

Perhaps you were surprised to learn that doctors at Mayo Clinic incorporate practices such as massage and meditation into their care plans for patients. Or perhaps you're interested in the research Mayo Clinic is doing in the realm of integrative medicine. Maybe you have a condition that you feel might benefit from an integrative health care approach.

Regardless of your reason, if you're interested in being seen as a patient at Mayo Clinic, here are some things that might be helpful to know.

- You don't have to be referred to Mayo Clinic by a physician — but it helps!

- To make an appointment at one of our three locations, these are the numbers to call: Arizona, 800-446-2279; Florida, 904-953-0853; Minnesota, 507-538-3270.

- Your visit will begin with a complete physical examination by a general internal medicine physician.

- The doctor who performs your physical examination will refer you to a specialist if he or she feels a specialist can help.

- If you're interested in alternative therapies, express this interest to your Mayo physician. You cannot make an appointment directly to receive treatments such as acupuncture, massage or meditation. You need to be referred for these services by a Mayo Clinic doctor.

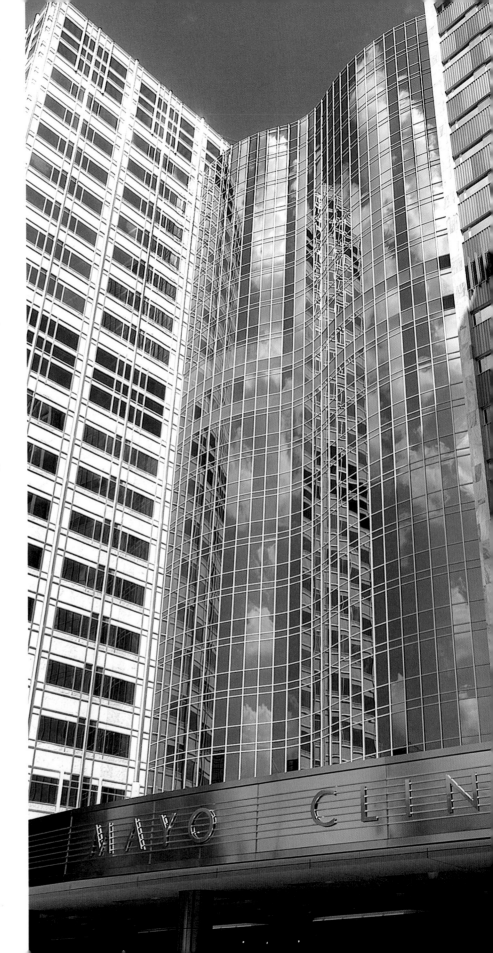

Additional Resources

Organizations

American Academy of Medical Acupuncture
1970 E. Grand Ave., Suite 330
El Segundo, CA 90245
310-364-0193
www.medicalacupuncture.org

American Academy of Osteopathy
3500 DePauw Blvd., Suite 1080
Indianapolis, IN 46268
317-879-1881
www.academyofosteopathy.org

American Association of Naturopathic Physicians
4435 Wisconsin Ave. NW, Suite 403
Washington, DC 20016
866-538-2267
www.naturopathic.org

American Association of Acupuncture and Oriental Medicine
P.O. Box 162340
Sacramento, CA 95816
866-455-7999
www.aaom.org

American Botanical Council
P.O. Box 144345
Austin, TX 78714
800-373-7105
www.herbalgram.org

American Chiropractic Association
1701 Clarendon Blvd.
Arlington, VA 22209
703-276-8800
www.acatoday.org

American Holistic Medical Association
23366 Commerce Park, Suite 101B
Beachwood, Ohio 44122
216-292-6644
www.holisticmedicine.org

American Massage Therapy Association
500 Davis St., Suite 900
Evanston, IL 60201
877-905-2700
www.amtamassage.org

American Osteopathic Association
142 E. Ontario St.
Chicago, IL 60611
800-621-1773
www.osteopathic.org

American Society of Clinical Hypnosis
140 N. Bloomingdale Road
Bloomingdale, IL 60108
630-980-4740
www.asch.net

Association for Applied Psychophysiology and Biofeedback
10200 W. 44th Ave., Suite 304
Wheat Ridge, CO 80033
800-477-8892
www.aapb.org

Consortium of Academic Health Centers for Integrative Medicine
D513 Mayo, Mail Code 505
420 Delaware St. SE
Minneapolis, MN 55455
612-624-9166
www.ahc.umn.edu/cahcim/home.html

ConsumerLab.com*

333 Mamaroneck Ave.
White Plains, NY 10605
888-502-5100
www.consumerlab.com

Food and Drug Administration

10903 New Hampshire Ave.
Silver Spring, MD 20993-0002
888-463-6332
www.fda.gov/Food/DietarySupplements/default.htm

Healing Touch International

445 Union Blvd., Suite 105
Lakewood, CO 80228
303-989-7982
www.healingtouchinternational.org

MayoClinic.com

www.MayoClinic.com

National Association for Holistic Aromatherapy

P.O. Box 1868
Banner Elk, NC 28604
828-898-6161
www.naha.org

National Cancer Institute

NCI Public Inquiries Office
6116 Executive Blvd., Room 3036A
Bethesda, MD 20892-8322
800-422-6237
www.cancer.gov/cancertopics/treatment/cam

National Center for Complementary and Alternative Medicine

NCCAM Clearinghouse
P.O. Box 7923
Gaithersburg, MD 20898
888-644-6226
www.nccam.nih.gov

National Center for Homeopathy

101 S. Whiting St., Suite 16
Alexandria, VA 22304
703-548-7790
www.homeopathic.org

Office of Cancer Complementary and Alternative Medicine

National Cancer Institute, NIH
6116 Executive Blvd., Suite 609, MSC 8339
Bethesda, MD 20892
301-435-7980
www.cancer.gov/cam

Databases

Natural Medicines Comprehensive Database*

www.naturaldatabaseconsumer.com

Natural Standard*

www.naturalstandard.com

* Subscription fee required for access to information

Index

MAYO CLINIC

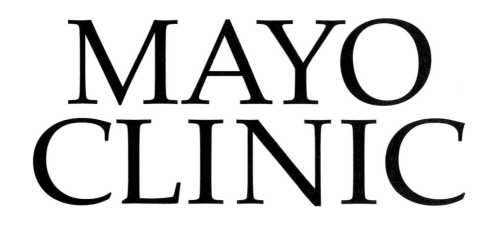

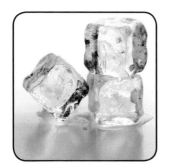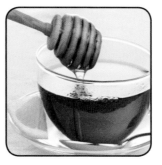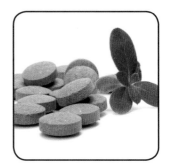

Book of
HOME
REMEDIES

WHAT TO DO FOR THE
MOST COMMON HEALTH PROBLEMS

Table of Contents

pg
Common cold 43

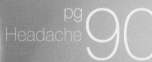
pg
Headache 90

Introduction

The idea for *Mayo Clinic Book of Home Remedies* came from many discussions with Mayo Clinic physicians, nurses, health educators and other health care providers about the questions and concerns they hear most frequently from visitors to Mayo. In other words, what are the main reasons why people go to a doctor?

Our goal was to develop a simple resource that could guide your health decisions, offer easy remedies to treat many of your problems and possibly reduce the need for a visit to a clinic or emergency room. The result is a book filled with reliable, practical information on more than 120 of the most common medical conditions and issues related to good health.

Today, greater responsibility has been placed on each of us to stay healthy and prevent illness. This has been triggered, in no small part, by the rising costs of health care and by growing concern over public health issues as diverse as obesity, diabetes, influenza and food safety.

Of course, things happen that you may have little control over — even after taking precautions, you may still catch colds, sprain ankles, have allergic reactions or develop high blood pressure. But *Mayo Clinic Book of Home Remedies* can show you how to minimize your risks of disease and injury and — in the event that something should happen — take necessary steps that help treat the condition until it's resolved or until you're able to see your doctor. It can help you detect illness before it becomes a serious and costly problem. Of course, this book is not intended to replace the advice of your doctor, and lets you know when you need to see a medical professional.

How this book is organized

Considering the broad spectrum of health issues included in *Mayo Clinic Book of Home Remedies,* we feel that the easiest way for you to access the information is by arranging topics alphabetically. Each topic is introduced in a summary that may include signs and symptoms, causes, and possible outcomes.

Accompanying each topic is a "Home Remedies" segment that describes simple actions you can take to help prevent, treat or manage the condition, whether it's straightforward advice on diet and exercise, or a change in behavior, or a supplement to help relieve signs and symptoms.

The "Medical Help" segment with each topic identifies serious signs and symptoms and advises you on when to contact a doctor or other health care provider and what kind of treatment you might expect.

At the back of the book is an Emergency Care section that provides quick referral to information you'll need in the event of an emergency, be it stroke, heart attack, poisoning or bone fracture. Your decisive action during an emergency can be the difference between life and death.

Mayo Clinic Book of Home Remedies is based on the premise that there are many things you can do at home to stay healthy, relieve symptoms, improve emotional health, feel invigorated and enjoy a higher quality of life. It's our sincere hope that this book provides you with an important resource in achieving this complete approach to good health.

Philip Hagen, M.D., Martha Millman, M.D.
Medical Editors

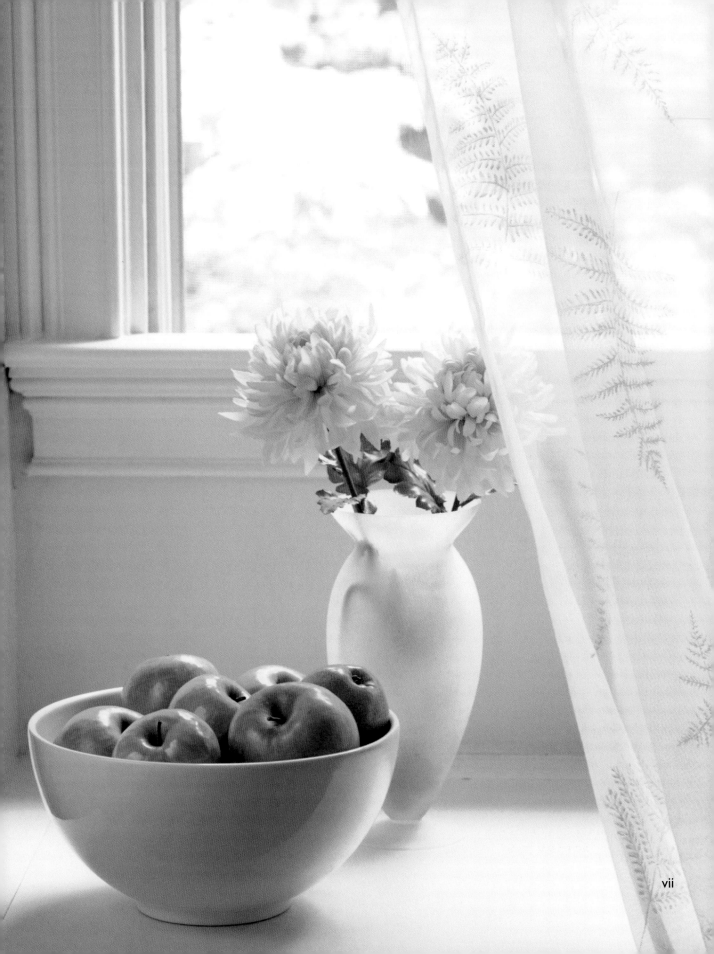

Medical supplies for your home

When an accident or health problem occurs, it's nice to have basic supplies on hand to treat the condition. That's why you want to have a medical supply kit ready for use — whether it's an actual first-aid kit or just your bathroom cabinet stocked with a variety of helpful items.

It's best to store medical supplies in a place that's easily accessible to adults but out of the reach of children. Remember to replace items after their use to make sure the kit is always complete. And check your supplies yearly for outdated items that may need replacing. Check expiration dates on medications twice yearly.

Here are key items that you should have on hand if you want to be prepared for accidents and common illnesses:

- *For general care.* Sharp scissors, tweezers, cotton balls, cotton-tipped swabs, tissues, soap, cleansing pads or instant hand sanitizer, plastic bags, safety pins, latex or synthetic gloves for use if blood or body fluids are present, anti-diarrheal drugs, and a medicine cup or spoon.
- *For cuts.* Bandages of various sizes, gauze, paper or cloth tape, antiseptic solution to clean wounds and antibacterial ointment to prevent infection.
- *For burns.* Cold packs, gauze, burn spray and antiseptic cream.
- *For aches, pain and fever.* Thermometer, aspirin (for adults only), other nonsteroidal anti-inflammatory drugs such as ibuprofen (Advil, Motrin, others), and acetaminophen (Tylenol, others).
- *For eye injuries.* Eyewash, such as saline solution, eyewash cup, eye patches and goggles.
- *For sprains, strains and fractures.* Cold packs, elastic wraps for wrapping injuries, finger splints and a triangular bandage for making an arm sling.
- *For insect bites and stings.* Cold packs to help reduce pain and swelling. Topical cream containing hydrocortisone (0.5 or 1 percent), calamine lotion or baking soda (combine baking soda with water to form a paste) to apply until symptoms subside. Antihistamines (Benadryl, Chlor-Trimeton, others) may help relieve itching. For individuals allergic to insect stings, include a kit with a syringe containing epinephrine (adrenaline). Your doctor can prescribe one. Check the expiration date regularly.
- *For ingestion of poisons.* Keep the number of your local poison control center and the national poison control center (800-222-1222) in your medicine kit or near your telephone. The national center can route you to a center that serves your local area.

Emergency items

Here are additional items you may want to have on hand in case of an emergency at home or while traveling:

- Cell phone and recharger that uses the accessory plug in your car dash
- Emergency phone numbers, including contact information for your family doctor and pediatrician, local emergency services, emergency road service providers and the regional poison control center
- Medical consent forms for each family member
- Medical history forms for each family member
- Small, waterproof flashlight and extra batteries
- Candles and matches for cold climates
- Sunscreen
- Mylar emergency blanket
- First-aid instruction manual

Acne

Acne occurs when hair follicles, the tiny openings in your skin from which hair grows, become plugged with oil and dead skin cells. The plugged follicles may produce:

- *Comedones (blackheads and whiteheads).* Comedones that occur at the skin surface are called blackheads due to their dark appearance. Comedones that are closed and just below the skin surface are called whiteheads.
- *Papules.* Papules are small, red and tender bumps that signal inflammation or infection in the hair follicles.
- *Pustules.* Pustules are red and tender bumps with white pus at their tips.
- *Nodules.* Nodules are large, solid painful lumps beneath the surface of the skin. They are the result of a buildup of secretions deep within the hair follicles.
- *Cysts.* These painful, pus-filled lumps beneath the surface of the skin are boil-like infections that can cause scars.

A number of factors — including hormones, bacteria, certain medications and heredity — play a role in the development of acne. Though acne is most common in teenagers, people of all ages can get acne.

🏠 Home Remedies

To reduce or prevent acne:

- *Be careful what you put on your face.* Avoid oily or greasy cosmetics or hairstyling products or acne coverups. Use products labeled water-based or noncomedogenic.
- *Keep your face clean.* Wash problem areas daily with a gentle cleanser that gently dries your skin. Products such as facial scrubs, astringents and masks generally aren't recommended because they tend to irritate skin, which can worsen acne.
- *Watch what touches your face.* Keep your hair clean and off your face. Avoid resting your hands or objects, such as telephone receivers, on your face. Tight hats also can pose a problem, especially if you sweat. Sweat and dirt can contribute to acne.
- *Care for yourself.* Consider whether lack of sleep or stress, or both, cause your acne to flare. Try to get enough sleep and manage stress.
- *Don't pick or squeeze blemishes.* Doing so can lead to infection or scarring.
- *Try over-the-counter products.* Look for acne lotions that contain benzoyl peroxide or salicylic acid as the active ingredient to help dry excess oil and promote peeling of dead skin cells.
- *Tea tree oil.* Some studies suggest that gels containing 5 percent tea tree oil are as effective as are lotions containing 5 percent benzoyl peroxide, although tea tree oil might work more slowly. There's some concern that topical products containing tea tree oil might cause breast development in young boys. Don't use tea tree oil if you have acne rosacea because it can worsen symptoms.
- *Zinc supplements.* The mineral zinc plays a role in wound healing and reduces inflammation, which may help improve acne.
- *Glycolic acid.* A natural acid found in sugar cane, glycolic acid applied to your skin helps remove dead skin cells and unclog pores.

➕ Medical Help

Persistent pimples, inflamed cysts or scarring may need medical attention and treatment with prescription drugs. Proper evaluation and treatment can prevent the physical and psychological scarring of acne. In rare cases, a sudden onset of severe acne in an older adult may signal an underlying disease requiring medical attention.

Airplane ear

The medical name for airplane ear is ear barotrauma or barotitis media. It refers to the stress exerted on your eardrum, eustachian tube and other ear structures when air pressure in your middle ear and air pressure in the environment are out of balance.

You may experience airplane ear at the beginning of a flight when the airplane is climbing and at the end of a flight when the airplane is descending. These rapid changes in altitude cause air pressure in the environment to also change rapidly. The air pressure in the middle ear does not adjust quickly enough.

Signs and symptoms may include pain in one ear, slight hearing loss or a stuffy feeling in both ears. This is caused by your eardrum bulging outward or retracting inward as a result of the change in pressure.

Ear barotrauma is also a common problem with scuba diving when water pressure on the outside of the ear becomes greater than air pressure in the middle ear.

Any condition that can interfere with the normal function of the middle ear can increase the risk of airplane ear. This would include a stuffy nose, allergy, cold or throat infection. A cold or ear infection isn't necessarily a reason to change or delay a flight, however.

♠ Home Remedies

To prevent or reduce airplane ear:

- *Use a decongestant.* Take a decongestant about 30 minutes to an hour before takeoff and 30 minutes to an hour before landing. This may prevent blockage of your eustachian tube. If you have heart disease, a heart rhythm disorder or high blood pressure or if you've experienced possible medication interactions, avoid taking an oral decongestant unless your doctor approves.
- *During the flight, suck candy or chew gum.* This encourages swallowing, which helps open your eustachian tube.
- *Don't sleep during ascents and descents.* If you're awake during ascents and descents, you can do the necessary self-care techniques when you feel pressure on your ears.
- *Try the Valsalva maneuver to unplug your ears.* Gently blow, as if blowing your nose, while pinching your nostrils and keeping your mouth closed. If you can swallow at the same time, it's more helpful. Repeat several times to equalize the pressure between your ears and the airplane cabin.
- *Look for specially designed filtered earplugs.* Theses earplugs slowly equalize the pressure against your eardrum during ascents and descents. You can purchase these at drugstores, airport gift shops or your local hearing clinic.
- *Give infants and children fluid.* Drinking fluids during ascent and descent encourages swallowing. Give the child a bottle or pacifier to encourage swallowing. Decongestants should not be used in infants or young children.

✚ Medical Help

Usually, you can do things on your own to treat airplane ear. If discomfort, fullness or muffled hearing lasts more than a few hours or if you experience any severe signs or symptoms, call your doctor.

Allergies

An allergy is an overreaction by your immune system to an otherwise harmless substance, such as pollen or pet dander.

Contact with this substance — called an allergen — triggers the production of antibodies to fight the invader. The antibodies, in turn, cause immune cells in the lining of your eyes and airways to release inflammatory substances, including histamine.

When these chemicals are released, they produce the familiar signs and symptoms of allergy: itchy, red and swollen eyes, stuffy nose, frequent sneezing, cough, and hives or bumps on the skin.

Many people mistake allergies for colds, but signs and symptoms of these two conditions are different (see page 14). A cold generally goes away in a few days, whereas an allergy often persists for a longer time.

Types

Substances found outdoors and indoors can cause allergic reactions.

The most common allergens are inhaled:

- *Pollen.* Spring, summer and fall are the pollen-producing seasons in many climates, when you're more exposed to airborne particles from trees, grasses and weeds.
- *Dust mites.* House dust harbors many allergens, including pollen and molds. But the main allergy trigger is the dust mite. Thousands of these microscopic insects are in a pinch of house dust. House dust can cause year-round allergy symptoms.
- *Pet dander.* Dogs and especially cats are the most common animals to cause allergic reactions. The animal's dander (skin flakes), saliva, urine and sometimes hair are the main culprits.
- *Molds.* Many people are sensitive to airborne mold spores. Outdoor molds produce spores mostly in the summer and early fall in northern climates and year-round in subtropical and tropical climates. Indoor molds shed spores all year long. People also may develop allergies to certain foods, insect stings, medications and latex or other things you touch.

Hayfever

Signs and symptoms generally include a stuffy or runny nose, frequent sneezing, and itchy eyes, nose, throat or mouth. Hayfever may also be accompanied by a cough. Seasonal hay fever triggers include:

- Tree pollen, common in spring
- Grass pollen, common in the late spring and summer
- Weed pollen, most common in the fall
- Spores from fungi and molds, which can be worse during warm-weather months

🏠 Home Remedies

The best approach for managing allergies is to know and avoid your allergy triggers.

Pollen

- *Rinse out your sinuses.* Sinus congestion and hay fever symptoms often improve with nasal lavage — rinsing out the sinuses with a saline solution. You can use a neti pot or a specially designed bulb syringe to flush out thickened mucus and irritants from your nose. See page 151.
- *Don't hang laundry outside.* Pollen can stick to the laundry. Also shower and change clothes upon entering your home after outdoor exposure.
- *Close windows and doors during pollen season.* Use an air conditioner with a good filter.
- *Use an allergy-grade filter.* Look for a high-efficiency particulate air (HEPA) filter for your ventilation and heating system. Change filters monthly.
- *Wear a pollen mask.* Use it outdoors for yardwork, or when you're around known triggers.

Dust or mold

- *Limit your exposure.* To prevent dust from building up, clean your home at least once a week. Wear a mask while cleaning, or have someone else clean for you.
- *Encase mattresses and pillows.* Place them in dust-proof or allergen-blocking covers.
- *Redecorate your house.* Consider replacing upholstered furniture with leather or vinyl, and carpeting with wood, vinyl or tile (particularly in the bedroom).

➕ Medical Help

See your doctor if you find your signs and symptoms aren't easily controlled by these steps. A number of prescription medications are available that can lessen or prevent your concerns.

- *Maintain indoor humidity between 30 and 50 percent.* Use kitchen and bathroom exhaust fans and a dehumidifier in the basement.
- *Clean humidifiers and dehumidifiers often.* It helps prevent mold and bacterial growth in the appliances.
- *Change furnace filters monthly.* Also consider installing a high-efficiency particulate air (HEPA) filter in your heating system.

Pets

- *Be selective about your pets.* Avoid pets with fur or feathers.
- *Keep pets out of the bedroom.* If you choose to keep a furry pet, keep it out of the bedroom and in an area of the home that's easily cleaned. Keep your pet outside as much as possible.
- *Bathe pets weekly.* Using wipes that are specially designed to reduce dander also may help.

Continued next page >

An allergy vs. a cold

If you tend to get "colds" that develop suddenly and occur at about the same time every year, it's possible that you actually have a seasonal allergy.

Although colds and seasonal allergies may share some of the same symptoms, they are very different conditions. Common colds are caused by viruses, while seasonal allergies are immune system responses that are triggered by exposure to an allergen.

Treating colds may include rest, pain relievers and over-the-counter cold remedies, such as decongestants. Treating allergies may include over-the-counter or prescription antihistamines, nasal steroid sprays and decongestants, and avoiding or reducing exposure to the allergens where possible.

Is it a cold or allergy?

Symptom	Cold	Allergy
Cough	Usually	Sometimes
General aches and pains	Sometimes	Never
Fatigue	Sometimes	Sometimes
Itchy eyes	Rarely	Usually
Sneezing	Usually	Usually
Sore throat	Usually	Sometimes
Runny nose	Usually	Usually
Stuffy nose	Usually	Usually
Fever	Rarely	Never

Adapted from National Institute of Allergy and Infectious Diseases 2008

Arthritis

Arthritis is one of the most common medical conditions in the United States. There are more than 100 different types of arthritis, which have varying causes, signs and symptoms and treatments. The most common types of arthritis are osteoarthritis and rheumatoid arthritis.

Osteoarthritis

Osteoarthritis is often associated with wear and tear on one or more of your joints, causing the cartilage to degenerate in your spine, hands, hips or knees. Obesity, aging, injury or genetics can increase your risk. Osteoarthritis is most often seen in people older than age 50. The signs and symptoms include:

- Pain in a joint after use
- Swelling and loss of flexibility in a joint
- Bony lumps at finger joints
- Aching

While the disease doesn't go away, the pain and other signs and symptoms may come and go.

Rheumatoid arthritis

Rheumatoid arthritis is a form of inflammatory arthritis. It most often develops in middle age, but can occur in any age group. The cause is unknown, but it's an autoimmune disease, meaning that your immune system triggers inflammation in the lining of your joints and in other areas. Signs and symptoms of rheumatoid arthritis include:

- Swelling in one or more joints
- Prolonged early-morning stiffness
- Recurring pain or tenderness in any joint
- Inability to move a joint normally
- Obvious redness and warmth in a joint

Continued next page >

Rub it in

Topical painkillers come as gels, creams, lotions or patches that are applied directly to the skin over your aching joints. Three types that you can purchase without a prescription include:

- *Hot or cold rubs.* Doctors call these products counterirritants because they contain ingredients that irritate your skin. Ingredients such as menthol, oil of wintergreen or eucalyptus oil produce a sensation of hot or cold that distracts you from your arthritis pain, giving you temporary pain relief. Examples include Bioreeze, Flexall and Icy Hot.
- *Aspirin-like pain rubs.* Topical analgesics contain salicylates, the same ingredients that give aspirin its pain-relieving quality. In addition, these products may reduce joint inflammation as they're absorbed into the skin. Examples include Bengay, Aspercreme, Mobisyl and Sportscreme.
- *Chili pepper seed rubs.* The seeds contain a compound called capsaicin, which causes the burning sensation. Creams made with capsaicin are most effective for arthritis pain in joints close to the skin surface, such as your fingers, knees and elbows. Examples include Capzasin and Zostrix.

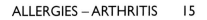

Treatments for arthritis include:

Rest

If you're experiencing pain or inflammation in a joint, rest it for 12 to 24 hours. Do activities that don't require you to use the joint repetitively. Try taking a 10-minute break every hour.

Exercise

Exercise is probably the one therapy that will do the most good for managing arthritis. Different types of exercise can achieve different goals. For better flexibility, try gentle stretching. Brisk walking, bicycling, swimming and dancing are good examples of aerobic exercise that puts low to moderate amounts of stress on your joints.

Don't continue any exercise beyond the point that's painful without the advice of your doctor.

Heat and cold

Both heat and cold can relieve joint pain. Heat also relieves stiffness, and cold can relieve muscle spasms. Apply heat for 20 minutes several times a day using a heating pad, hot water bottle or warm bath. Cool joint pain with cold treatments, such as with ice packs. You can use cold treatments several times a day, but don't use them if you have poor circulation or numbness.

Many people with rheumatoid arthritis find relief by soaking their joints in warm water for four minutes and then in cool water for a minute. Repeat the cycle for a half-hour, ending with a warm-water soak.

Lose weight

Being overweight or obese increases the stress on weight-bearing joints, such as your knees and hips. Managing even a small amount of weight loss can relieve some pressure and reduce pain.

Relaxation

Relaxation techniques such as hypnosis, visualization, deep breathing, muscle relaxation and others may help decrease joint pain.

Tai chi and yoga

These movement therapies involve gentle stretches combined with deep breathing. Several small studies have found they may help relieve osteoarthritic pain. Avoid any movements that cause pain.

Glucosamine and chondroitin

Glucosamine and chondroitin are natural compounds found in cartilage. Supplements of both compounds are used to treat osteoarthritis, and individuals with severe symptoms seem to benefit the most. Although long-term effectiveness requires further study, glucosamine and chondroitin may help and appear to be safe, so it may not hurt to give them a try.

SAMe

SAMe occurs naturally in the human body. A synthetic version of this compound has become a popular dietary supplement in the United States. Several trials indicate that SAMe can relieve pain from osteoarthritis. However, it may take up to 30 days before you notice an improvement in symptoms. The supplement is generally well tolerated in smaller doses. Don't take SAMe if you take antidpressant medications.

Devil's claw

Studies suggest this herb may help decrease osteoarthritic pain. It's used extensively in Europe as an anti-inflammatory agent.

➕ Medical Help

If you have swelling or stiffness in your joints that lasts for more than two weeks, make an appointment with your doctor.

Asthma

Asthma occurs when the main air passages of your lungs, called bronchial tubes, become inflamed and constricted, or narrowed. The muscles in the bronchial walls tighten, and the passageways produce extra mucus, reducing the flow of air.

Common signs and symptoms are wheezing, shortness of breath, chest "tightness" and coughing. In emergencies, you may have extreme difficulty breathing, a high pulse rate, sweating and severe coughing.

Millions of Americans — adults and children — have asthma. It isn't clear why some people get asthma and others don't, but it's probably due to a combination environmental and genetic (inherited) factors.

Common asthma triggers

A family history of asthma, frequent childhood respiratory infections, exposure to secondhand smoke and a low birth weight may increase your risk of developing asthma. Common causes, or triggers, of asthma attacks include:

- Air pollutants such as smoke or fumes
- Chemical smells
- Cockroaches
- Cold air or air conditioning
- Colds or flu (influenza)
- Dust or dust mites
- Exercise, physical activity or sports
- Foods, such as peanuts or shellfish
- Heartburn
- Medications, such as aspirin or beta blockers
- Menstrual cycle
- Mold or mildew
- Perfume or deodorants
- Pet allergy
- Stress or strong emotional reactions, like crying
- Sulfites (preservatives in some foods and beverages)
- Tobacco smoke
- Weather, such as high humidity

Continued next page >

These tips can help control your asthma symptoms by trigger-proofing your environment:

- *Avoid allergens that might be causing your symptoms.* If you're allergic to cats or dogs, consider removing them from your home and avoid contact with other people's pets. Avoid buying clothing, furniture or rugs made from animal hair.
- *Use your air conditioner.* Air conditioning helps reduce the amount of airborne pollen from trees, grasses and weeds that somehow finds its way indoors. Air conditioning also lowers indoor humidity and can reduce your exposure to dust mites. If you don't have air conditioning installed in your house, keep your windows closed during pollen season and use a fan.
- *Check your furnace.* If you have a forced-air heating system and you're allergic to dust, use a filter for dust control. Change or clean filters on heating and cooling units monthly. The best filter is a high-efficiency particulate air (HEPA) filter. Wear a mask when you remove dirty filters.

- *Clean weekly.* Avoid dust build-ups in your house. Use a vacuum cleaner with a small-particle filter. Avoid projects that raise dust.
- *Don't smoke and avoid second-hand smoke.* Avoid all types of smoke, even the type from a fireplace or burning leaves. Smoke irritates the eyes, nose and bronchial tubes.
- *Avoid activities that might contribute to your symptoms.* For example, home improvement projects might expose you to triggers that lead to an asthma attack, such as paint vapors, wood dust, mold or similar irritants.

Exercise

Years ago if you had asthma, doctors told you not to exercise. Now they believe well-planned regular workouts are beneficial, especially if you have mild to moderate symptoms. If you're fit, your heart and lungs don't have to work as hard to expel air.

However, because vigorous exercise can trigger an attack, make sure you choose suitable activities and exercise at a moderate pace. Consider talking with your doctor about an appropriate exercise schedule.

Maintain a healthy weight

Being overweight can worsen asthma symptoms, and the excess pounds put you at higher risk of other health problems.

Control heartburn and GERD

It's possible that the acid reflux causing your heartburn may also be damaging your lungs and worsening asthma symptoms. Avoid foods, beverages or activities, including overeating, that seem to cause heartburn. If your heartburn is frequent or constant, discuss treatment options with your doctor. You may need treatment for gastroesophageal reflux disease (GERD) before your asthma symptoms improve.

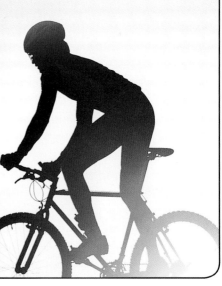

✚ Medical Help

See your doctor if you think that you have asthma or if your symptoms or peak flow readings seem to be getting worse. In case of a severe asthma attack, seek emergency medical help.

Athlete's foot

Athlete's foot is a fungal infection that develops between your toes and sometimes on other parts of your foot. Mold-like fungi called dermatophytes cause athlete's foot. These fungi live on the outer layer of your skin.

Dermatophytes thrive in moist, close environments created by thick, tight shoes that squeeze the toes together, creating warm areas between them. Damp socks and shoes and warm, humid conditions also favor the organisms' growth. Plastic shoes in particular provide a welcoming environment for fungal infection.

Athlete's foot usually causes itching, stinging and burning with redness, especially between your toes. Sometimes the sole and sides of the foot are affected, appearing thickened and leathery in texture. Sections of skin may become excessively dry and cracked.

Although locker rooms and public showers are often blamed for spreading athlete's foot, the environment inside your shoes is probably more important. Athlete's foot becomes more common with age.

⌂ Home Remedies

To manage and prevent athlete's foot:

- *Treat your feet.* Try over-the-counter antifungal creams (Lotrimin AF, Tinactin, others) or a drying powder two to three times a day until the rash disappears.
- *Keep your feet dry.* This is particularly important for the areas between your toes. Go barefoot to let your feet air out as much as possible when you're home.
- *Wear well-ventilated shoes.* Avoid shoes made of synthetic materials, especially ones that are tightly closed.
- *Alternate shoes.* Don't wear the same shoes every day, and don't store them in plastic.
- *Wear waterproof sandals or shoes.* Do this around public pools and showers and in locker rooms where infection can spread.
- *Don't borrow shoes.* Borrowing risks spreading a fungal infection.
- *Wear good socks.* Buy socks that are made of natural material, such as cotton or wool, or a synthetic fiber designed to draw moisture away from your feet. If your feet sweat a lot, change socks twice a day.

✚ Medical Help

See a doctor if your symptoms last longer than four weeks or they worsen. Seek medical help sooner if you notice excessive redness, swelling, drainage or fever. In addition, if you have diabetes and suspect you have athlete's foot, see your doctor.

Back pain

Almost everyone has a back problem at some point in his or her lifetime. Muscle tone and strength tend to decrease with age, making your back more prone to injury.

Your spine may stiffen, the intervertebral disks wear out, and the spaces between the vertebrae narrow, allowing bone to rub on bone. These changes are common but don't have to be painful.

Back pain also may result from an injury, strain or overdoing an activity. Often, it's hard to pinpoint the cause of back pain due to the back's complex structure.

Because your lower back carries most of your weight, it tends to be the site of most back pain. However, sprains and strains can injure any part of your back.

Common causes

Causes of back pain include:
- Improper lifting
- Sudden, strenuous physical effort
- Trauma from an accident, fall or sports injury
- Lack of muscle tone
- Excess weight, especially around your middle
- Daily stress and tension
- Sleeping position, especially if you sleep on your stomach
- Poor sitting and standing postures
- Sitting in one position for a long time or with a thick wallet in your back pocket
- Carrying a heavy briefcase, shoulder bag or backpack
- Holding a forward-bending position for a long time
- Relaxation of muscles and ligaments during pregnancy

Listen up!

When your back starts hurting, it's warning you to slow down to prevent further injury.

A severe muscle spasm may last 48 to 72 hours, followed by several days or weeks of less severe pain. Most back pain disappears within a few weeks. Even after you start feeling a little better, strenuous use of the muscle during the three to six weeks after the initial injury may continue causing pain.

Regular exercise to maintain your flexibility and strength and keeping your abdominal muscles strong are your best bets to avoid back problems.

Cold vs. hot

When do you apply cold and when do you apply heat to treat an injury?

	Cold	Hot
What it does	Cold reduces inflammation, constricts blood vessels to limit bruising, and relieves pain by acting as a local anesthetic.	Heat improves circulation to speed healing, reduces pain by relaxing tight or sore muscles, and helps restore range of motion.
When to use it	Use cold for one to three days after an injury. Apply cold for 15 minutes at a time every two to three hours.	Use heat once the swelling is gone. Apply heat for 20 minutes at a time several times a day.

♠ Home Remedies

Healing occurs most quickly if you're able to continue going about your daily routine in a gentle manner and at the same time avoiding any movements or actions that may have caused the back pain in the first place.

With proper care of a strain or sprain, you should improve within the first two weeks. Most forms of acute back pain improve in four to six weeks. Sprained ligaments or severe muscle strains may take up to 12 weeks to heal.

Apply ice
Use cold packs initially to relieve pain. Wrap an ice pack or bag of frozen vegetables in cloth. Hold it on the sore area for 15 minutes and repeat every two to three hours. To avoid frostbite, never place ice directly on your skin.

Rest up, but move
Getting plenty of rest allows your back to heal, but avoid prolonged bed rest — lying in bed for more than a day or two may actually slow recovery. Moderate movement helps keep your muscles strong. Avoid the activity that caused the injury. Avoid lifting, pushing, pulling, repetitive bending, and twisting.

Apply heat
After 48 hours, or once the swelling is gone, you may use heat to relax sore or knotted muscles. Use a warm bath, warm packs, heating pad or heat lamp. Be careful not to burn your skin with extreme heat. If you find that applying cold provides more relief than heat does, continue using cold, or try a combination of the two methods.

Stretch
Do gentle stretching exercises. Avoid jerking, bouncing, or any movements that increase pain or require straining. Spending 10 to 15 minutes a day doing gentle exercises also can help prevent back problems (see page 22).

Get a massage
If back pain is caused by tense or overworked muscles, massage may help loosen knotted muscles and promote relaxation.

Progressive relaxation
This relaxation technique involves systematically tensing and relaxing different muscle groups in your body. Progressive relaxation boosts your ability to recognize and counteract muscle tension as soon as it starts.

Yoga
Studies indicate that yoga can help relieve back pain, with the improvement in symptoms lasting several months.

Stand, sit and lift smart
Stand up straight. Don't stand with your shoulders and back hunched. Sit up straight, with your lower back against the back of the chair. Use chairs that support your lower back. When lifting, let your legs do the work. Bend at the knees and keep your back straight.

Continued next page >

✚ Medical Help

Although uncommon, back pain can result from serious problems such as cancer, inflammatory arthritis and other diseases. Pain that worsens or remains constant for a month or more should be investigated by a doctor. Seek medical care immediately if your pain:

- Is severe, progressive or prolonged (lasting more than a month).
- Results from an injury. Don't try to move someone who has severe pain or can't move his or her arms or legs after an accident.
- Produces weakness, pain or numbness in your legs or arms.
- Is new and accompanied by an unexplained fever or weight loss.
- Is constant and worse at night.
- Is accompanied by poorly controlled blood pressure, abdominal aortic aneurysm, cancer, or sudden loss of bowel or bladder control.

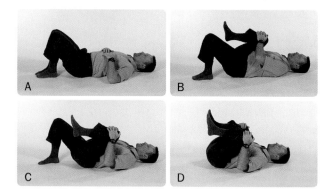

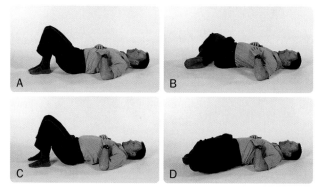

Knee-to-chest stretch

Lie on your back with your knees bent and your feet flat on the floor (A). Using both hands, pull up one knee and press it to your chest (B). Hold for 15 to 30 seconds. Return to the starting position and repeat with the opposite leg (C). Return to the starting position and repeat with both legs at the same time (D).

Lower back rotational stretch

Lie on your back with your knees bent and your feet flat on the floor (A). Keeping your shoulders firmly on the floor, roll your bent knees to one side (B). Hold for five to 10 seconds. Return to the starting position (C). Repeat on the opposite side (D).

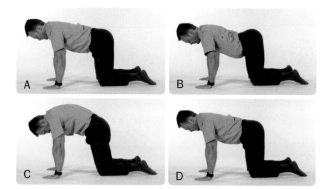

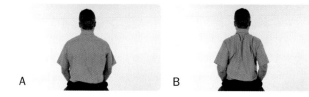

Shoulder blade squeeze

Sit on an armless chair or stool (A). Keeping your chin tucked in and your chest high, pull your shoulder blades together (B). Hold for five seconds, then relax. Repeat.

Cat stretch

Position yourself on your hands and knees (A). Slowly let your back and abdomen sag toward the floor (B). Then slowly arch your back, as if you're pulling your abdomen up toward the ceiling (C). Return to the starting position. Repeat (D).

Bad breath

There are many causes of bad breath. Your mouth itself may be a source. The breakdown of food particles and other debris by bacteria in and around your teeth can cause a foul odor.

If your mouth becomes dry, such as occurs during sleep or after smoking, dead cells can accumulate and decompose on your tongue, gums and cheeks, causing odor.

Eating foods containing oils with a strong odor, such as onions and garlic, can lead to bad breath. Foul-smelling breath may also be a symptom of illness, such as lung disease, diabetes or liver failure.

♠ Home Remedies

The following steps may help improve or prevent bad breath:

- *Brush your teeth after you eat.* Keep a toothbrush at work to brush after eating. Be sure to brush at least twice a day for two to three minutes at a time.
- *Brush your tongue.* Give your tongue a gentle brushing to remove dead cells, bacteria and food debris. Use a soft-bristled toothbrush or flexible tongue scraper. Try to clean as far back as you can because bacteria tend to collect toward the back of your mouth.
- *Floss daily.* Proper flossing removes food particles and plaque from between your teeth.
- *Clean your dentures well.* If you wear a bridge or a partial or complete denture, clean it thoroughly at least once a day or as directed by your dentist.
- *Avoid strong foods that cause bad breath.* This includes onions, garlic and hot peppers. The odors from these types of foods generally linger in your mouth.
- *Drink plenty of water.* To keep your mouth moist, be sure to consume plenty of water, and not coffee, soft drinks or alcohol.
- *Grab some gum or a mint.* Chewing a piece of gum (preferably sugarless) or sucking on candy (preferably sugarless) stimulates saliva, washing away food particles and bacteria. If you have chronic dry mouth, your dentist or doctor may prescribe an artificial saliva preparation or an oral medication that stimulates the flow of saliva.
- *Chew fresh parsley.* Chewing on parsley may temporarily improve bad breath.

✚ Medical Help

After trying these approaches and your breath is still bad, talk to your doctor or dentist.

Bedbugs

Bedbugs have feasted on sleeping humans for thousands of years. After World War II, they were eradicated from most developed nations with the use of DDT. This pesticide has since been banned because it's so toxic to the environment.

Spurred perhaps by an increase in international travel, bedbugs are becoming a problem once again. The risk of encountering bedbugs increases if you spend time in locations with a high turnover of nighttime guests — such as hotels, hospitals or homeless shelters.

Bedbugs are small, reddish brown, oval and flat. During the day, they hide in the cracks and crevices of beds, box springs, headboards and bed frames.

What to look for

It can be difficult to distinguish bedbug bites from other kinds of insect bites. In general, bedbug bites are:

- Red, often with a darker red spot in the middle
- Itchy
- Arranged in a rough line or in a cluster
- Located on the face, neck, arms and hands

Some people have no reaction at all to bedbug bites, while others experience an allergic reaction that may include severe itching, blisters or hives.

🏠 Home Remedies

The redness and itching associated with bedbug bites usually goes away within a week or two. You might speed recovery by using:

- Skin cream containing hydrocortisone
- Oral antihistamine, such as diphenhydramine (Benadryl)

Treating your home

Once your symptoms are treated, you must tackle the underlying infestation. This can be difficult because bedbugs hide so well and can live for months without eating. Nonchemical treatments include:

- *Vacuuming.* A thorough vacuuming of cracks and crevices can physically remove bedbugs from an area. But vacuum cleaners can't reach all hiding places.
- *Hot water.* Washing clothes and other items in water at least 120 F can kill bedbugs.
- *Clothes dryer.* Placing sheets, pillowcases and other bedding in a clothes dryer set at medium to high heat for 20 minutes will kill bedbugs and their eggs.
- *Enclosed vehicle.* If it's summer, bag up infested items and leave them in a car parked in the sun with the windows rolled up for a day. The target temperature is at least 120 F.
- *Freezing.* Bedbugs are vulnerable to temperatures below 32 F, but you'd need to leave the bedding and other items outdoors or in the freezer for several days.

Prevention

To prevent infestations and bites:

- *Inspect secondhand items.* Check used mattresses or upholstered furniture carefully before bringing them into your home.
- *Use hotel precautions.* Check mattress seams for bedbug excrement and don't place your luggage on the floor.
- *Cover up.* Because bedbugs don't tend to burrow under clothing, you may be able to avoid bites by wearing pajamas that cover as much skin as possible.

➕ Medical Help

If you experience allergic reactions or severe skin reactions to your bedbug bites, see your doctor.

Bed-wetting

Bed-wetting isn't a sign of toilet training gone bad. It's often just a childhood developmental stage.

Generally, bed-wetting before age 6 or 7 should not be a cause for concern. At this age, nighttime bladder control simply may not be established.

If bed-wetting continues past age 7, treat the concern with patience and understanding. Bladder training, moisture alarms and other steps may help reduce bed-wetting.

Often, bed-wetting occurs for simple reasons, such as forgetting to go to the bathroom before bedtime. Other causes may include stress, constipation or an inability to recognize when the bladder is full.

Several underlying factors associated with the increased risk of bed-wetting include:

- *Sex.* Bed-wetting is more common in boys than in girls.
- *Family history.* If both parents wet the bed as children, their child has an increased risk of wetting the bed.
- *Attention-deficit/hyperactivity disorder (ADHD).* Bed-wetting is more common in children who have ADHD.

🏠 Home Remedies

Changes you can make at home that may reduce bed-wetting include:

- *Limit your child's fluid intake in the evening.* Around 8 ounces or so of fluid in the evening is generally enough, but be careful when you limit fluid intake for yourself or your child. Some experts feel a good rule of thumb is for children to have 40 percent of their daily fluids between 7 a.m. and noon, another 40 percent between noon and 5 p.m. and just 20 percent after 5 p.m. However, don't limit fluids if your child participates in evening sports, either practices or games. Check with your doctor to find out what's right for your child.
- *Avoid caffeinated drinks and foods in the evening.* Caffeine may increase the need to urinate, so don't give your child caffeinated drinks, such as cola, or snacks, such as chocolate, in the evening.
- *Encourage double voiding before bed.* Double voiding is urinating at the beginning of the bedtime routine — for example, before changing into pajamas — and then again just before lights out. Remind your child that it's OK to use the toilet during the night if needed. Use small night lights so that your child can easily find the way between the bedroom and bathroom.
- *Encourage regular urination throughout the day.* During awake hours, suggest that your child urinate once every two hours, or at least enough to avoid a feeling of urgency.
- *Treat constipation.* If constipation is a problem for your child, treating that problem may also reduce bed-wetting.
- *Experiment with foods.* Some people believe that certain foods negatively affect bladder function and that removing these foods from your child's diet may decrease bed-wetting. More study on this idea is necessary. However, if you think a food may be a problem, avoid it for awhile (only one food at a time) and see what happens.

➕ Medical Help

Most children outgrow bed-wetting on their own, but sometimes bed-wetting may indicate an underlying condition that requires medical attention. Consult your child's doctor if:

- Your child regularly wets the bed after age 7
- Your child starts wetting the bed after a period of being dry at night
- The bed-wetting is accompanied by painful urination, unusual thirst, pink urine or snoring

Black eye

An injury or trauma to the face or head may cause bleeding beneath the skin around your eye.

The so-called black eye is due to discoloration from the collected blood as well as swelling of the soft tissue around the eye socket.

Most black eyes are not serious injuries and the eye itself is usually not damaged. Generally, they heal within a few days. However, a black eye may indicate a more extensive injury, even a skull fracture — particularly if the area around both eyes is bruised or there has been head trauma.

Sometimes, there's an accompanying injury to the eyeball that's sufficient to cause bleeding within the eye. This condition, called a hyphema, can be serious, reducing vision and damaging the cornea. For this reason, it's advisable to have an eye specialist examine your eyeball if there has been enough of an injury to cause a black eye.

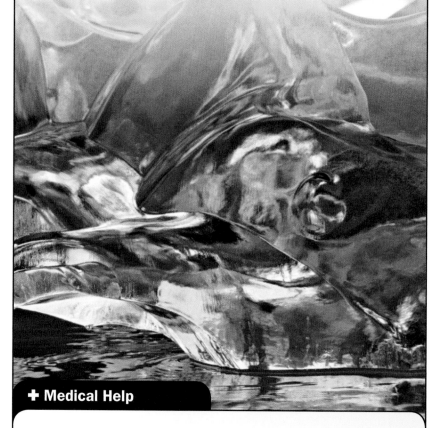

♠ Home Remedies

To reduce bruising and swelling around the eye:
- Using gentle pressure, apply ice or a cold pack to the area around the eye for 15 minutes several times a day. Apply cold as soon as possible after the injury. Don't apply ice directly to your skin — first wrap it in a small towel or washcloth.
- Take care not to press on the eye itself when you're applying ice or cleaning the area around the injury.
- Continue using ice or cold packs for 24 to 48 hours.
- Take acetaminophen (Tylenol, others) for pain associated with the black eye. Don't take aspirin, which may delay blood from clotting and make the bruised area even larger.

✚ Medical Help

Seek medical care immediately if you experience vision problems (double vision, blurring), severe pain, bleeding in the eye or from the nose, or loss of consciousness.

Bladder infection

Bladder infections, also known as urinary tract infections (UTIs), are usually caused by bacteria that have entered the tract from the anal region. The condition is common among women, especially in their reproductive years.

Your urinary system is composed of the kidneys, ureters, bladder and urethra. Any part of your urinary system can become infected, but most infections involve the lower urinary tract — the urethra and the bladder.

With the beginning of sexual activity, women have a marked increase in the number of infections. Sexual intercourse, pregnancy and urinary obstruction all contribute to the likelihood of such an infection.

Signs and symptoms include pain or a burning sensation during urination, an increase in the number of times you need to urinate, and a feeling of urgency every time you urinate.

🏠 Home Remedies

The following steps may ease the discomfort of a bladder infection until antibiotics prescribed by your doctor can clear the infection:

- *Drink plenty of water.* Water dilutes your urine and helps flush out bacteria. Avoid coffee, alcohol, and soft drinks containing citrus juices and caffeine until your infection has cleared. These kinds of beverages may irritate your bladder and increase the frequency or urgency of urination.
- *Use a heating pad.* Place the pad on your abdomen at low to moderate heat to minimize bladder pressure or discomfort. If you don't have a heating pad, a hot water bottle or washcloth soaked in hot water may work just as well.

Prevention

Take these steps to reduce your risk of a bladder infection:

- *Drink plenty of liquids.* Water is best to flush bacteria from your urinary tract, reducing the risk of infection.
- *Try cranberry juice.* There's some indication, though still not proven in rigorous study, that cranberry juice may have infection-fighting properties and drinking the juice daily may help prevent bladder infection. Don't drink cranberry juice if you're taking the blood-thinning medication warfarin. Possible interactions between cranberry juice and warfarin cause bleeding.
- *Wipe from front to back.* Doing so after urinating and after a bowel movement helps prevent bacteria in the anal region from spreading to the vagina and urethra.
- *Go to the bathroom as soon as possible after intercourse.* Emptying your bladder helps flush bacteria from your urinary tract.
- *Avoid potentially irritating feminine products.* Using deodorant sprays or other feminine products, such as douches and powders, in the genital area can irritate the urethra.

➕ Medical Help

If you have symptoms of a bladder infection, contact your doctor.

Blisters

A blister is a pocket of fluid that forms under your skin, commonly caused by friction or rubbing, burning or freezing. The blister can be painful, especially when pressure is applied to the site.

To reduce risk of infection, try keeping the pocket intact. Unbroken skin over a blister provides a natural barrier to bacteria. Don't puncture a blister unless it's very painful or prevents you from walking or using your hands.

Cover a small blister with an adhesive bandage, and cover a large one with a porous, plastic-coated gauze pad that absorbs moisture and allows the wound to breathe. If you're allergic to the adhesive used in some tape, use paper tape.

You may protect the blister with moleskin, a soft, plush fabric with adhesive backing that's sold in many drugstores and pharmacies. Cut a piece of moleskin into a doughnut shape and place the pad so that it encircles the blister, with the open center directly over the blister pocket. The moleskin cushions the blister and protects it from further friction and rubbing.

♠ Home Remedies

Priorities in the treatment of blisters are, first, avoiding the source of friction or rubbing and, second, protecting the injury until your skin has had time to heal. To relieve blister-related pain, drain the fluid while leaving the overlying skin intact. Here's how:

- Wash your hands and the blister site with soap and warm water.
- Swab the blister with iodine or rubbing alcohol.
- Sterilize a clean, sharp needle by wiping it with rubbing alcohol.
- Use the needle to puncture the blister. Aim for several spots near the blister's edge. Let the fluid drain, but leave the overlying skin in place.
- Apply an antibiotic ointment to the blister and cover with a bandage or gauze pad.
- Cut away all the dead skin after several days, using tweezers and scissors sterilized with rubbing alcohol. Apply more ointment and a bandage.

Shoe-shopping tips

Poorly fitting shoes are a common cause of blisters on your feet. Remember the following when you shop for shoes:

- Shop during the middle of the day. Your feet swell throughout the day, so a late-day fitting will probably give you the best fit.
- Wear the same socks you'll wear when walking, or bring them with you to the store.
- Measure your feet. Shoe sizes change throughout adulthood.
- Measure both feet and try on both shoes. If your feet differ in size, buy the larger size.
- Go for flexible, but supportive, shoes with cushioned insoles.
- Leave toe room. Be sure that you can comfortably wiggle your toes.
- Avoid shoes with seams in the toe box, which may irritate bunions or hammertoes.

✚ Medical Help

Call your doctor if you see signs of infection around a blister — pus, redness, increasing pain or warm skin. If you have diabetes or poor circulation, call your doctor before treating the blister yourself.

Boils

A boil is a skin infection that often appears suddenly as a painful pink or red bump, generally between ½ inch to ¾ inch in diameter. The surrounding skin may be red and also swollen.

Boils usually form when one or more hair follicles become infected with staph bacteria (*Staphylococcus aureus*). The bacteria, which normally inhabit your skin's surface, may enter through a cut, scratch or other break in your skin.

Within a few days, the bump fills with pus. It grows larger and more painful, sometimes reaching golf ball size before developing a yellow-white tip that finally ruptures and drains.

Boils usually clear completely in a couple weeks, though it can take a month or more. Small boils generally heal without scarring, but a large boil may leave a scar.

Boils can occur anywhere on your skin, but appear mainly on your face, neck, armpits, buttocks or thighs — hair-bearing areas where you're most likely to sweat or experience friction.

🏠 Home Remedies

To avoid spreading infection from a boil and to minimize discomfort, follow these measures:

- *Soak the area with a warm washcloth or compress.* Do this for at least 10 minutes every few hours. Doing so may help the boil burst and drain much sooner. Use warm salt water. (Add 1 teaspoon of salt to 1 quart of boiling water and let it cool.) Prevent the drained matter from contacting other areas of skin.
- *Gently wash the boil two to three times a day with antibacterial soap.* Then apply an over-the-counter antibiotic ointment and cover with a bandage.
- *Never squeeze or lance a boil.* You might spread the infection.
- *Wash your hands thoroughly after treating a boil.* Also, launder towels, compresses and clothing that have touched the infected area.

➕ Medical Help

Contact your doctor if the infection is located on your spine, groin or face, worsens rapidly or causes severe pain, isn't gone within two weeks, or is accompanied by a fever or reddish lines that radiate out from the boil.

Breast tenderness

Generalized tenderness in both breasts may be common for many women, especially during the week before a menstrual period. These changes can be a symptom of premenstrual syndrome (see page 142). Breast tenderness may also be caused by vigorous exercise or by an inflamed cyst.

If redness develops in breast tissue and fever occurs, then infection of the breast, or mastitis, is a concern. The infection usually occurs in only one breast. Mastitis most commonly affects women who are breast-feeding.

♠ Home Remedies

To reduce breast tenderness:
- Use hot or cold compresses on your breasts.
- Wear a firm support bra, fitted by a professional if possible.
- Wear a sports bra during exercise and while sleeping, especially when your breasts may be more sensitive.
- Experiment with relaxation therapy, which can help control the high levels of anxiety associated with severe breast pain.
- Limit or eliminate caffeine — a dietary change many women swear by, although medical studies of caffeine's effect on breast pain and other premenstrual symptoms have been inconclusive.
- Decrease the amount of fat in your diet to less than 20 percent of total calories, which may help relieve breast pain by altering the fatty acid balance.
- Use a pain reliever, such as acetaminophen (Tylenol, others) or ibuprofen (Advil, Motrin, others), to alleviate breast pain.
- Though not proven, vitamins and dietary supplements may lessen breast pain. Evening primrose oil appears to change the balance of fatty acids in your cells, which may reduce breast pain. Studies of vitamin E show a possible beneficial effect on breast pain, but the medical literature to date remains inconclusive.
- See other tips in the section on premenstrual syndrome (page 142).

✚ Medical Help

Breast tenderness alone rarely signifies breast cancer. Still, if you have unexplained breast pain that persists for more than a couple of weeks, causes worry about breast cancer or otherwise disrupts your life, get checked by your doctor. Also see your doctor if tenderness is associated with a lump or change in breast texture.

Bronchitis

Bronchitis is an inflammation of the lining of your bronchial tubes, or bronchi, which carry air to and from your lungs. It's usually caused by a viral infection, producing a deep cough that, in turn, brings up yellowish gray matter from your lungs.

A common condition, acute bronchitis often develops from a cold or other respiratory infection. Chronic bronchitis, a more serious condition, is a constant irritation or inflammation of the bronchi, often due to smoking.

Signs and symptoms of bronchitis may include:
- Cough
- Production of mucus, either clear or white, or yellowish gray or green in color
- Shortness of breath, made worse by mild exertion
- Wheezing
- Fatigue
- Slight fever and chills
- Chest discomfort

♠ Home Remedies

Besides the basic guidelines of getting plenty of rest and drinking plenty of fluids, the following suggestions can help make you more comfortable, speed recovery, prevent complications and help control symptoms:

- *Avoid exposure to irritants, such as tobacco smoke.* Don't smoke. Wear a mask when the air is polluted or if you're exposed to irritants, such as paint or household cleaners with strong fumes.
- *Use a humidifier in your room.* Warm, moist air helps relieve coughs and loosens mucus in your airways. But be sure to clean the humidifier according to the manufacturer's recommendations to avoid the growth of bacteria and fungi in the water container.
- *Use over-the-counter medications.* To relieve pain and lower a high fever, acetaminophen (Tylenol, others) and ibuprofen (Advil, Motrin, others) may help.
- *Consider a face mask outside.* If cold air aggravates your cough and causes shortness of breath, put on a cold-air face mask before you go outside.
- *Try pursed-lip breathing.* If you have chronic bronchitis, you may breathe too fast. Pursed-lip breathing helps slow your breathing, and may make you feel better. Take a deep breath, then slowly breathe out through your mouth while pursing your lips (hold them as if you're going to kiss someone.) Repeat. This technique increases the air pressure in your airways.

✚ Medical Help

Short-lived (acute) bronchitis usually disappears in a matter of days. Contact a doctor if you experience shortness of breath or a fever of 101 F or higher for more than three days. If your cough lasts for more than 10 days with no end in sight, seek medical attention.

Bruises

A bruise forms when a blow or impact breaks blood vessels near your skin's surface, allowing a small amount of blood to leak into the tissues under your skin. The trapped blood appears as a black-and-blue mark.

Symptoms may include pain and swelling. Eventually your body resorbs the blood, and the mark disappears. The color of the bruise can change to light blue or greenish yellow before returning to normal skin color.

Bruising more common with age

Some people — especially women — are more prone to bruising than are others. As you get older, several factors may contribute to increased bruising, including:

- *Aging capillaries.* Over time, the tissues supporting these vessels weaken, and capillary walls become more fragile and prone to rupture.
- *Thinning skin.* With age, your skin becomes thinner and loses some of the protective fatty layer that helps cushion your blood vessels against injury. Excessive exposure to the sun accelerates the aging process in the skin.

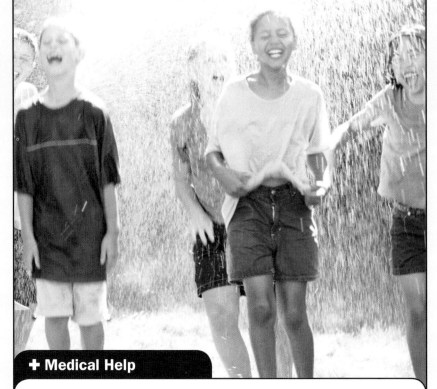

♠ Home Remedies

You can enhance bruise healing with these simple techniques:
- Elevate the injured area, if possible. This may help reduce the amount of blood that pools in the area.
- Apply ice, cold pack or cold compress for 20 minutes at a time several times daily for a day or two after the injury.
- Rest the bruised area, if possible.
- Consider acetaminophen (Tylenol, others) for pain relief, or ibuprofen (Advil, Motrin, others) for pain relief and to reduce swelling.

✚ Medical Help

These signs and symptoms may indicate a more serious problem. See your doctor if:
- You have unusually large or painful bruises — particularly if your bruises seem to develop for no known reasons.
- You bruise easily and you're experiencing abnormal bleeding elsewhere, such as from your nose or gums, or you notice blood in your eyes, stool or urine.
- You have no history of bruising, but suddenly experience bruises.

Burns

Burns are traumatic injuries, often to the outer layers of your skin, that can result from a variety of sources: fire, the sun, chemicals, hot liquids, steam electricity and other means. A burn can be a minor medical problem or a life-threatening emergency.

Treatment depends on the size and severity of the burn. Distinguishing a minor burn from a more serious burn involves your understanding how much damage has occurred to the skin and underlying tissues.

The following three categories and accompanying illustrations on this page can help determine how you should respond to a burn.

First-degree burn

The least serious burns are those in which only the outer layer of skin (epidermis) is burned. The skin is usually reddened, and there may be swelling and pain, but the outer layer of skin hasn't been burned through.

Unless such a burn involves substantial portions of the hands, feet, face, groin, buttocks or a major joint, it may be treated as a minor burn with the self-care remedies listed on page 34.

Chemical burns may require additional follow-up. If the burn was caused by exposure to the sun, see "Sunburn," page 165.

Second-degree burn

When the first layer of skin has been burned through and the second layer of skin (dermis) also is burned, the injury is called a second-degree burn. Blisters form, and the skin takes on an intensely reddened, splotchy appearance. Second-degree burns usually produce swelling and moderate to severe pain.

If a second-degree burn is limited to an area no larger than 3 inches wide, follow the home remedies listed on page 34. If the burned area of the skin is larger, or if the burn is on the hands, feet, face, groin, buttocks or over a major joint or encircles your limb, seek urgent care immediately.

Third-degree

The most serious burns involve all layers of the skin. Fat, nerves, muscles and even bones may be affected. Usually some areas are charred black or appear a dry white. There may be severe pain or, if nerve damage is substantial, no pain at all.

It's important to take quick action in all cases of third-degree burns. For more information on the treatment of severe burns while waiting for help to arrive, see page 187.

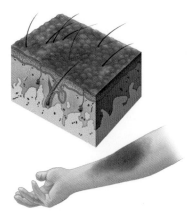

First-degree burn

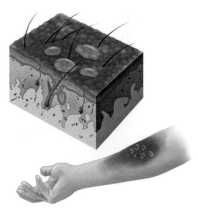

Second-degree burn

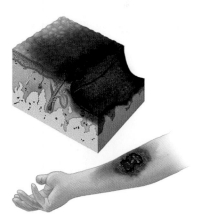

Third-degree burn

For minor burns, including second-degree burns limited to an area no larger than 3 inches wide, take the following actions:

Cool the burn

Hold the burned area under cold running water until the pain subsides. If this step is impractical, immerse the burn in cold water or apply cold compresses. Cooling the burn reduces pain and swelling.

Consider a lotion

Once a burn is completely cooled, applying a lotion, such as one containing aloe vera, or a moisturizer prevents drying and increases your comfort. For sunburn, try 1 percent hydrocortisone cream.

Bandage a burn

Cover the burn with a sterile gauze bandage (not fluffy cotton). Wrap it loosely to avoid putting pressure on burned skin. Bandaging keeps air off the area, reduces pain and protects blistered skin.

Take an over-the-counter pain reliever

These include aspirin, ibuprofen (Advil, Motrin, others), naproxen (Aleve) or acetaminophen (Tylenol, others). Don't give aspirin to children younger than age 12.

Don't use ice

Ice on a burn can cause frostbite and do more damage.

Don't break blisters

Fluid-filled blisters protect against infection. If blisters break, clean the area daily by rinsing with water (mild soap is optional). Apply an antibiotic ointment. But if a rash appears, stop using the ointment.

Watch for signs of infection

Minor burns will usually heal in about one to two weeks without further treatment, but watch for indications of infection.

➕ Medical Help

Seek emergency medical help if the burn appears severe or covers a large area. For minor burns, see a doctor if the burn does not improve or new symptoms develop, such as a fever or light-headedness.

Bursitis

Bursitis is a painful condition affecting small fluid-filled pads (bursae) that lubricate and cushion pressure points for your bones, tendons and muscles near your joints. Bursitis occurs when a bursa becomes inflamed.

The most common locations for bursitis are in the shoulders, elbows or hips. But you can also have bursitis at your knee, heel and base of your big toe.

Bursitis often occurs in joints that perform frequent repetitive motion. It's commonly caused by overuse, trauma, repeated bumping or prolonged pressure such as kneeling for an extended period. It may even result from an infection, arthritis or gout.

If you have bursitis, the affected joint may:

- Feel achy or stiff
- Hurt more when you move it or press on it
- Look swollen and red

🏠 Home Remedies

To treat symptoms of bursitis:

- Use over-the-counter pain medications.
- Keep pressure off the joint. Use an elastic bandage, sling or soft foam pad to protect it until the swelling goes down.
- Ease the joint back into activity slowly.

Prevention

While not all types of bursitis can be prevented, you can reduce your risk and reduce the severity of flare-ups by changing the way you perform certain tasks. Examples include:

- *Strengthen your muscles to help protect the joint.* But don't start exercising a joint that has bursitis until the pain and inflammation are gone.
- *Take frequent breaks from repetitive tasks.* Alternate repetitive tasks with rest or other activities. Follow ergonomic principles for desk work and lifting.
- *Cushion the joint before applying pressure.* Use knee pads or elbow pads. For bursitis in a hip, cushion a hard mattress with a foam pad or soft mattress cover.
- *Avoid elbow pressure.* Stop leaning on your elbows. If you push up from your elbows to get out of bed, consider tying a rope to the end of your bed so that you can pull yourself up that way.
- *Lift properly.* Bend your knees when you lift. Failing to do so puts extra stress on the bursae in your hips.
- *Avoid heavy loads.* Carrying heavy loads puts stress on the bursae in your shoulders. Use a dolly instead.

➕ Medical Help

Consult your doctor if you have:

- Disabling joint pain, or pain that lasts more than two weeks
- Excessive swelling, redness, bruising or a rash in the affected area
- Sharp or shooting pain, especially when you exercise or exert yourself
- Fever

Canker sores

A canker sore is an ulcer on the soft tissue inside your mouth — the tongue, soft palate, inner lips or inner cheeks. Typically, you notice a burning sensation and round whitish spot surrounded by a red edge or halo.

Despite a great deal of research on the condition, the cause of canker sores remains a mystery. Current thinking suggests that stress or tissue injury may cause the eruption of common canker sores.

Some researchers believe certain nutritional deficiencies or food sensitivities may complicate the problem. In addition, some gastrointestinal and immune deficiency disorders have been linked to canker sores, as well as agents such as sodium lauryl sulfate — an ingredient in some brands of toothpaste.

Types

There are two types of canker sore: simple and complex. Simple canker sores may appear three or four times a year and last four to seven days. The first occurrence is usually between the ages of 10 and 40, but also can happen in younger children. As a person reaches adulthood, the sores occur less frequently. Women seem to get them more often than do men, and they seem to run in families.

Complex canker sores are less common but much more of a problem. As old sores heal, new ones appear.

🏠 Home Remedies

There's no cure for either simple or complex canker sores, and effective treatments are limited. To relieve pain and speed healing:

- *Rinse your mouth.* Use salt water; baking soda (dissolve 1 teaspoon of soda in 1/2 cup warm water); hydrogen peroxide diluted by half with water; or a mixture of 1 part diphenhydramine (Benadryl) to either 1 part bismuth subsalicylate (Kaopectate, Pepto Bismol, others) or 1 part simethicone (Maalox). Be sure to spit out the mixtures after rinsing.
- *Cover lesions.* Use a paste made of baking soda.
- *Try over-the-counter products.* Look for ones that contain a numbing agent, such as Anbesol and Orajel.
- *Avoid abrasive, acidic or spicy foods.* They can cause further irritation and pain.
- *Apply ice to your canker sores.* Or allow ice chips to slowly dissolve over the sores.
- *Brush your teeth gently.* Use a soft brush and toothpaste without foaming agents, such as TheraBreath.
- *Try milk of magnesia.* Dab a small amount of milk of magnesia on your canker sore a few times a day. This can ease the pain and may help the sore heal more quickly.

➕ Medical Help

In severe cases, your dentist or doctor may recommend a prescription mouthwash, salve or solution. Contact your doctor if you have:
- Significant difficulty eating or drinking due to canker sores
- High fever with canker sores
- Spreading sores or signs of spreading infection
- Pain that's not controlled with the measures listed above
- Sores that don't heal completely within a week

See your dentist if you have sharp tooth surfaces or dental appliances that are causing sores.

Carpal tunnel syndrome

The carpal tunnel is a narrow passageway through your bony wrist that protects the primary nerves and tendons to your hand. When tissues in the passage become swollen or inflamed, they put pressure on a nerve that affects the movement of your thumb and index, middle and ring fingers. Too much pressure may cause carpal tunnel syndrome. If left untreated, permanent nerve and muscle damage can occur.

Risk factors for carpal tunnel syndrome include various occupations, activities and hobbies that involve awkward wrist positions, pressure on the palm of the hand, and repetitive lifting or grasping actions. Pregnancy, obesity and conditions such as diabetes, thyroid disease and arthritis also are risk factors.

Signs and symptoms of the condition include:

- Tingling or numbness in your thumb, index and middle fingers (but not your little finger). This sensation may occur at night, waking you up. It may also occur while you're driving or holding a phone or newspaper.
- Pain radiating or extending from your wrist up your arm to your shoulder or down into your palm or fingers, especially after forceful or repetitive use.
- Sense of weakness in your hands and a tendency to drop objects.

🏠 Home Remedies

To relieve carpal tunnel symptoms:

- *Take frequent breaks.* Every hour take a 5-minute break and gently stretch your wrists and hands.
- *Vary your activities.* Alternate tasks when possible.
- *Watch your form.* Avoid bending your wrist all the way up or down.
- *Relax your grip.* Avoid using a hard grip when driving your car, bicycling or writing. Oversized grips on pens, pencils and tools may allow a softer grasp.
- *Keep your hands warm.* You're more likely to develop hand pain and stiffness if you work in a cold environment. If you can't control the temperature at work, put on fingerless gloves that keep your hands and wrists warm.
- *Use a wrist splint at night.* A wrist splint may help ease pain or numbness in your wrists and hands. The splint should be snug but not tight.
- *Use nonprescription pain relievers.* Nonsteroidal anti-inflammatory drugs (NSAIDs), such as ibuprofen (Advil, Motrin, others), can help relieve both pain and swelling.
- *Try yoga and other relaxation techniques.* Yoga postures designed for strengthening, stretching and balancing joints in the upper body, as well as the upper body itself, may help reduce pain and improve the grip strength of people with carpal tunnel syndrome.

➕ Medical Help

If the symptoms continue for more than a couple of weeks, see your doctor. Splints, therapy, injection or prescription medications may be recommended. Occasionally, surgery is necessary.

Chronic pain

Physical pain is a part of life. Maybe you've slammed your finger in a door, burned your hand while touching a hot skillet on the stove or twisted your ankle while playing basketball. The result is a sensation of sharp or aching pain.

Chronic pain is persistent pain lasting long after the normal healing process, or when there doesn't seem to be any injury or bodily damage that could cause the ongoing sensation. Generally, chronic pain is considered to be pain that lasts more than three to six months.

Chronic pain can be overwhelming. But you can learn how to manage the pain so that it doesn't interfere with your life. Your outlook and positive attitude also are important.

Pain and your emotions

Pain isn't only a physical experience but also an emotional one.

People perceive pain differently and react to it in different ways. When you experience pain over a long period of time, you may find yourself overwhelmed by intense, often negative, emotions, including panic, fear, grief, anxiety and anger. Chronic pain can cause frustration and irritability. These emotions can affect you physically, sapping your energy and intensifying the symptoms.

Finding healthy ways to cope with pain can have both physical and emotional benefits.

Pain relievers: Matching the pill to the pain

For pain relief, the difference among nonprescription pain relievers is generally more subtle than significant. All over-the-counter pain relievers relieve mild to moderate pain associated with common conditions such as headache, muscle aches and arthritis. They also reduce fever. The difference among the various products is that some relieve inflammation while others don't:

- *NSAIDs.* These products, which include aspirin, ibuprofen and naproxen sodium, reduce inflammation. NSAID stands for nonsteroidal anti-inflammatory drugs. They're most helpful for pain associated with arthritis and tendinitis.
- *Acetaminophen.* The most common brand of acetaminophen is Tylenol. Acetaminophen doesn't relieve inflammation but does relieve pain.

With all nonprescription pain relievers, you need to be careful about how many you take. They all have side effects that can be serious if the medications are taken in excessive amounts.

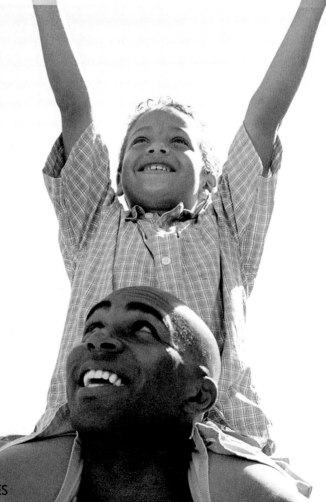

🏠 Home Remedies

There are many methods for relieving chronic pain. Experiment with different therapies to find which ones work best for you.

Exercise

Physical activity can stimulate the release of endorphins, your body's own natural painkillers. Endorphins are morphine-like pain relievers that send "stop pain" messages to your sensitive nerve cells.

The duration of exercise seems more important than the intensity. Low-intensity aerobic exercise — for example, brisk walking — for 30 to 45 minutes on five or six days a week may have a positive effect. (Be sure to build up slowly.) You can even benefit from only three days of exercise a week.

If you want to start an exercise program that's more vigorous than walking, have a medical evaluation, especially if:

- You're older than age 40
- You've been sedentary
- You have risk factors for coronary artery disease
- You have chronic health problems

Hot and cold

Heat and ice are used most often to treat acute pain following an injury but may also help relieve some forms of chronic pain. For more on the use of hot and cold for injury, see page 20.

Weight loss

It's easier to manage pain when you're not overweight. That's because excess weight saps your energy, increases stress on your muscles and joints and decreases flexibility. You don't have to become thin, but losing just a few pounds may help reduce your pain level.

Sleep

You're better equipped to deal with pain if you've had a good night's sleep. Sleep gives you energy and helps you fight off fatigue and stress, which can worsen pain. For tips on better sleep, see page 115.

Topical medications

Several medications are available without a prescription that may help relieve pain for a short time.

Capsaicin (Capzasin-P, Zostrix) is a nonprescription cream made from the seeds of hot chili peppers. Rub the product on your skin three to five times a day.

Some people find capsaicin helpful for arthritic pain in joints close to your skin's surface, such as fingers and elbows. It may also help relieve pain after shingles. However, the cream can temporarily irritate your skin and produce a burning sensation, which may be painful.

Counterirritants, such as Bengay and IcyHot, include ingredients such as menthol and oil of wintergreen that stimulate nerve endings to produce feelings of cold or warmth. These responses, which may be mildly painful, can counter, or block, more intense pain sensations.

Benzocaine is a local anesthetic that deadens your nerve endings — relieving pain and itching — where the cream or gel is applied to your skin. Lidocaine has a similar effect but is available only with a prescription from your doctor.

Continued next page >

➕ Medical Help

If your pain changes in character — for example, it grows from mild to severe — or if you develop new symptoms, such as a tingling or numb sensation, it might be a good idea to see your doctor and have your condition re-evaluated.

Stress reduction

When you're dealing with pain, you're less able to cope with the stress of everyday living. Stress may also cause you to do things that end up intensifying pain, such as tensing your muscles. In short, pain causes stress and stress tends to makes pain worse.

To better manage stress, you can learn and practice various relaxation techniques, such as:

- *Relaxed breathing*. Get in a relaxed position and close your eyes. Inhale slowly to the count of six. Hold the air in your lungs as you slowly count to four. Release the air slowly through your mouth as you count to six. Repeat three to five times.
- *Meditation*. This technique appears to reduce pain and stress by helping you relax and respond to the flow of emotions and thoughts you face in challenging situations.

Massage

A growing body of literature is beginning to validate the many benefits of massage. Studies suggest that it can decrease headache and fibromyalgia pain and, possibly, back pain.

Yoga

Studies indicate yoga may relieve back pain, with symptom improvement lasting several months. Yoga has also been found to reduce headache pain.

Tai chi

Tai chi involves gentle exercises combined with deep breathing. It may relieve some types of pain by strengthening muscles and improving joint flexibility.

Cold sores

Cold sores are small, painful, fluid-filled blisters that may appear on your mouth, lips, nose, cheeks or fingers. While cold sores occur most often in adolescents and young adults, they can occur at almost any age. Outbreaks decrease after age 35.

The herpes simplex virus causes cold sores. There are two types of this virus: Type 1 usually causes cold sores, while type 2 is most often responsible for genital herpes. However, either type can cause sores in the facial area or on the genitals.

You can get cold sores from contact with another person who has an active condition. Eating utensils, razors, towels or direct skin contact are common means of spreading this infection.

Symptoms may not start for up to 20 days after you were first exposed to the virus. The blisters develop on a raised, red, painful area of skin. Pain or tingling often precedes blister formation by one to two days. Cold sores typically clear up in seven to 10 days.

After the initial infection, the virus periodically re-emerges at or near the original site. Fever, menstruation and exposure to the sun may trigger the recurrence.

🏠 Home Remedies

Cold sores generally clear up without treatment. These steps may provide relief:

- Rest and take nonprescription pain relievers if you have a fever or the cold sore is painful. Children and teens should avoid aspirin use because of the risk of Reye's syndrome. Nonprescription pain creams also may provide comfort, but they won't speed healing.
- Don't squeeze, pinch or pick at any blister.
- Avoid kissing and skin contact with people while blisters are present.
- Try applying ice or warm compresses to the blisters to ease pain.
- Wash your hands carefully before touching another person.
- Use sunblock on your lips and face before prolonged exposure to the sun — during winter and summer — to prevent cold sores.

+ Medical Help

If you have frequent bouts of cold sores, an antiviral medication may help. These medications inhibit the growth of the herpes virus. Talk to your doctor about a prescription.

Caution: If you have a cold sore, take special care to avoid contact with infants or anyone who has eczema (see page 70). They're more susceptible to infection. Also, avoid people who are taking medications for cancer and organ transplantation because they have decreased immunity. Herpes simplex viral infections can lead to potentially serious eye complications.

Colic

Generations of families have had to dealt with colic. This frustrating and largely unexplainable condition affects babies who otherwise seem healthy. Colic usually peaks at six weeks of age and disappears sometime in the baby's third to fifth month.

Although the term *colic* is used widely for any fussy baby, true colic is determined by the following factors:

- *Predictable crying episodes.* A colicky baby cries about the same time each day, usually in the late afternoon or evening. Colic episodes may last from a few minutes to three or more hours on any given day.
- *Posture changes.* Many colicky babies pull their legs to their chests, clench their fists or thrash around during episodes as if they are in pain.
- *Intense or inconsolable crying.* Colicky crying is intense and often high pitched. The babies can be extremely difficult — if not impossible — to comfort.

Studies of colic have focused on several possible causes: allergies, an immature digestive system, gas, hormones, mother's anxieties, and handling. Still, it's unclear why some babies have colic and other babies don't.

🏠 Home Remedies

If your doctor determines that your baby has colic, these measures may help you and your child find some relief:

- *Feed your baby.* If you think your baby may be hungry, try feeding. Sometimes more frequent — but smaller — feedings are helpful. Try to hold your baby as upright as possible, and burp your baby often. If you're breast-feeding, it may help to empty one breast completely before switching sides. This will give your baby more hindmilk, which is richer and potentially more satisfying than foremilk, which is present at the beginning of a feeding.
- *Offer a pacifier.* For many babies, sucking is a soothing activity. Even if you're breast-feeding, it's OK to offer a pacifier.
- *Hold your baby.* Cuddling helps some babies. Others quiet when they're held closely and swaddled in a lightweight blanket. Don't worry about spoiling your baby by holding him or her too much.
- *Keep your baby in motion.* Gently rock your baby in your arms or in an infant swing. Lay your baby tummy down on your knees and then sway your knees slowly. Take a walk with your baby, or buckle your baby in the car seat for a drive.
- *Turn up the background noise.* Some babies cry less when they hear steady background noise. When holding or rocking your baby, try making a continuous "shssss" sound. Turn on a kitchen or bathroom exhaust fan, or play soothing music or nature sounds, such as ocean waves or gentle rain. Sometimes the tick of a clock or metronome does the trick.
- *Use gentle heat or touch.* Give your baby a warm bath. Softly massage your baby, especially around the tummy.
- *Consider dietary changes.* If you breast-feed, see if eliminating certain foods from your own diet — such as dairy products, citrus fruits, spicy foods or drinks containing caffeine — has an effect on your baby's crying.

➕ Medical Help

There are no medications to relieve colic. In general, consult with your doctor before giving your baby any medication. If you're worried that your baby is sick or if you or others caring for the baby are becoming frustrated or angry because of the crying, call your doctor or bring the baby to the doctor's office or emergency room.

Common cold

The common cold is a viral infection of your upper respiratory tract — your nose and throat. A common cold is usually harmless, although it may not feel that way. If it's not a runny nose, sore throat and cough, it's watery eyes, sneezing and congestion — or maybe all of the above.

Most adults likely experience a cold two to four times a year. Children, especially preschoolers, may get a cold as many as six to 10 times annually.

Don't waste your money

Over-the-counter cold preparations won't cure a common cold or make it go away any sooner. Here's what's known about common cold remedies:

- *Pain relievers.* Products such as acetaminophen (Tylenol, others) and ibuprofen (Advil, Motrin, others) may relieve fever, sore throat and headache. Overuse of these products can cause side effects. Be careful when giving acetaminophen to children because the dosing guidelines can be confusing. For instance, the infant-drop formulation is much more concentrated than is the syrup commonly used in older children. Don't give aspirin to children. It has been associated with Reye's syndrome — a rare but potentially fatal illness.
- *Decongestant nasal sprays.* Adults shouldn't use decongestant drops or sprays for more than three days because

prolonged use can cause chronic inflammation of the mucous membranes. And children shouldn't use decongestant drops or sprays at all. There's little evidence that they work in young children, and may cause side effects.
- *Cough syrups.* The American College of Chest Physicians strongly discourages the use of cough syrups because they don't effectively treat the underlying cause of cough due to colds. Some syrups contain ingredients that may alleviate coughing, but the amounts are too small to do much good and may actually be harmful for children. The college recommends against using over-the-counter cough syrups or cold medicines for anyone younger than age 14. The Food and Drug Administration strongly recommends against giving nonprescription cough and cold medicines to children younger than age 2.

Continued next page >

Is it a cold or the flu?

Cold	Flu (influenza)
Runny nose, sneezing, nasal congestion	Runny nose
Sore throat (usually scratchy)	Sore throat and headache
Cough	Cough
No fever or low fever	Fever, usually over 101 F, chills
Mild fatigue	Moderate to severe fatigue and weakness
	Achy muscles and joints

You may not cure the common cold but you can make yourself more comfortable with these tips:

Drink lots of fluids

Water, juice and tea are all good choices. They help replace fluids lost during mucus production or fever. Avoid alcohol and caffeine, which can cause dehydration, and cigarette smoke, which can aggravate your symptoms.

Try chicken soup

Generations of parents have spooned chicken soup into their sick children, and scientists have found that it does seem to help relieve symptoms in two ways.

First, it has anti-inflammatory properties that help reduce mucus production in your respiratory tract.

Second, it temporarily speeds up the movement of mucus through the nose, helping relieve congestion and limiting the time that viruses are in contact with the nasal lining.

Get some rest

If possible, stay home from work if you have a fever or bad cough, or are drowsy from medications. Rest is important to speeding recovery.

Adjust your room's humidity

If the air is dry, a cool-mist humidifier or vaporizer can moisten the air and help ease sinus congestion and coughing. Be sure to keep the humidifier clean and regularly change the filter to prevent the growth of bacteria and molds.

Soothe your throat

Gargling with warm salt water several times a day or drinking warm lemon water mixed with honey may help soothe your sore throat and relieve the coughing spells.

Use saline nasal drops

Saline drops are effective, safe and non-irritating — even for children — for the relief of nasal congestion. The drops can be purchased over-the-counter in most drugstores. To use in babies, put several drops into a nostril, then immediately bulb suction that nostril.

Try andrographis

There is some evidence this Indian herb can reduce the severity and duration of upper respiratory infections. It may also reduce your risk of getting a cold. The herb seems safe when used short-term.

Try echinacea

While no studies have shown that this herb can prevent a cold, there is some evidence that it can modestly relieve cold symptoms or shorten the duration of a cold. Echinacea seems most effective when taken soon after cold symptoms appear.

Get your vitamin C

Despite popular belief, there's no evidence that taking large doses of vitamin C reduces your risk of a cold. However, there's evidence that high doses of vitamin C — up to 6 grams a day — may have a small effect in reducing the duration of cold symptoms.

Consider zinc

There's some evidence that zinc lozenges taken at the beginning of a cold may help reduce symptoms. The claim that zinc nasal sprays are helpful is controversial. In general, the use of these sprays is discouraged because many people have experienced permanent loss of smell following use.

✚ Medical Help

Most people recover from a common cold in about a week or two. If symptoms don't improve, see your doctor.

Constipation

You have constipation when you have infrequent bowel movements (generally, fewer than three stools a week), you pass hard stools or you have to strain during bowel movements. You may feel a bloated sensation and crampy discomfort. This common problem is often improperly treated.

Like a fever, constipation is a symptom, not a disease. The problem occurs when the passage of food through your large intestine slows down. Contributing factors include: not drinking enough fluids, a diet low in fiber, irregular bowel habits, older age, lack of activity, pregnancy and illness. Some types of medication also may cause constipation.

Constipation can be extremely bothersome but is usually not serious. If it persists, however, constipation can lead to complications such as hemorrhoids and cracks in the anus, called fissures.

Constipation in kids

Young children sometimes experience constipation because they neglect to take the time to use the bathroom. Toddlers may become constipated out of anxiety during toilet training. Stress also plays a role in bowel changes. However, as few as one bowel movement a week may be normal for your child.

♠ Home Remedies

To lessen your chance of constipation:
- Eat on a regular schedule (including breakfast), and eat plenty of high-fiber foods, including fresh fruits, vegetables, and whole-grain cereals and breads.
- Drink plenty of water or other liquids to soften stool.
- Increase physical activity. Exercise stimulates bowel activity.
- Don't ignore the urge to have a bowel movement.
- Don't rely on laxatives. Overuse of certain laxatives can be harmful and make constipation worse. Overuse can cause your body to flush out vitamins and other nutrients before they're properly absorbed, and interfere with other medications you're taking. Excessive use can also cause lazy bowel syndrome, a condition in which your bowels don't function properly and rely on laxatives for stimulation.

The effectiveness of each type of laxative will vary from person to person. In general, bulk-forming laxatives, or fiber supplements, such as Citrucel and Metamucil, are the gentlest on your body and the safest to use long term. Stimulant laxatives such as Ex-lax and Senokot are the harshest and not for long-term use. However, use of any laxative, unless prescribed, can be habit-forming.

Remedies for kids

Have your child drink plenty of fluids to soften stools. Warm baths also may help relax your child and encourage bowel movements. A diet rich in high-fiber foods, such as beans, whole grains, fruits and vegetables, will help your child's body form soft, bulky stools. Limit foods that have little or no fiber, such as cheese, meat and processed foods.

✚ Medical Help

Contact your doctor if your constipation is severe or lasts longer than three weeks. In rare cases, constipation may signal more-serious medical conditions such as cancer and hormonal disturbances. Chronic use of certain laxatives add risk if you have heart or kidney failure.

Corns and calluses

Corns and calluses are thick, hardened layers of skin that develop as your skin tries to protect itself against friction and pressure. They typically appear on your hands and feet.

Corns are small and often cone-shaped with a hard center surrounded by inflamed skin. They tend to develop on parts of your feet that don't bear weight, such as the tops or sides of your toes. Corns can be painful when pressure is applied to them.

Calluses usually develop on the soles of your feet, on the palms of your hands, or on your knees. Calluses are rarely painful and vary in size and shape. They're often larger than corns.

Although corns and calluses can be unsightly, treatment may be necessary only if they cause discomfort. For most people, eliminating the source of friction or pressure will help corns and calluses disappear.

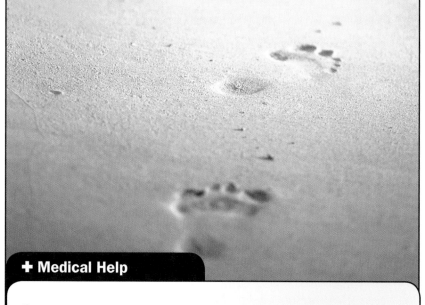

♠ Home Remedies

To relieve symptoms and prevent corns and calluses:
- *Wear properly fitted shoes with adequate toe room.* Have a shoe store stretch your shoes at any point that rubs or pinches your feet. Place pads under your heels if your shoes rub. Try using a shoe insert to cushion or soften the corn while wearing shoes.
- *Wear padded gloves when using hand tools.* Or try padding your tool handles with cloth tape or covers.
- *Soak your hands or feet.* Soaking your hands or feet in warm, soapy water softens corns and calluses. This makes it easier to remove the thickened skin.
- *Use a pumice stone.* During or after bathing, rub your corn or callus with a pumice stone, metal nail file or washcloth to gradually thin some of the thickened skin. This advice isn't recommended if you have diabetes or poor circulation.
- *Try corn dissolvers containing salicylic acid.* These over-the-counter products are available as plaster-pad disks or solutions.
- *Trim corns and calluses carefully.* Don't cut or shave them with a sharp edge.
- *Use a moisturizer.* Apply moisturizing cream daily to your hands and feet to keep them soft.

✚ Medical Help

If a corn or callus becomes very painful or inflamed, contact your doctor.

Cough

A cough is a reflex — just like breathing. It's actually a way of protecting your lungs against irritants, such as dust or smoke. When there's a buildup of fine particles or mucus in your breathing passages (bronchi), you cough to clear the passages, allowing easier breathing.

A small amount of coughing is normal and even healthy as a way to keep the passages clear. However, strong or persistent coughing can become an irritant. Repeated coughing causes your bronchi to narrow, which can irritate the interior walls of the breathing passages.

Causes of persistent cough

Persistent coughing is frequently a symptom of a viral infection in the upper respiratory tract, which includes your nose, sinuses and airways. Colds and flu (influenza) are common examples of this kind of infection. Your voice box may become inflamed from the infection (laryngitis), causing pain and hoarseness.

Coughing also results from throat irritation caused by the drainage of mucus down the back of your throat, a condition known as postnasal drainage. Coughing may also occur with various chronic disorders.

People with allergies and asthma often have bouts of involuntary coughing, as do people who smoke. Many irritants in the environment, such as smog, dust, and second-hand smoke, as well as meteorological conditions, such as cold or dry air, can produce coughing.

Sometimes coughing is caused by stomach acid that backs up into your esophagus or, in rare cases, your lungs. This condition is called gastroesophageal reflux. Some people may develop a "habit" cough, which can often occur despite the lack of any underlying condition.

Continued next page >

Take these steps to help relieve a persistent cough:

Drink plenty of fluids

Fluids help keep your throat clear. Drink water or fruit juices — not soda or coffee.

Use a humidifier

The air in your home can get very dry, especially during the winter. Dry air irritates your throat when you have a cold. Using a humidifier to moisturize the air will make breathing easier.

Suck on hard candy or lozenges

Hard candy or medicated throat lozenges may help to soothe simple throat irritation and prevent coughing if your throat is dry or sore.

Try honey

Drink a cup of warm tea or warm lemon water that is sweetened with honey. Mix 2 teaspoons of honey with the warm liquid.

A study of children age 2 and older found honey at bedtime seemed to reduce nighttime coughing and improve sleep.

Due to the risk of infant botulism, a rare but serious form of food poisoning, never give honey to a child younger than age 1.

Elevate your bed

Sleep with the head of your bed elevated. Raise your bed 4 to 6 inches if your cough is caused by a backup of stomach acid. Also avoid food and drink within two to three hours of bedtime.

Avoid cough syrups

Don't waste your money on over-the-counter cough medicines because they aren't effective. See page 43.

➕ Medical Help

Contact a doctor if your cough lasts more than two or three weeks, or if it's accompanied by fever, increased shortness of breath or bloody phlegm. Managing a chronic cough requires careful evaluation.

Cramps and charley horses

A cramp, sometimes called a charley horse, is actually a muscle spasm — a sudden, involuntary contraction of one or more muscles into a painful knot. Overuse or strain of a muscle, dehydration or simply holding a single position for a prolonged period may result in the muscle cramp.

Almost everyone gets a cramp at some point in the course of day-to-day activities. For example, people who become fatigued and dehydrated while participating in sports in warm weather often complain of muscle cramps.

Writer's cramp affecting the thumb and first two fingers of your writing hand results from using the same muscles to grip a pen or pencil for long periods. At home, you can develop cramps in your hand or arm after spending long hours using a paintbrush or garden tool.

A common type of cramp — nocturnal cramps — occurs in your calf muscles or toes during sleep. The cause of this type of cramp is unknown but frequency seems to increase with age.

♠ Home Remedies

If you have a cramp, these actions may provide relief:
- Gently stretch and massage a cramping muscle.
- For lower leg (calf) cramps, put your weight on the leg and bend your knee slightly.
- For upper leg (hamstring) cramps, straighten your legs and lean forward at your waist. Steady yourself with a chair.
- Apply heat to relax tense, tight muscles.
- Apply cold to sore or tender muscles.
- Drink plenty of water. Fluid helps your muscles function normally.

Prevention
To prevent muscle cramps:
- Stretch your leg muscles daily, using the stretches for the Achilles tendon and calf as shown on page 97.
- Stretch your muscles carefully and gradually warm up before participating in vigorous activity.
- Stop exercising as soon as a cramp begins.
- Drink plenty of liquids every day. Fluids help your muscles contract and relax and keep muscle cells hydrated and less irritable. Drink fluids before any exercise activity.

✚ Medical Help

Muscle cramps usually disappear on their own, and are rarely serious enough to require medical care. However, if you experience frequent and severe muscle cramps or if your cramps disturb your sleep, see your doctor.

Croup

Croup, marked by a harsh, repetitive cough, is a viral infection that develops most often in young children. The cough is similar to the noise of a seal barking, which can be frightening for both the children and their parents.

The harsh sounds of coughing are the result of swelling around the vocal cords (larynx) and windpipe (trachea). When the cough reflex forces air through this narrowed passage, the vocal cords vibrate with the barking sound. Because children have smaller air passages, those younger than age 5 are more susceptible to the symptoms of croup.

In addition to the coughing, a child with croup may have difficulty breathing in. The child may become agitated and begin crying — actions that make inhaling even more difficult.

Croup typically lasts five or six days. During this time, symptoms may fluctuate back and forth between mild and severe. Symptoms are usually worse at night.

♠ Home Remedies

Keep your child comfortable with a few simple measures:

- *Stay calm.* Comfort or distract your child — cuddle, read a book or play a quiet game. Crying only makes breathing more difficult.
- *Moisten the air.* Use a cool-air humidifier in your child's bedroom or have your child breathe warm, moist air in a steamy bathroom. Researchers have questioned the benefits of humidity as part of emergency treatment for croup, but moist air seems to help children breathe easier — especially when croup is mild.
- *Get cool.* Sometimes breathing fresh, cool air helps. If it's cool outdoors, wrap your child in a blanket and walk outside for a few minutes.
- *Hold your child in an upright position.* Sitting upright can make breathing easier. Hold your child on your lap, or place your child in a favorite chair or infant seat.
- *Offer fluids.* For babies, water, breast milk or formula is fine. For older children, warm soup or frozen fruit pops may be soothing.
- *Encourage your child to rest.* Sleep can help your child fight infection.

✚ Medical Help

Seek immediate medical attention if your child:
- Makes noisy, high-pitched breathing sounds when inhaling
- Begins drooling or has difficulty swallowing
- Seems agitated or extremely irritable
- Struggles to breathe
- Has a fever of 103.5 F (39.7 C) or higher

Call 911 or your local emergency number for help if the child is in severe distress, unresponsive, blue or dusky.

Cut and scrapes

Everyday cuts and wounds often don't require a trip to the emergency room. Yet proper care is essential to avoid infection and other complications. The guidelines on page 52 can help you in caring for simple wounds.

What about puncture wounds?

A puncture wound doesn't usually result in excessive bleeding. Often in fact, little blood flows, and the wound seems to close quickly. This doesn't mean that treatment is unnecessary. You may require medical attention.

A puncture wound — such as from stepping on a nail, tack, wood splinter or glass — may be dangerous because of the risk of the infection. The object that caused the puncture may carry spores of tetanus or other bacteria, especially if the object has been exposed to dirt. For shallow wounds, follow the self-care steps and advice on seeking medical help on page 52. A puncture wound may need to be cleaned by a doctor.

What about scarring?

No matter how you treat cuts, all wounds that penetrate deeper than the first, or outermost layer of skin will form a scar when healed. Even small, superficial wounds can change skin tone or form a scar if infection or re-injury occurs. Following the self-care guidelines on page 52 may help minimize these complications.

When a healing wound is exposed to sunlight, it can darken permanently. This darkening can be prevented by covering the area with clothing or sunblock with a sun protection factor (SPF) over 30 whenever you're outside during the first six months after the injury occurred.

A scar usually thickens about two months into the healing process. Within six months to a year, the scar tissue thins out.

Scar tissue that continues to enlarge is called a keloid. Surgical incisions, vaccinations, burns or even a scratch can cause keloids. The tendency to develop keloids is often inherited, and the darker the skin, the greater the likelihood of this happening.

Continued next page >

When was your last tetanus shot?

A cut, laceration, bite or other wound that penetrates the skin, even if minor, can lead to a tetanus infection. Tetanus is a serious bacterial disease caused by a toxin that leads to muscle stiffness, especially of the jaw muscles. Tetanus is sometimes called lockjaw.

Immunization is vital. The tetanus vaccine usually is given to children as part of the diphtheria, tetanus and acellular pertussis (DTaP) shot. Adults generally need a tetanus booster every 10 years.

If a wound is deep and dirty, your doctor may recommend an additional booster even if your last one was within 10 years. Boosters should be given within two days of the injury.

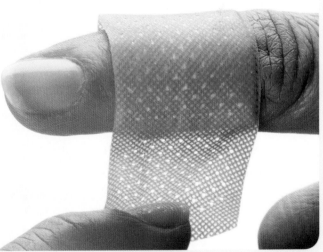

If you are the person treating a wound, it's important to have washed your hands with soap and water or an alcohol-based hand sanitizer beforehand to help avoid infection or other complications. The following guidelines can help you care for simple wounds:

Stop the bleeding

Minor cuts and scrapes usually stop bleeding on their own. If not, apply gentle pressure with a clean cloth or bandage.

Keep the wound clean

Rinse the wound with clear water. Clean the area around the wound with soap and a washcloth. Keep soap out of the wound, as it can cause irritation.

If dirt or debris remains in the wound after washing, use tweezers cleaned with alcohol to remove the particles. If debris still remains embedded in the wound, don't attempt to remove it by yourself – contact your doctor.

Thorough wound cleaning reduces the risk of infection and tetanus. There's no need to use hydrogen peroxide, iodine or an iodine-containing cleanser, which can be irritating to injured tissue.

Consider the source

Puncture wounds or other deep cuts, animal bites or particularly dirty wounds put you at higher risk of infections, including tetanus. If the wound is serious, you may require antibiotics or an additional tetanus booster (see page 51).

Prevent infection

After cleaning the wound, if desired, you can apply a thin layer of an antibiotic cream, such as Neosporin or Polysporin. These products don't make the wound heal faster, but they can discourage infection and allow the wound to close more efficiently. Certain ingredients in some ointments may cause a mild rash in some people. If a rash appears, stop using the ointment.

Cover the wound

Exposure to air will speed healing, but bandages can help keep the wound clean, keep harmful bacteria out and protect the wound from additional irritation. Blisters that are opened and draining are vulnerable to infection and should be covered until a scab forms.

Change the dressing

Change the bandage at least once a day or whenever it becomes wet or dirty to help prevent infection. If you're allergic to tape adhesive, switch to sterile gauze and paper tape or pressure netting. These supplies generally are available at pharmacies and drug stores.

✚ Medical Help

If bleeding persists — if blood spurts or continues to flow after several minutes of direct pressure — emergency care is necessary. Are stitches needed? A deep, gaping or jagged-edged wound with exposed fat or muscle will require stitches to hold it together. Was this an animal bite? Seek medical care.

Dandruff

Dandruff is a chronic scalp condition, marked by intensive itching and flaking skin on your scalp. Although dandruff isn't contagious and is rarely serious, it can be embarrassing.

The causes of dandruff are many, including dry skin, irritated and oily skin (seborrheic dermatitis), psoriasis, eczema, a yeast-like fungus called malassezia, not shampooing enough, and scalp sensitivity to hair care products (contact dermatitis).

Babies get dandruff too

A type of dandruff called cradle cap can affect babies. This disorder, which causes a scaling, crusty scalp, is most common in newborns, but it can occur anytime during infancy. Although it can be alarming for parents, cradle cap isn't dangerous and usually clears up on its own by the time a baby is a year old. To treat cradle cap:

- Gently rub your baby's scalp with your fingers or rough washcloth to loosen the scales.
- Wash your baby's hair once a day with mild baby shampoo.
- If the scales don't loosen easily, rub petroleum jelly or a few drops of mineral oil onto your baby's scalp. Let it soak into the scales for a few minutes, and then brush and shampoo your baby's hair as usual. If you leave the oil in your baby's hair, the scales may accumulate and worsen the cradle cap.

♠ Home Remedies

To treat dandruff:

- *Shampoo regularly.* Start with a mild, nonmedicated shampoo. Gently massage your scalp to loosen flakes. Rinse thoroughly.
- *Use medicated shampoo for stubborn cases.* Look for shampoos containing zinc pyrithione, salicylic acid, coal tar or selenium sulfide in brands such as Head & Shoulders, Neutrogena T/Sal or T/Gel, Denorex or Selsun Blue. The medicated shampoo Nizoral 1% is intended to kill dandruff-causing fungi that live on your scalp. This shampoo is available over-the-counter or by prescription.
- *If you use tar-based shampoos, use them carefully.* These products can leave a brownish stain on light-colored or gray hair and make the scalp more sensitive to sunlight.
- *Cut back on styling products.* Hair sprays, styling gels, mousses and hair waxes can all build up on your hair and scalp, making them oilier.
- *Eat a healthy diet.* A diet that provides enough zinc, B vitamins and certain types of fats may help prevent dandruff.
- *Get a little sun.* Sunlight may be good for dandruff. But because exposure to ultraviolet light damages your skin and increases your risk of skin cancer, don't sunbathe. Instead, just spend a little time outdoors. And be sure to wear sunscreen on your face and body.
- *Try tea tree oil.* This herbal product seems to reduce dandruff. The oil comes from the leaves of the Australian tea tree and has been used for centuries as an antiseptic, antibiotic and antifungal agent. It's now included in some shampoos found in natural foods stores. The oil may cause allergic reactions in some people.

✚ Medical Help

If dandruff persists or your scalp becomes irritated or severely itchy, you may need a prescription shampoo, or you may have some other skin condition. See your doctor.

Depression

Many people experience the blues from time to time — a period of several days or a week in which you seem to be in a funk. This feeling usually goes away, and you're able to regain your normal outlook on life.

Having the blues isn't the same as having depression. While the blues are temporary, depression is not something you simply "snap out" of. Depression is a chronic illness that can lead to a variety of serious emotional and physical problems. It typically requires long-term treatment, involving medications and psychological counseling.

If you're depressed, you may find little, if any, joy in life. You may have no energy, feel unworthy or guilty for no reason, find it difficult to concentrate, and become irritable. You might wake up after only a few hours of sleep or experience changes in your appetite — eating either too little or too much. You may experience a sense of hopelessness and deep anxiety, or even feel as if life isn't worth living.

Depression or the blues?

Signs of depression	Signs of the blues
• Persistent lack of energy • Lasting sadness • Irritability and mood swings • Recurring sense of hopelessness • Continual negative view of the world and of others • Overeating or loss of appetite • Feelings of unworthiness or guilt • Inability to concentrate • Recurrent early morning awakening or other changes in sleep patterns • Inability to enjoy pleasurable activities • Feeling as though you'd be better off dead	• Feeling down for several days but still able to function normally in daily activities • Occasional lack of energy, or a mild change in sleeping patterns • Ability to enjoy some recreational activities • Stable weight • Quickly passing sense of hopelessness

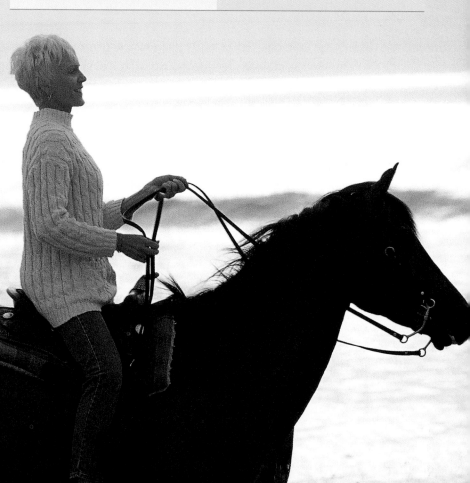

To help ease depression, try these tips:

- *Share your feelings.* Talk to a trusted friend, partner, family member or spiritual counselor. He or she can offer support, guidance and perspective.
- *Spend time with other people.* Social interaction generally is good, but make sure to spend your time with positive people, not those who may make your symptoms worse.
- *Do things you enjoy.* Engage in activities that have interested you in the past, but also don't be afraid to try something new.
- *Exercise regularly.* Physical activity can reduce the symptoms of depression. Consider walking, jogging, swimming, gardening or taking on active projects that you enjoy.
- *Avoid alcohol and illicit drugs.* It may seem like alcohol or drugs lessen symptoms of depression, but in the long run they generally make them worse and make your condition that much harder to treat.
- *Get plenty of sleep.* A good night's sleep is especially important when you're depressed. If you're having trouble sleeping, talk to your doctor about what you can do.
- *Don't take on too much responsibilty all at once.* If you have large tasks, divide them into smaller ones. Set simple goals you can accomplish.
- *Look for opportunities to be helpful.* You feel better about yourself when you can help others, even in a small way.

St. John's wort

Studies suggest that St. John's wort may be beneficial in treating mild to moderate depression, but not major depression. The greatest concern with using this herb is the potential for serious interactions with other medications. Don't take this herb if you take prescription medications.

SAMe

SAMe occurs naturally in the human body, and a synthetic version of the compound is a popular dietary supplement in the United States. Studies indicate SAMe may be effective for treating depression in some individuals.

Omega-3 fatty acids

Eating a diet rich in omega-3s or taking omega-3 supplements may help ease depression, along with providing other health benefits. These healthy fats are found in certain foods, such as cold-water fish, flaxseed, flax oil and walnuts.

Relaxation therapies

A number of relaxation therapies may help relieve some symptoms of depression by helping you deal with stress and anxiety — conditions that can heighten depression. These therapies include massage, yoga, meditation, relaxed breathing and self-expression through music and art.

➕ Medical Help

If depressive symptoms last more than a few weeks, or if you're feeling hopeless or suicidal, it's important to seek help. For many people, the most effective treatment is a combination of therapies. Contact your family doctor or ask for a referral to a psychiatrist, who is trained as a medical doctor and can help you find out if a medical illness might be contributing to your symptoms. If your symptoms are mild but persistent, a psychologist may be helpful. Psychologists are trained in psychotherapy, which is effective in treating both depression and anxiety.

Diabetes

Diabetes (diabetes mellitus) is a disease that affects the way your body uses blood sugar, or blood glucose — which is your body's main source of energy.

Your body breaks down the food you eat and converts it into glucose, which is absorbed into the bloodstream. Insulin,which is made by the pancreas, helps move the glucose from the bloodstream into your cells, where it's burned for energy. If you have diabetes, your body produces little or no insulin. Or, the insulin doesn't work very well, so too much glucose remains in your blood.

The most common forms of diabetes are known as type 1 and type 2. Other forms include gestational diabetes, which can occur during pregnancy.

Type 1 vs. type 2

Type 1 diabetes is an autoimmune disease. Your own immune system attacks your pancreas, destroying cells, so little if any insulin is made. Without insulin to help move glucose into your cells, glucose stays in your bloodstream. Daily insulin shots are needed. The disease most often develops when you're young, although adults also can develop type 1 diabetes.

Type 2 diabetes is by far the most common form of the disease. Your pancreas may make some insulin, but your cells become resistant to it, so too much glucose stays in your bloodstream. Being overweight makes it harder for your body to use insulin. Type 2 diabetes usually develops in adults, but as more children and teens become overweight, the incidence of type 2 diabetes is increasing.

What's prediabetes?

Prediabetes means that your blood glucose level is higher than normal but not high enough for you to be diagnosed with type 2 diabetes. Long-term damage associated with diabetes — especially to your heart and blood vessels — may already be starting if you have prediabetes.

But you can prevent or delay type 2 diabetes by making healthy changes to your lifestyle. In a major study on diabetes prevention, those in the lifestyle-treatment group (who ate a healthy diet and engaged in moderately intense physical activity) cut their risk of diabetes in half.

Diabetes warning signs

Often, prediabetes has no signs or symptoms, so it's important to know your blood glucose level. Watch for two classic signs of diabetes:
- Excessive thirst
- Frequent urination

Other signs and symptoms may include:
- Constant hunger
- Unexplained weight loss
- Weight gain (more common in type 2)
- Flu-like symptoms, including weakness and fatigue
- Blurred vision
- Slow-healing cuts or sores
- Tingling or loss of feeling in the hands and feet
- Recurring infections of gums and skin
- Recurring vaginal or bladder infections

If you want to play an active role in your health, take control of your diabetes with these steps:

Exercise

Regular physical activity and exercise is essential to lowering your blood glucose level and improving your body's ability to use insulin or other diabetes medications. Getting plenty of exercise may even reduce the amount of diabetes medication you need to take.

In addition, taking part in regular physical activity and exercise helps promote weight loss, improves blood circulation, lowers risk of heart disease and reduces stress.

You can become more physically active in many small ways, such as taking the stairs instead of the elevator. Learn how to avoid blood glucose problems while exercising. Before you start a fitness program, discuss precautions you may need to take with your doctor.

Monitor your blood sugar

Good management of your blood glucose level is key to feeling your best and preventing the complications of diabetes. Knowing how often and when to test your blood glucose will depend on which type of diabetes you have and on your treatment plan. If you have type 1 diabetes and take insulin, test your blood glucose at least twice a day. Your doctor may advise testing more often.

If you have type 2 diabetes and don't need insulin, test your blood glucose as often as needed to be sure it's under control. This can mean daily testing or twice a week. Discuss the schedule with your doctor.

Eat healthy foods

Follow these basic tips:

- *Stick to a schedule.* Eat three meals a day. Be consistent in the amount of food you eat and the timing of your meals. If you're hungry after dinner, choose a food low in calories or carbohydrates before going to bed, such as raw vegetables.
- *Focus on fiber.* Eat a variety of fresh fruits, vegetables, legumes and whole-grain foods. These high-fiber foods help control blood glucose and are low in fat and rich sources of vitamins and minerals.
- *Limit foods that are high in saturated and trans fat.* Choose lean cuts of meat and use low-fat or fat-free dairy products. Use small amounts of healthy oils and trans fat-free spreads instead of shortening and butter.
- *Choose proteins low in saturated fat.* If you eat too much protein, your body stores the extra calories as fat. Choose fish and poultry more often than red meat.
- *Eat fewer sweets.* Candy, cookies and other sweets aren't forbidden but they're often high in fat and calories. Count them in your total carbohydrate intake.

Lose weight

Being overweight is by far the greatest risk factor for type 2 diabetes. If you're overweight, losing even a few pounds can improve your blood glucose level.

Continued next page >

Diabetes requires expert care. If you think you may have diabetes, see your doctor. Also see a doctor if you have diabetes and your symptoms seem to be worsening.

Diabetes and your feet

Good foot care is essential if you have diabetes. Diabetes can impair blood flow to your feet and cause severe nerve damage. Left untreated, minor foot injuries can quickly develop into open sores (ulcers) that may be difficult to treat — even leading to tissue death (gangrene). Put your best foot forward with these simple foot-care tips:

- *Wash your feet daily.* Wash your feet in lukewarm water once a day. Dry them gently, especially between the toes. Sprinkle talcum powder or cornstarch between your toes to keep the skin dry. Use a moisturizing cream or lotion on the tops and bottoms of your feet to keep the skin supple and soft.
- *Inspect your feet daily.* Check your feet for blisters, cuts, sores, redness or swelling once a day. If you have trouble bending over, use a hand mirror to inspect the bottoms of your feet, or ask someone to help you.
- *Trim your toenails carefully.* Trim your nails straight across. If you have any nail problems or numbness in your feet, ask your doctor about profes- sional nail trimming.
- *Don't go barefoot.* Protect your feet from injury with comfortable socks and shoes, even indoors. Make sure new shoes fit well, too. Even a single blister can lead to an infection that won't heal.
- *Wear clean, dry socks.* Wear socks made of fibers that pull (wick) sweat away from your skin, such as cotton and special acrylic fibers — not nylon. Avoid socks with tight elastic bands that reduce circulation or that are thick or bulky. Bulky socks often fit poorly, and a poor fit can irritate your skin.
- *Use foot products cautiously.* Don't use a file or scissors on calluses, corns or bunions. You can injure your feet that way. Also, don't put chemicals on your feet, such as wart removers. See your doctor or foot specialist (podia- trist) for problem calluses, corns, bunions or warts.
- *Don't smoke or use other types of tobacco.* Smoking reduces blood flow to your feet. Talk to your doctor about ways to quit smoking or to stop using other types of tobacco.
- *Schedule regular foot checkups.* Your doctor can inspect your feet for early signs of nerve damage, poor circulation or other foot problems. You may be referred to a podiatrist.
- *Take foot injuries seriously.* Contact your doctor if you have a sore or other foot problem that doesn't begin to heal within a few days. Your doctor may prescribe antibiotics to treat infection. In other cases, infected tissue may be drained or removed. Sometimes, surgery is needed to remove infected bone or increase blood flow to the affected area.

Diaper rash

Diaper rash causes reddish, puffy, irritated skin in the diaper area. The rash generally is caused by a combination of moisture, acid in urine or stool, and chafing of diaper fabric on your baby's skin. Some babies also get a rash from the detergent used to launder cloth diapers, or from plastic pants, elastic, or certain types of disposable diapers and wipes. Sometimes a yeast infection may be the cause of rash.

Diaper rash may alarm parents and irritate babies, but most occurrences can be resolved with simple at-home treatments.

Cloth or disposable diapers?

Many parents wonder about which kind of diaper to use for their babies. When it comes to preventing diaper rash, there's no compelling evidence that cloth diapers are better than disposable ones or vice versa, although disposables may keep baby's skin slightly drier. Because there's no clearcut "best" diaper, use whatever works best for you and your baby. If one brand of disposable diaper seems to irritate your baby's skin, then try out another brand.

🏠 Home Remedies

To treat or prevent diaper rash:

- Change your baby's diapers frequently to minimize the exposure of sensitive skin to urine and stool.
- If using cloth diapers, use softened water for washing and rinsing and make sure that all the detergent is rinsed out.
- Wash and pat the skin dry at each diaper change, using plain water or a mild soap and water.
- Apply a thin barrier of cream or ointment. Various diaper rash medications are available without a prescription. Talk to your doctor or pharmacist for specific recommendations. Some popular over-the-counter creams, including Balmex and Desitin, contain zinc oxide as the active ingredient. These products are usually applied in a thin layer to the irritated region throughout the day to soothe and protect the skin. Zinc oxide products can also be used on healthy skin to prevent diaper rash.
- Allow your child to go without a diaper for short periods of time. Exposing skin to air is a natural and gentle way to let it dry. To avoid messy accidents, try laying your baby on a large towel and engage in some playtime while he or she is bare-bottomed.
- Try switching to a different brand if you use disposable diapers.
- Avoid diaper wipes because many contain perfume and alcohol. Use a washcloth with plain water instead.

➕ Medical Help

See your doctor if the above tips don't help, if the rash is crusty, blistered or weepy, or if your baby has a fever.

Diarrhea

Diarrhea is loose, watery stools, often accompanied by abdominal cramps. You also may notice abdominal pain and other flu-like signs and symptoms, such as low-grade fever, achy or cramping muscles, and headache.

The most common cause is a viral infection of the digestive tract. Bacteria and parasites also can cause diarrhea, sometimes with bloody stools and high fever. Infection-induced diarrhea can be extremely contagious. Nausea and vomiting may precede it.

Diarrhea also can be a sign of irritable bowel syndrome or lactose intolerance. It can be a side effect of many medications, particularly antibiotics, or from the use of products made with artificial sweeteners, such as sorbitol and mannitol.

Acute diarrhea is something that nearly everyone experiences at some time, and it usually clears up within days. Chronic diarrhea generally lasts longer than four weeks and may signal a serious underlying medical problem such as chronic infection, inflammatory bowel disease, microscopic colitis or certain kinds of cancer.

🏠 Home Remedies

Diarrhea caused by infections typically clears on its own without medications. Over-the-counter anti-diarrheal products, such as Imodium A-D, Pepto Bismol and Kaopectate, may slow bowel movements, but won't speed recovery. Focus your attention on preventing dehydration and easing the symptoms of diarrhea as you recover:

- Drink plenty of clear liquids, including water, clear sodas (caffeine-free), broths and weak tea.
- Add semisolid and low-fiber foods gradually as your bowel movements return to normal. Try soda crackers, toast, eggs, rice or chicken.
- Avoid eating dairy products, fatty foods or highly seasoned foods for a few days.
- Avoid caffeine, alcohol and nicotine.

Probiotics

Probiotics can help maintain a proper microorganic balance in your intestinal tract. Food sources of probiotics include yogurt, miso, tempeh and some juices and soy drinks. Probiotic supplements may help manage diarrhea, especially following treatment with antibiotics.

Diarrhea in infants

Diarrhea in infants should be closely monitored. Contact your doctor if diarrhea persists for more than 12 hours and if your child:

- Hasn't had a wet diaper in eight hours
- Has a temperature of more than 102 F
- Has bloody stools
- Has a dry mouth or cries without tears
- Is unusually sleepy, drowsy or unresponsive

✚ Medical Help

Contact your doctor if diarrhea persists for more than a week, or if you become dehydrated or see traces of blood in your stool or in the toilet bowl. Also seek medical attention if you have severe abdominal or rectal pain, a temperature of more than 101 F, or signs of dehydration despite drinking fluids. Your doctor may prescribe antibiotics for diarrhea caused by some bacteria and parasites. However, not all bacterial diarrhea requires treatment with antibiotics, and antibiotics don't help viral diarrhea.

Dizziness

Lightheadedness, weakness, loss of balance, faintness, wooziness and unsteadiness on your feet are signs and symptoms associated with dizziness. You may feel that you or your surroundings are rotating — a condition known as vertigo. You may need to support yourself or hold on to something to maintain your balance.

Dizziness is one of the most common reasons why people visit their doctors. Although it may be disabling, dizziness rarely signals a serious, life-threatening condition. Treatment depends on the cause and on your symptoms, but it's usually effective.

Fainting is a sudden, brief loss of consciousness that may accompany dizziness. Fainting may be caused by a variety of medical disorders, including heart disease, severe coughing spells and circulatory problems. It may also be related to:

- Blood pressure and heart rhythm medications
- Excessive sweating, vomiting or diarrhea causing fluid loss
- Upsetting news or sights
- Rapid drop in blood pressure, for example, when you stand quickly from a sitting or reclining position

🏠 Home Remedies

If you feel faint or dizzy, find a safe place to lie down or sit down. If you lie down, elevate your legs slightly to return blood to your heart. If you can't lie down, then sit leaning forward and put your head between your knees.

Prevention of dizziness

- Stand and change positions slowly — particularly when turning from side to side or when changing from lying down to standing up. Before standing up in the morning, sit on the edge of the bed for a minute or two.
- Pace yourself. Take breaks when you are active in heat and humidity.
- Dress appropriate to weather conditions to avoid overheating.
- Drink enough fluids to avoid dehydration. Aim to drink at least 48 to 64 ounces a day, unless your doctor tells you to limit fluids.
- Avoid caffeine, alcohol, smoking and tobacco products. Excessive use of these substances can restrict your blood vessels and worsen signs and symptoms of dizziness.
- Don't drive a car or operate dangerous equipment if you feel dizzy.
- Check your medications. Your doctor may need to adjust your prescriptions.

➕ Medical Help

Seek medical care if symptoms of dizziness persist for weeks or become severe. Seek emergency care for fainting or when dizziness is accompanied by symptoms such as pain in the chest or head, trouble with breathing, numbness or continuing weakness or paralysis, irregular heartbeat, confusion, decreased responsiveness, memory loss, seizure, trouble talking, problems with vision or coordination, blood in stools (sometimes indicated by black tarry stools) or other signs of blood loss, or nausea or vomiting.

Dry eyes

Healthy eyes are continuously covered by a thin layer of fluid — a tear film that remains stable between the blinks of your eyelids. The tear film lubricates the eyes and helps maintain clear vision.

Dry eyes occur when the tear film is destabilized, often due to decreased fluid production from your tear glands. This allows dry spots to form on the surface of your eyes. Poor tear quality can also cause dry eyes.

Dry eyes are a common source of discomfort. The condition usually affects both eyes, especially in women after menopause. Some drugs — such as antihistamines, sleep medications and some high blood pressure medications — also can cause dry eyes or make them worse.

Signs and symptoms of dry eyes may include:

- Stinging, burning or scratchy sensations
- Stringy mucus in or around your eyes
- Increased eye irritation from smoke or wind
- Eye fatigue after short periods of reading
- Sensitivity to light
- Difficulty wearing contact lenses
- Tearing
- Blurred vision, often worsening at the end of the day

♠ Home Remedies

To help reduce dryness in your eyes:

- Try over-the-counter artificial tears that don't contain a redness remover (these may worsen symptoms). If you're sensitive to preservatives, try single-use preservative-free lubricants. If your eyes are dry overnight, use a gel-type lubricant at bedtime. Ask your doctor which option might work best for you.
- Avoid air blowing in your eyes. Don't direct hair dryers, car heaters, air conditioners or fans toward your eyes.
- Consciously blinking repeatedly helps spread your tears more evenly across the surface of your eyes.
- Avoid rubbing your eyes.
- Wear glasses on windy days and goggles while swimming.
- Add moisture to the air. In winter, a humidifier can improve the dry indoor air. Some people use specially designed glasses that form a moisture chamber around the eye, creating additional humidity.
- Don't smoke and avoid secondhand smoke. Avoid all types of smoke, even the type from a fireplace or burning leaves.

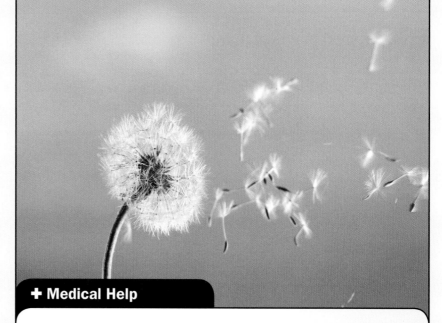

✛ Medical Help

Seek medical care if the condition continues despite self-care efforts. Your doctor may prescribe a medication for chronic dry eyes or refer you to a specialist if needed.

Dry mouth

Saliva is a clear liquid mixture that moistens your mouth and helps with digestion. It's produced in your salivary glands. When there's a lack of saliva, your mouth feels dry and the saliva seems thick and stringy. Your lips crack, and splits in the skin appear at the corners of your mouth. A sore throat may develop, and you may have difficulty speaking and swallowing.

Dry mouth may seem like little more than a nuisance, but it can have a very negative impact on your enjoyment of food and the health of your teeth. The medical term for dry mouth is xerostomia.

Without enough saliva, the food in your mouth will seem dry and difficult to swallow. You won't be able to taste properly because of a dry tongue. In addition, there are enzymes in saliva that aid in digestion. Saliva also helps prevent tooth decay by limiting the growth of bacteria and washing away food and plaque.

Although the treatment of dry mouth depends on the cause, it's often a side effect of medication. Dry mouth is also more common as you age.

♠ Home Remedies

If the cause of dry mouth either can't be determined or can't be resolved, the following tips may help improve your symptoms and keep your teeth healthy:

- Chewing sugar-free gum or sucking on sugar-free hard candies helps stimulate saliva production.
- Limit your caffeine intake. Caffeine can make your mouth drier.
- Avoid sugary or acidic foods and candies because they increase the risk of tooth decay.
- Brush with a fluoride toothpaste. Ask your dentist if you might benefit from prescription fluoride toothpaste.
- Use a fluoride rinse or brush-on fluoride gel before bedtime.
- Don't use a mouthwash that contains alcohol because this can make your mouth drier.
- Stop all tobacco use.
- Sip water regularly.
- Try over-the-counter saliva substitutes. Look for ones containing carboxymethyl cellulose or hydroxyethyl cellulose, such as Biotene Oral Balance.
- Avoid using over-the-counter antihistamines and decongestants because they can make symptoms worse.
- Breathe through your nose, not your mouth.
- Add moisture to the air at night with a room humidifier.

✚ Medical Help

If you've noticed persistent signs and symptoms of dry mouth, make an appointment with your family doctor or your dentist.

Dry skin

Dry skin is often a temporary or seasonal problem — one that you experience only in winter or summer, for example — but the problem may remain a lifelong concern. Patches of itchy, irritated skin announce its arrival.

Although your skin is often driest on your arms, lower legs and sides of your abdomen, the locations where these dry patches form can vary considerably from one person to the next.

Signs and symptoms of the condition will depend on your age, health status, living environment, the amount of time you spend outdoors, and the specific cause of your problem.

With dry skin, you may have one or more of the following:

- Sensation of skin tightness, especially after showering, bathing or swimming
- Skin that appears shrunken or dehydrated
- Skin that feels and looks rough rather than smooth
- Itching that sometimes may be intense

- Slight to severe flaking, scaling or peeling skin
- Fine lines or cracks in the skin
- Redness

Causes

Dry skin is caused primarily by your amount of exposure to certain environments, particularly when the air is dry and has low humidity. Common causes of dry skin include:

- *Weather.* In general, your skin is driest in the winter, when temperatures and humidity levels plummet. Winter conditions also tend to make many existing skin conditions worse. But the reverse may be true if you live in desert regions, where temperatures can soar but humidity levels remain low.
- *Interior heating and air conditioning.* Central heating and cooling systems, as well as wood-burning stoves, space heaters and fireplaces all reduce humidity and dry your skin.

- *Hot baths and showers.* Frequent cleaning and rinsing, especially if you like hot water and long soaks, breaks down the lipid barriers in your skin and dries you out. So does frequent swimming, particularly in chlorinated pools.
- *Harsh soaps and detergents.* Many popular soaps and detergents strip lipids and water from your skin. Deodorants and antibacterial soaps are usually the most damaging, as are many shampoos, which dry out your scalp.
- *Sun exposure.* Like any type of heat, the sun dries your skin. Yet damage from ultraviolet (UV) radiation penetrates far below the top layer of skin. The most significant damage occurs deep, where collagen and elastin fibers break down much more quickly than they should, leading to deep wrinkles and loose, sagging skin (solar elastosis). Sun-damaged skin may have the appearance of dry skin.

Consider this: It's more important to prevent moisture from leaving your skin than it is to try adding moisture back into your skin. Although it may not be possible to achieve flawless skin, the following measures can help keep it moist and healthy:

Moisturize your skin

Moisturizers form a seal over your skin that helps keep water from evaporating from its surface. Thicker moisturizers work best, such as over-the-counter brands Eucerin and Cetaphil. Also consider using cosmetics that contain moisturizers. If your skin is extremely dry, you may want to apply an oil, such as baby oil, while your skin is still moist. Oil has more staying power on the skin than moisturizers do.

Avoid harsh, drying soaps

If you have dry skin, it's best to use cleansing creams, gentle skin cleansers, and bath or shower gels with added moisturizers. Choose mild soaps that have added oils and fats, such as Neutrogena, Basis or Dove. Avoid deodorant and antibacterial detergents, which are especially harsh. You might want to experiment with several brands until you find one that works well for you. A good rule of thumb is that your skin should feel soft and smooth after cleansing, never tight or dry.

Limit bath time

Hot water and long showers or baths remove oils from your skin. Limit your bath or shower time to about 15 minutes or less, and use warm, rather than hot, water.

Moisturize after bathing

After washing or bathing, gently pat or blot your skin dry with a towel so that some moisture remains on the skin. Immediately moisturize your skin with an oil or cream to help trap water in the surface cells.

Use a humidifier

Hot, dry indoor air can parch sensitive skin and worsen itching and flaking. A portable home humidifier or one attached to your furnace adds moisture to the air inside your home. Choose a humidifier that meets your budget and special needs. Be sure to keep the humidifier clean to ward off bacteria and fungi growth.

Choose natural fabrics

Natural fibers such as cotton and silk allow your skin to breathe. Wool, although it certainly qualifies as natural, can irritate even normal skin. When you wash your clothes, try to use detergents without dyes or perfumes.

Suppress itching

If dry skin causes itching, apply cool compresses to the area. To reduce inflammation, use a non-prescription hydrocortisone cream or ointment, containing at least 1 percent hydrocortisone.

Most cases of dry skin respond well to lifestyle changes and home remedies. See your doctor if:
- Your skin doesn't improve in spite of your best efforts
- Dry skin is accompanied by redness
- Dryness and itching interfere with sleeping
- You have open sores or infections from scratching
- You have large areas of scaling or peeling skin

Ear infection

A middle ear infections (otitis media) is one of the most common conditions of early childhood. Studies show that 3 out of 4 children have had at least one middle ear infection by age 3. Many have multiple episodes. Though less common, adults also can get ear infections.

The condition often starts with a respiratory infection, such as a cold, which is caused by a virus. Colds may cause swelling and inflammation in the narrow passageways (eustachian tubes) that connect the middle ear to the nose. Inflammation may block one of the tubes completely, trapping fluid in the middle ear and causing infection.

Signs and symptoms include earache, feeling of blockage in the ear, fever of 100 F or higher, and temporary hearing loss. Children may tug or pull at their ears, cry more than usual, have trouble sleeping, and be unusually irritable. Clear discharge may drain from the ear.

Your doctor will examine your child and study the symptoms. Many cases of ear infection won't need treatment such as antibiotics. The next steps depend on many factors, including your child's age and medical history.

Before prescribing antibiotics, many doctors may recommend a wait-and-see approach for the first 72 hours, especially if the child has few symptoms. Most ear infections cause discomfort and worry but generally clear up on their own in just a few days.

Some doctors believe people who have a middle ear infection with discharge should also be given antibiotics. However, it's not universally agreed that the antibiotics are necessary or will work to prevent the infection.

If the medication is effective, your child should start feeling better in a few days. Be sure to take the antibiotic for the full length of the prescription. Remember, antibiotics won't help an infection caused by a virus — and the overuse of antibiotics contributes to strains of bacteria that resist the medications.

What about recurrent infections?

Many ear infections resolve on their own after about three days. However, some long-lasting or recurrent ear infections may lead to complications. Usually, fluid buildup from an ear infection disappears in a few weeks. But sometimes it remains in the middle ear for months, which can damage the eardrum and bones of the middle ear, causing long-term hearing loss.

Can you prevent ear infections?

Preventing ear infections is difficult, but these approaches may help reduce your child's risk:
- Breast-feed your baby for as long as possible.
- When bottle-feeding, hold your baby in an upright position.
- Avoid exposing your child to tobacco smoke.

- Keep immunizations up to date. Certain vaccines, such as the flu (influenza) vaccine, can reduce the risk of middle ear infections in your child.

Do children outgrow ear infections?

For many parents, coping with the ear infections of their young children is almost as routine as changing wet diapers. But most children stop having ear infections by age 4 or 5. As your child matures, the eustachian tubes become wider and more angled, making it harder for inflammation to block the passageway and easier for fluid to drain out of the ear. Although ear infections still may occur in adults, they probably won't develop as often.

To find relief from ear infections, try the following:

- *Over-the-counter medications.* If your child is uncomfortable, ask the doctor about using an over-the-counter pain reliever such as acetaminophen (Tylenol, others) or ibuprofen (Advil, Motrin, others). Use the correct dose for your child's age and weight. Don't give aspirin to children, due to the risk of Reye's syndrome — a rare but serious condition.

Giving over-the-counter cough or cold medications also isn't recommended for children age 2 and younger.

- *Warm compress.* It may help to place a warm, moist cloth over the affected ear.
- *Nonprescription eardrops with a local anesthetic.* The drops won't prevent or stop infection but may reduce pain. Don't use drops if there's drainage from the ear. To administer the eardrops, warm the bottle slightly in water and place the child safely on a flat surface (not in your arms or on your lap) with the infected ear up. Apply the eardrops and then insert a small cotton wick to help retain the drops.
- *Distractions.* When caring for your child, plan low-key activities, such as reading books aloud, singing or playing board games. And don't underestimate the benefits of some extra cuddling.

✚ Medical Help

Contact your child's doctor if pain lasts more than a day or so or it's associated with fever. About 80 percent of children's ear infections resolve on their own, without using antibiotics. But antibiotics may be used if your child is under 2 years old, has recurrent middle ear infections or has a high-risk medical condition. Keep immunizations up to date: Some may help reduce the risk of middle ear infections.

Ear ringing

Some people may hear a persistent ringing or buzzing sound in their ears when no other sounds are present. The noise, known as tinnitus, seems to originate in their heads and not come from their surroundings.

Although bothersome, tinnitus usually isn't a sign of something seriously wrong. The cause of the sound is often unknown. Sometimes, however, tinnitus may be treated if an underlying cause can be identified: Earwax buildup or a foreign object in the ear, infection or exposure to loud noise. The sound also may be caused by high doses of aspirin or large amounts of caffeine.

Persistent ringing in one or both ears may also be a symptom of a more serious ear disorder, particularly if it's accompanied by hearing loss or dizziness.

🏠 Home Remedies

Strategies to help you cope with a persistent ringing or buzzing sound in your ear include:

- If aspirin in high doses has been recommended to you, ask your doctor about alternatives. If you're taking aspirin on your own, try lower doses or another kind of over-the-counter pain medication.
- Avoid nicotine, caffeine and alcohol, which may aggravate the condition.
- Manage stress. Stress can make tinnitus worse. Stress management, whether through relaxation therapy, biofeedback or exercise, may provide some relief.
- Try to determine a cause for the tinnitus, such as exposure to loud noise, and avoid the cause, if possible.
- Wear earplugs or some form of hearing protection when you're exposed to loud noise, such as when you're working with yard equipment (snow blower, leaf blower, lawn mower or power tools).
- Some people benefit from covering up the ringing sound with another, more acceptable sound, such as soft music or listening to a radio as you fall asleep.
- Some people may benefit by wearing a masker, a device that fits in the ear and produces white noise that masks the ringing.

➕ Medical Help

If ringing in your ear gets worse, persists or is accompanied by hearing loss or dizziness, consider getting a full evaluation from your doctor. The doctor may pursue further testing. Although most causes of tinnitus are benign and not life-threatening, it can be a difficult and frustrating condition to treat.

Earwax blockage

Earwax is part of your body's natural defenses. It helps protect the ear canal by trapping dirt and slowing the growth of bacteria. At times, though, blockage of the ear canal occurs if you produce too much earwax or a buildup of earwax becomes too hard to wash away naturally. This may give you an earache or feeling of fullness in the affected ear, or cause ear noise (tinnitus).

Note of caution

The safest way to have earwax removed is to have it done by your doctor. Your ear canal and eardrum are extremely delicate structures that can be damaged easily. Don't poke them with objects such as cotton swabs, paper clips or bobby pins, especially if you've had ear surgery, have a hole in your eardrum, or are having ear pain or drainage. These objects may push the wax deeper, damaging the ear canal lining and eardrum.

Flushing wax out of the ears should be avoided if you've had an eardrum perforation or ear surgery, unless your doctor approves. If infection is a concern, don't flush your ears.

Some people use ear candling, a technique that involves placing a lighted, hollow, cone-shaped candle into the ear, to remove earwax. This procedure doesn't work and may cause additional injury, such as burns or perforations.

🏠 Home Remedies

If you think you may have earwax blockage — and your eardrum doesn't contain a tube or have a hole (perforation) in it — this procedure may help you remove excess earwax:

- Soften the earwax by applying a few drops of baby oil, mineral oil or glycerin with an eyedropper twice a day, for no more than four to five days.
- When the wax is softened, fill a bowl with water heated to body temperature. If the water is colder or hotter, it may make you feel dizzy during the procedure.
- With your head upright, grasp the top of your ear and pull upward. With your other hand, squirt the water gently into your ear canal with a 3-ounce rubber-bulb syringe. Then, tilt your head and drain the water into the bowl or sink.
- You may need to repeat this process several times before the extra wax falls out.
- Gently dry your outer ear with a towel or a hand-held hair dryer. Earwax removal kits sold in stores can be effective. If you're unsure which one is right for you, ask your doctor.

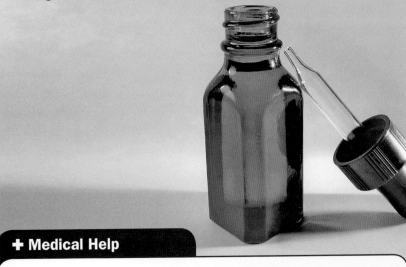

➕ Medical Help

Many people have difficulty washing wax out of their ears, even after following the procedure described above. Asking your doctor to remove earwax may seem unnecessary, but excess earwax can damage your eardrum. Your doctor can remove the excess wax safely and effectively using a similar procedure.

Eczema

The terms *eczema* and *dermatitis* are both used to describe inflammation of the skin. The condition occurs in many forms but usually involves patches of dry, swollen, reddened and itchy skin. Patches may thicken and develop blisters or weeping sores in severe cases.

The skin inflammation can make you feel uncomfortable and self-conscious, but it's generally not life-threatening or contagious.

Contact dermatitis results from the direct contact of skin with an irritant, which includes poison ivy, rubber, metals, jewelry, perfume and cosmetics.

Neurodermatitis can occur when something such as a tight garment rubs or scratches (or causes you to scratch) your skin.

Seborrheic dermatitis (known as cradle cap in infants) appears on the scalp and face as itchy dandruff or areas of greasy scales.

Stasis dermatitis may cause the skin at your ankles to discolor, thicken and itch. This condition can lead to infection.

Atopic dermatitis causes itchy, thickened, cracking skin, most often in the folds of the elbows or backs of the knees. It frequently runs in families and is often associated with allergies.

♠ Home Remedies

To relieve symptoms of eczema and prevent the condition from worsening:

- *Try to identify and avoid triggers.* Irritants may include rapid changes of temperature, sweating and stress. Some people should avoid direct contact with wool products, such as rugs, bedding and clothes, as well as harsh soaps and detergents.
- *Apply an anti-itch cream or calamine lotion to the affected area.* A nonprescription hydrocortisone cream, containing at least 1 percent hydrocortisone, can temporarily relieve itching. A nonprescription oral antihistamine (Benadryl, others), may be helpful if the itching is severe.
- *Avoid scratching whenever possible.* Cover the itchy area if you can't keep from scratching it. Trim nails and wear gloves at night.
- *Apply cool, wet compresses.* Covering the area with bandages and dressings can help protect the skin and prevent scratching.
- *Take a warm bath.* Sprinkle the bath water with baking soda, uncooked oatmeal or colloidal oatmeal — a finely ground oatmeal made for the bathtub (Aveeno, others). Or add 1/2 cup of bleach to a 40 gallon bathtub filled with warm water. The diluted bleach bath is thought to kill bacteria that grow on the skin.
- *Choose mild soaps without dyes or perfumes.* Be sure to rinse the soap completely off your body.
- *Moisturize your skin.* Use an oil or cream to seal in moisture while your skin is still damp from a bath or shower. If your skin is already dry, consider using a lubricating cream.
- *Use a humidifier.* Hot, dry indoor air can parch sensitive skin and worsen itching and flaking. A portable home humidifier or one attached to your furnace adds moisture to the air inside your home.
- *Wear cool, smooth-textured cotton clothing.* Avoid clothing that's rough, tight, scratchy or made from wool.

✚ Medical Help

See your doctor if:

- You're so uncomfortable that you're losing sleep or distracted from your daily routines
- Your skin is painful
- You suspect your skin is infected
- You've tried self-care steps without success

Elbow pain

Most elbow pain results from overuse injuries, often from activities requiring repetitive hand, wrist or arm movements.

- *Bursitis and tendinitis* are common sources of pain in your elbow. Bursitis may produce a small, egg-shaped, fluid-filled sac at the tip of your elbow. Keep pressure off the elbow, such as using a soft foam elbow pad.
- *Dislocated elbow* occurs when the ends of the joint bones are forced from their natural positions. Dislocation is very painful and severely limits movement.
- *Hyperextended elbow* occurs when your elbow is pushed beyond its normal range of motion, often as a result of a fall or misplay during the swing of a racket or bat.
- *Tennis elbow and golfer's elbow* are two similar conditions. Tennis elbow affects the outer side of your elbow, while golfer's elbow affects the inner side. Common causes include swinging a racket or club, pitching a baseball, painting, using a screwdriver or hammer, raking, typing, or any movement requiring twisting arm motions or repetitive gripping.

🏠 Home Remedies

If pain and swelling occurs in your elbow and in the tissues beneath your elbow, try these tips:

- *Practice R.I.C.E.* (see page 157). Support your elbow with a splint or sling for a few days.
- *Take an anti-inflammatory medication.* It may take six to 12 weeks of treatment for the pain to disappear.

Pain prevention while participating in sports

- *Use proper technique.* Ask a trainer to review your technique to see if you're using the proper motion.
- *Warm up.* Prepare for repetitive work-related tasks by participating in fitness and strengthening routines. Gently stretch the forearm muscles before and after use.
- *Get in shape.* Prepare for any sport with appropriate preseason conditioning. Do strengthening exercises with a hand weight by flexing and extending the wrists.
- *Try support bands.* Wear forearm support bands just below your elbow.
- *Heat up.* Try applying a warm pack for five minutes before activity and an ice pack after heavy use.
- *Lift properly.* When lifting anything — including free weights — keep your wrist rigid and stable to reduce the force transmitted to your elbow.

➕ Medical Help

If the pain hasn't improved in a day or two, or your elbow is hot and inflamed and you have a fever, see your doctor. Seek medical care immediately if:

- Your elbow seems deformed, or dislocated
- The area around your elbow is very sensitive to pressure
- Your arm or hand becomes numb
- Your elbow is very stiff and has limited range of motion after a fall
- The pain in your arm is severe

Enlarged prostate gland

The prostate is a walnut-sized gland in males, tucked beneath the bladder, which produces semen. Testosterone, the male sex hormone, causes the prostate to enlarge as men get older.

As the prostate enlarges, some men develop bothersome urinary symptoms. Untreated prostate gland enlargement can block the flow of urine out of the bladder and can cause bladder, urinary tract or kidney problems.

Signs and symptoms of an enlarged prostate gland (benign prostatic hyperplasia, or BPH) may include a weak or slow urine stream, trouble starting urination, stopping and starting during urination, dribbling at the end of urination, frequent and sometimes urgent need to urinate, frequent nighttime urination, and not being able to completely empty the bladder.

Having an enlarged prostate doesn't necessarily mean your symptoms will get worse. Only about half the men with prostate gland enlargement have symptoms that become noticeable or bothersome enough for them to seek medical treatment. In some men, symptoms eventually stabilize and may even improve over time.

♠ Home Remedies

Lifestyle changes can often help control the symptoms of an enlarged prostate and prevent your condition from getting worse.

- Avoid drinking fluids an hour or two before bedtime.
- Limit your intake of caffeine and alcohol.
- When you first feel the urge to urinate, go. Waiting too long may damage your bladder muscle.
- Schedule bathroom visits. Try to urinate regularly during the day, such as every four to six hours.
- Keep moving. Even a small amount of physical activity can help reduce urinary problems caused by an enlarged prostate.
- Limit decongestants or antihistamines. These drugs tighten the band of muscles around your urethra that controls urine flow, which makes it harder to urinate.
- Consider saw palmetto. In some men, this herb may be an effective treatment for managing mild to moderate symptoms. (However, some studies have not found the herb to be effective.) Because saw palmetto is generally safe, it doesn't hurt to give it a try.

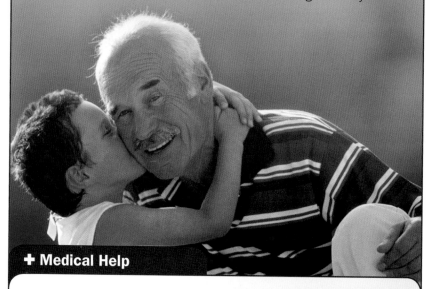

✛ Medical Help

If you're having urinary problems, it's best to see your doctor for an evaluation. If your symptoms aren't too burdensome, self-care measures may be all you need. If self-care measures don't work, you may benefit from prescription medications that shrink the prostate gland or improve urine flow. Surgery can reduce the size of the prostate.

Eye scratch

The most common types of eye injury involve the cornea — the clear, protective dome of tissue that covers the iris and pupil at the front of the eye. The cornea can be scratched when it comes in contact with dirt, sand, wood shavings, metal particles or even the edge of a piece of paper.

Usually the scratch is superficial, and this is called a corneal abrasion. Everyday activities may lead to abrasions, for example, getting a wood chip caught in your eye while doing home repairs, or being scratched by a child who accidentally brushes your cornea with a fingernail.

Because the cornea is extremely sensitive, an abrasion can be painful. A scratched cornea might make you feel like you have sand and grit in your eye. You may also have tears, blurred vision, light sensitivity, and redness in and around the eye.

Some corneal abrasions become infected and result in a corneal ulcer, which is a serious problem. Abrasions that are caused by plant matter, such as a pine needle, can cause a delayed inflammation that develops inside the eye.

🏠 Home Remedies

Immediate steps you may take to treat a corneal abrasion include:

- *Rinse your eye with clean water (use a saline solution, if available).* You can use an eyecup or small, clean drinking glass positioned with its rim resting on the bone at the base of your eye socket. If your work site has an eye-rinse station, use it. Rinsing the eye may wash out a foreign object.
- *Blink several times.* This movement may remove small particles of dust or sand.
- *Pull the upper eyelid over the lower eyelid.* The lashes of your lower eyelid can brush a foreign object from the undersurface of your upper eyelid.
- *Don't rub your eye after an injury.* Touching or pressing on your eye can worsen a corneal abrasion.
- *Don't touch your eyeball with cotton swabs, tweezers or other instruments.* This can aggravate the abrasion.
- *Don't try to remove an object that's embedded in your eyeball.* Avoid trying to remove a large object that makes closing the eyelid difficult.

➕ Medical Help

In case of any injury to the eye, seek prompt medical attention.

Eyestrain

Eyestrain occurs when your eyes tire from intense use, such as driving a car or reading for extended periods, exposure to bright lights or glare, or spending long hours in front of a computer monitor. Signs and symptoms may include:

- Sore, tired or burning eyes
- Watery or dry eyes
- Blurred or double vision
- Headache
- Sore neck
- Increased sensitivity to light

Although eyestrain is often fatiguing and annoying, it usually isn't serious. Typically, the strain goes away once you're able to rest your eyes. In some cases, the signs and symptoms of eyestrain indicate an underlying eye condition that needs treatment.

Using a computer for long periods of time is one of the most common causes of eyestrain. Although you may not be able to change the nature of your job or avoid all the factors that cause eyestrain, you can take steps to reduce its effects.

🏠 Home Remedies

Simple adjustments in how you read, work or surf the Internet may help give your eyes a much-needed rest.

- For close-up work, use light that's directed on what you're doing.
- When reading, position the light source behind you and direct the light onto the page. When reading at a desk, use a shaded light positioned in front of you.
- Take frequent eye breaks throughout the day. Try to stand up and move around at least once every hour or so.
- Blink often to help refresh and lubricate your eyes. Because many people blink less than normal when working at a computer, dry eyes often result from prolonged computer use.
- Consider using artificial teardrops. These over-the-counter products can help relieve dry eyes from prolonged computer work. Lubricating drops that don't contain preservatives may be used as often as you need. If the drops contain preservatives, don't use them more than four times a day. Avoid eyedrops with a redness remover, as these ingredients may worsen dry eye symptoms.

Tips for computer work

Make sure your work space is set up in an eye-friendly way.

- Position your monitor directly in front of you about 20 to 28 inches from your eyes.
- Check the lighting and reduce glare. Bright lighting and too much glare can make it difficult to see objects on your screen
- Place your keyboard directly in front of your monitor.
- Get proper computer eyewear.

➕ Medical Help

If self-care doesn't relieve your eyestrain symptoms, see your eye doctor if you have ongoing symptoms that include:

- Eye discomfort
- Noticeable change in vision
- Double vision

Eye sty

A sty is a red, painful lump that forms on the outer edge of your eyelid — although sometimes it can form on the inner surface of the eyelid. A sty may resemble a boil or pimple. Usually the lump is filled with pus, develops gradually over several days, and ruptures in about a week.

The cause of a sty is bacterial infection, usually from staphylococcus, or "staph." Due to the swelling, it may become difficult to see clearly because you can't fully open your eye.

More than one sty can occur at a time, leading to a widespread inflammation of your eyelid — a condition known as blepharitis. Fortunately, most sties disappear on their own after a few days. In the meantime, you may be able to relieve the pain and discomfort with simple self-care treatments.

♠ Home Remedies

Until the sty goes away on its own, self-care usually involves:

- Leaving the sty alone. Don't try to pop the sty or squeeze the pus from the sty.
- Applying a clean, warm compress four times a day for 10 minutes to help encourage the sty to burst. Once the sty has ruptured, rinse your eye thoroughly and keep the area clean.

Prevention

To prevent recurrent infections:

- *Wash your hands*. Practice good hand-washing techniques and keep your hands away from your eyes. If you have children, make sure they practice proper hand-washing techniques because they may be more prone to sties.
- *Take care with cosmetics*. You can help prevent recurrent infections by not using old cosmetics or sharing makeup with anyone.
- *Make sure your contact lenses are clean*. If you wear contact lenses, follow your doctor's advice on disinfecting your lenses and wash your hands thoroughly before inserting your contacts.

✚ Medical Help

Most sties are harmless to your eye. Still, you should see your doctor if a sty causes one of the following problems:

- Interferes with your vision
- Recurs frequently with successive infections
- Doesn't disappear on its own
- Doesn't respond to self-care
- Develops redness or swelling that extends beyond the lid into your face or cheek

Fatigue

Almost everyone experiences fatigue at some time. After a long weekend of yard work or a hectic day with the children, it's natural to feel tired and worn out. This kind of physical and emotional fatigue is normal. You can usually restore your energy with a little rest or exercise.

If you feel tired all the time, or if exhaustion becomes overwhelming, you may worry that your condition is more serious than just being worn out. In some cases, fatigue is a symptom of an underlying condition that may require medical treatment.

Most of the time, however, fatigue can be traced to one or more of your daily habits or routines. Chances are you know what's causing your fatigue. And with a few lifestyle changes, it's likely that you'll find the resources to revitalize your life.

Fatigue isn't the same thing as sleepiness, although you often have a desire to sleep. Nor is it a lack of motivation. Fatigue can result from physical or emotional factors. Physical fatigue usually strengthens later in the day, while emotional fatigue often improves as the day progresses.

Common causes of physical fatigue
- Poor eating habits
- Lack of sleep
- Being out of shape
- Over-the-counter drugs, such as pain relievers, cough and cold medicines, antihistamines and allergy remedies
- Prescription drugs, such as tranquilizers, muscle relaxants, sedatives and blood pressure medications
- Dehydration
- Warm interior environments

Medical causes of fatigue
Fatigue may also be an early symptom of the following medical conditions:
- Low red blood cell count
- Cancer
- Low thyroid activity
- Diabetes
- Various acute or chronic infections
- Alcoholism
- Heart disease
- Rheumatoid arthritis
- Sleep disorder
- Electrolyte imbalance (when the blood levels of minerals, such as sodium and potassium, are too high or too low)

Many of these illnesses are accompanied by other signs and symptoms, such as muscle aches, pain, nausea, weight loss, sensitivity to cold and shortness of breath.

What is chronic fatigue syndrome?
Chronic fatigue syndrome is a complicated disorder characterized by extreme fatigue that may worsen with physical or mental activity, but doesn't improve with rest. Besides fatigue, symptoms include memory loss, sore throat, joint or muscle pain, painful lymph glands, abdominal pain or bloating, headaches and unrefreshing sleep.

Although there are many theories about what causes the condition, in most cases the cause is unknown. There's no specific treatment for chronic fatigue syndrome. In general, doctors aim to simply relieve signs and symptoms.

Before discussing concerns with your doctor, consider the possibility that your fatigue may be resolved with one or more of these lifestyle changes:

- *Get an adequate night's sleep.* Aim for seven to eight hours of uninterrupted sleep.
- *Follow a sleep schedule.* Regularly go to bed and wake up at about the same time each day.
- *Give yourself time to relax.* Ask others for help if you're feeling overworked or overwhelmed.
- *Organize your daily schedule.* Prioritize the most important activities. Don't try to do everything.
- *Identify the factors that cause stress.* And then try to reduce your stress level.
- *Include more physical activity and exercise in your day.* Exercise gives you more energy. Increase activity gradually, especially if you've recently been inactive. If you're over age 40, it might be a good idea to consult your doctor before beginning a vigorous exercise program.
- *Increase daily exposure to fresh air at home and at work.* Fresh air gives you more energy.
- *Eat a balanced diet.* Include plenty of fruits, vegetables and whole grains. Steer clear of high-fat foods. Eat a healthy breakfast and don't skip other meals.
- *Create a plan to lose weight if you're overweight.* But avoid very low calorie diets that don't provide enough nutrients and increase fatigue.
- *Drink plenty of water.* If your urine is clear or pale yellow, you're probably getting enough fluid. If it's dark yellow, you probably need to drink more.
- *Review your medications.* This includes both over-the-counter and prescription drugs. Fatigue may be a side effect.
- *Quit smoking.* Smoking increases fatigue.
- *Reduce or eliminate the use of substances such as alcohol and caffeine.* These substances are known to affect sleep or cause fatigue.

➕ Medical Help

If fatigue persists even after you've had ample rest and the fatigue lasts for two weeks or longer, you may have a problem that requires medical care.
See your doctor.

Fever

Even when you're well, your body temperature varies, and that variation is normal. In the morning your temperature is generally a little lower, and in the afternoon it's somewhat higher. The average healthy body temperature is around 98.6 F (37 C).

Temperatures under 100.4 F (38 C) are still considered normal. If they are 100.4 F or higher, it's often considered a fever.

Fever signals that something out of the ordinary is going on inside your body. It's not necessarily an illness, but it may be a sign of one. Fever may be accompanied by other symptoms, such as sweating, shivering, headache, muscle ache and weakness.

Most likely, when you have a fever, you're fighting a bacterial or viral infection. Rarely, it's the sign of a reaction — either to a medicine or to an inflammatory condition. Sometimes, it's difficult to identify the cause of fever.

Don't automatically try to lower your temperature if you have a fever. Over-the-counter medications may help, but sometimes it's better to leave it untreated. Fever seems to play a role in helping your body fight off infections. And lowering your temperature may mask other symptoms, making it harder to identify the cause. Usually fever goes away within a few days.

Fever in children

Signs of fever in small children include irritability, disinterest and inability to feed or sleep well. Children under age 6 may have a sudden change in temperature accompanied by a seizure (febrile seizure). Although alarming, the seizure typically lasts less than five minutes and has no lasting effects.

If a seizure happens, lay your child on his or her side. Don't put anything in the mouth or try to stop the convulsions. Call 911 or emergency medical help if it's the first febrile seizure or it lasts more than five minutes.

Sometimes a low-grade fever accompanies teething or a recent immunization. Fever with ear pulling may indicate a middle ear infection. If you're concerned, don't hesitate to call your doctor.

If medication is needed, it's usually provided in liquid form. For a small child, use a syringe (without a needle) to gently squirt the medicine in the back corners of the child's mouth.

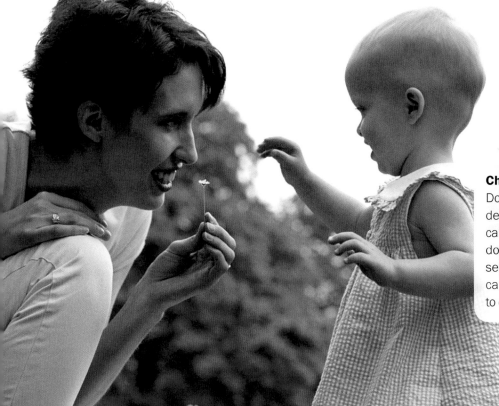

Children and aspirin
Don't give aspirin to anyone under 18 years old, unless specifically recommended by the child's doctor. Rarely, aspirin causes a serious or even fatal disease called Reye's syndrome if given to children during a viral infection.

🏠 Home Remedies

Here are steps you can take to make yourself or your child more comfortable during a fever:

Drink plenty of fluids
Fever can cause fluid loss and de-hydration. Drink water, juices or rehydration drinks such as Gato-rade or Pedialyte (for infants). A child may want to suck on frozen fruit pops. Pedialyte ice pops also are available.

Rest
Rest is necessary for recovery. By contrast, physical activity can raise your body temperature and, if moderately intense, sap some of your energy.

Take medication
Take acetaminophen (Tylenol, others) and ibuprofen (Advil, Mo-trin, others) according to label instructions or as recommended by your doctor. Don't use these medications at the same time or alternate doses unless you are instructed to do so by your doctor.

Avoid taking too much medica-tion. High doses or long-term use of acetaminophen may cause liver or kidney damage, and acute over-doses can be fatal.

For temperatures below 102 F (38.9 C), don't use fever-lowering drugs unless advised by your doc-tor. Sometimes a low-grade fever helps the body eliminate a virus, such as a cold.

If you're not able to get your child's fever down, don't continue to give more medication. Call your doctor instead.

Soak in lukewarm water
Especially for fevers with high tem-peratures, a lukewarm five- to 10-minute soak in the bathtub can be cooling. Giving a sponge bath to a small child has the same effect. If the sponge bath causes shivering, stop the bathing and dry your child. Shivering raises the body's internal temperature — shaking muscles generate heat.

✚ Medical Help

Call your doctor in the following situations, especially if accompanied by a cough that produces phlegm, side pain, reddened skin, painful urination, or diarrhea:
- Temperature of more than 104 F (40 C)
- Temperature of more than 102 F (38.9 C) for 48 hours or more
- Fever over 100.4 F (38 C) for more than three days or one that returns after it was gone for 24 hours
- Older adult or anyone with lowered immunity who has a fever over 101 F (38.3 C)

A fever is only one sign of illness. Inform your doctor of any contagious diseases that people around you have had, including flu, colds, measles and mumps.

Call 911 or emergency medical help immediately if any of these occur in addition to fever:
- Severe headache or unusual eye sensitivity to bright light
- Severe swelling of the throat
- Significant stiff neck and pain when the head is bent forward
- Persistent vomiting or difficulty breathing
- Mental confusion or extreme listlessness or irritability

Call 911 or emergency medical help if your baby has a fever along with a bulging soft spot on the head. Call your doctor immediately if your baby is 3 months old or younger with a rectal temperature of 100.4 F (38 C) or higher.

Fibromyalgia

Fibromyalgia is a chronic condition characterized by widespread pain in your muscles, ligaments, tendons and soft tissue. But even after extensive tests, your doctor is unable to find anything specifically wrong with you.

The type of pain varies but is often described as a constant dull ache. Women are more likely to develop the disorder than are men. You're more likely to have it if a relative also has the condition. And it tends to develop in early or middle adulthood.

Signs and symptoms of fibromyalgia often include:

- Widespread aching, lasting more than three months
- Fatigue and non-restorative, nonrestful sleep
- Tender points — where slight pressure can cause pain — at multiple locations, usually where muscle is attached to the bone
- Associated problems such as headaches, irritable bowel syndrome and pelvic pain

Signs and symptoms may vary depending on the weather, level of stress, physical actvity or even time of day. Many people awaken tired, even after sufficient sleep.

Although people with fibromyalgia feel pain in their muscles, this is not a disease of the muscles.

The science of fibromyalgia is still emerging, but the condition may eventually be found to be a disorder of the nervous system. Medications used for this condition affect chemical receptors in the brain and spinal cord — they don't treat your muscles.

Depression or depressive feelings often accompany fibromyalgia and often require specific treatment. Similarly, stress usually worsens the symptoms of fibromyalgia.

Self-care and coping strategies are critical elements in the management of fibromyalgia.

Reduce stress

Develop a plan to avoid or limit overexertion and emotional stress. Allow yourself time each day to relax. But don't change your routine totally. People who quit work or drop all activity tend to do worse than those who remain active. Try stress management techniques, such as deep-breathing exercises or meditation.

Get enough sleep

Because fatigue is a common symptom of fibromyalgia, getting sufficient sleep is essential. Practice good sleep habits, such as going to bed in the evening and getting up in the morning at the same time each day. Try to limit daytime napping.

Exercise regularly

At first, exercise may increase pain, but doing it regularly often decreases symptoms. Appropriate exercises include walking, biking, swimming and water aerobics. Strengthen supportive muscles, especially abdominal muscles, to help improve your posture. Stretching and relaxation exercises also are helpful. A physical therapist can help you develop an exercise program.

Pace yourself

Develop a routine that alternates work with rest. Avoid long hours of repetitive activity. If you try to do too much on your good days, you may end up having more bad days.

Seek support

Find a support group that emphasizes maintaining health. Ask your family and friends for support.

Learn relaxation techniques

There are a broad range of therapies you can choose from. Most are low-risk techniques that may provide some benefits. Set aside time to practice them in your daily schedule. Relaxation techniques include:

- *Deep-breathing exercises.* Breathe in slowly and deeply through your nose to a count of five. Hold the air in your lungs for a count of five and then breathe out slowly through your mouth to a count of 10.
- *Progressive muscle relaxation.* Gently tighten and then relax muscle groups in your body one at a time, starting at either your head or your feet.
- *Meditation.* Focus on a single object or repeat a particular sound to help quiet your mind and relax your muscles.
- *Visualization.* Take an imaginary trip to a beautiful place. Use all of your senses to experience the location as fully as possible. Feel the sun's warmth and the gentle breeze. Listen to birds singing.

✚ Medical Help

If you feel that you have excessive stress or depression from trying to cope with fibromyalgia, discuss your concerns with your doctor or a mental health provider.

Flu

Influenza — commonly called the flu — is a viral infection that attacks your respiratory system, including your nose, throat, bronchial tubes and lungs.

If you're generally healthy and you catch influenza, you're likely to feel rotten for a few days, but you probably won't develop complications or need hospital care. If you have a weakened immune system or chronic illness, though, influenza can be fatal.

Initially, the flu may seem like a common cold with a runny nose, sneezing and sore throat (see page 43). But colds usually develop slowly, while the flu tends to strike suddenly. While a cold feels like a nuisance, you usually feel much worse with the flu. Signs and symptoms of the flu include:

- Fever
- Chills and sweats
- Headache
- Dry cough
- Muscular aches and pains, especially in your back, arms and legs
- Fatigue and weakness
- Nasal congestion
- Loss of appetite
- Diarrhea and vomiting in children

Flu viruses travel through the air in droplets when someone with the infection coughs, sneezes or talks. You can inhale the droplets directly, or you can pick up the germs by touching an object where the droplets have landed, such as a telephone or computer.

Not all flu is the same

The flu is caused by three types (strains) of viruses — influenza A, B and C. Type A can be responsible for the deadly influenza pandemics (worldwide epidemics) that strike every 10 to 40 years. Type B can lead to smaller, more localized outbreaks. Either type A or B can cause the flu that circulates almost every winter. Type C has never been connected with a large epidemic.

🏠 Home Remedies

If you do come down with the flu, these measures may help ease your symptoms:

- *Drink plenty of liquids.* Choose water, juice and warm soups to prevent dehydration. Drink enough so that your urine is clear or pale yellow.
- *Rest.* Get more sleep to strengthen your body and help your immune system fight against the infection.
- *Try chicken soup.* It's not just good for your soul — chicken soup really can relieve flu symptoms by helping to break up sinus congestion.
- *Consider pain relievers.* Use an over-the-counter pain reliever such as acetaminophen (Tylenol, others) or ibuprofen (Advil, Motrin, others) cautiously, as needed. Remember, pain relievers may make you feel more comfortable, but they won't make your symptoms go away any faster. They may also have side effects.

For example, ibuprofen may cause stomach pain, bleeding and ulcers. If taken for a long period of time or in higher than recommended doses, acetaminophen can be toxic to your liver. Don't give aspirin to children or teens because of the risk of Reye's syndrome, a rare but potentially fatal disease.

Prevention

To reduce your risk of the flu:

- *Get an annual flu vaccination.* The best time to be vaccinated is October or November. This allows ample time for your body to develop antibodies to the flu virus before the peak flu season starts, which is typically between December and March in the Northern Hemisphere. However, getting a flu shot later is better than not getting one at all, and may still protect you. It takes up to two weeks to build immunity following a flu shot.

- *Wash your hands.* Thorough and frequent hand washing is the best way to prevent many common infections. Scrub your hands vigorously for at least 15 seconds, rinse well and turn off the faucet with a paper towel. Or use an alcohol-based hand gel containing at least 60 percent alcohol.
- *Eat right, sleep tight.* Both poor diet and poor sleep can lower your immunity and make you more vulnerable to infections. A balanced diet emphasizing fresh fruits and vegetables, whole grains, and small amounts of lean protein works best for most people. The amount of sleep needed for a healthy immune system varies. In general, adults seem to do best on seven to eight hours of sleep a night. Older children and teens need more rest – between nine and ten hours every night.

➕ Medical Help

If you have flu symptoms and are at risk of complications, see your doctor right away. Taking antiviral drugs within the first 48 hours after you first notice symptoms may reduce the length of your illness by a day or two and may help prevent more serious problems. Seek immediate medical care if you have signs and symptoms of pneumonia. These include a severe cough that brings up phlegm, a high fever and a sharp pain when you breathe deeply. If you have bacterial pneumonia, you'll need treatment with antibiotics.

Foot and ankle pain

The foot is made up of 26 bones, 33 joints, and hundreds of muscles, nerves and ligaments. The ankle is the intricate, bony joint where the foot and leg meet. Given this complex structure and the amount of punishment that your feet and ankles have to endure every day, it's no wonder that pain can be so common. See also pages 96–97 regarding heel pain.

Sprains and strains

A sprain is an injury to a ligament — when the band of fibrous tissue connecting one bone to another in your joints is stretched or torn. The most common location for a sprain is in your ankle. A strain is an injury to a muscle or tendon — when the cord of tissue connecting muscle to bone is stretched or torn. See pages 156–157 for more information.

Fractures

A stress fracture in the foot is really a hairline crack in the bone. It's often caused by the repetitive application of force, typically by overuse — such as repeatedly jumping up and down or running in high-impact activities such as basketball or track and field.

Achilles tendinitis

This is an inflammation of the Achilles tendon, which connects your calf muscles in the lower leg to your heel bone. It's often a running or other sports-related injury caused by overuse or intensive exercise, which strains the tendon. You'll feel a dull ache or pain, especially when you run or jump. The tendon may also be mildly swollen or tender.

Bunions

A bunion is an abnormal, bony bump that forms at the base of your big toe. The big toe joint becomes enlarged, forcing the toe to crowd against your other toes. The base of your big toe is pushed outward, extending beyond your foot's normal profile. Ill-fitting footwear or an inherited structural defect are often the cause of this condition. Shoe pressure over a bunion can be very painful and lead to callus formation. Arthritis of the big toe joint can develop as a result of bunion deformity.

Hammertoe and mallet toe

Unlike a bunion, hammertoe may occur in any toe (most commonly the second toe). The toe becomes bent, giving it a claw-like appearance, and may be painful. Hammertoe can result from wearing shoes that are too short, but also can occur in people with muscle and nerve damage from diseases such as diabetes. A mallet toe is a deformity in which the very end of the toe is bent downward.

Flatfeet

You have flatfeet when the arch on the inside of your foot is flattened, allowing your entire foot to touch the floor when you stand up. A common and usually painless condition, flatfeet may occur when the arches don't develop during childhood. It can also happen due to injury or from simple wear and tear. Flatfeet can become a problem if the condition forces your ankle to turn inward, throwing off the alignment of your leg.

Burning feet

Burning feet — the sensation that your feet are painfully hot – can be mild or severe. Burning feet can occur simply because your feet are tired. Infections, such as athlete's foot, also can cause burning feet or changes in the nerves in your feet.

Does the shoe fit?

You can avoid many foot and ankle problems with shoes that fit properly. Here's what to look for:

- Adequate toe room — height, width and length. Avoid shoes with pointed toes.
- Low heels, which will help you avoid back problems.
- Laced shoes, which are roomier and more adjustable.
- Comfortable athletic shoes, strapped sandals or soft pumps with cushioned insoles. Avoid vinyl and plastic shoes. They don't breathe when your feet perspire, trapping moisture.

Buy shoes in the afternoon and evening. Your feet are smaller in the morning and swell throughout the day. Measure both feet. As you age, your shoe size (length and width) may change.

For foot and ankle pain
- Follow the instructions for R.I.C.E. (see page 157).

For a stress fracture
- Allow at least one month for healing. A cast or walking boot may be necessary, based on the location of the stress fracture.
- Avoid high-impact activities anywhere from six weeks to several months, based on stress fracture location and advice from your doctor.

For Achilles tendinitis
- Wear soft-soled running shoes, and avoid running or walking up or down hills.
- Avoid any impact on your heel for several days.
- Use gentle calf stretches daily (see page 97).

For bunions
- Wear shoes with adequate toe width that are made of soft leather.

- Have your shoes stretched in the area of the bunion.
- Wear sandals or lightweight shoes in the summer.
- Larger deformities may require special shoes.

For flatfeet
- Arch supports in well-fitting shoes may give you a better weight-bearing position.

For hammtertoe
- Special toe pads or cushions help protect the toe. Metatarsal pads may reduce pain in the ball of the foot behind the hammertoe.

For burning feet
- Wear nonirritating cotton or cotton-synthetic blend socks and shoes of natural materials that "breathe." A specially fitted insole also may help.
- Eliminate aggravating activities, such as standing for long periods.
- Bathe your feet in cool water.

Seek medical care immediately if:
- Your foot pain is severe and the area is swollen after an injury
- Your foot is hot and inflamed or you have a fever following the injury
- Your foot or ankle is deformed or bent in an abnormal position
- The pain is so severe that you can't move your foot
- You can't bear weight 72 hours after any injury

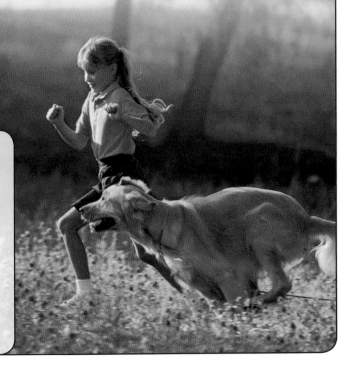

Frostbite

Frostbite occurs when skin and underlying tissues freeze. The most common cause of frostbite is direct exposure to cold-weather conditions, but exposure to freezing materials, such as ice, also can cause frostbite. In subfreezing temperatures, the tiny blood vessels in your skin tighten, reducing the flow of blood and oxygen. Eventually, tissue cells are destroyed.

Frostbite can affect any part of your body. Your hands, feet, nose and ears are most susceptible because they are delicate and often exposed to cold.

Frostnip, the first stage of frostbite, irritates the skin but doesn't cause permanent damage. The first sign of frostnip may be a slightly painful, tingling sensation. With continued exposure, the skin becomes numb, feels hard and cold, and may turn deathly pale in color. Frostbitten areas, as they thaw, may burn with pain.

When frostbite is severe, the area will probably remain numb until it heals completely. Healing can take months, and the damage to your skin can permanently change your sense of touch.

Frostbite can damage deep layers of tissue. As deeper layers of tissue freeze, blisters may form. The blistering usually occurs over one to two days.

♠ Home Remedies

Gradually warming the affected skin is the key to treating frostbite. To do so:

- *Protect your skin from further exposure.* If you're outside, warm your frostbitten hands by tucking them into your armpits. Protect your face, nose or ears by covering the area with dry, gloved hands. Don't rub the affected area and never rub snow on frostbitten skin.
- *Get out of the cold.* Once you're indoors, remove wet clothes.
- *Gradually warm frostbitten areas.* Put frostbitten hands or feet in warm water — 104 to 107.6 F (40 to 42 C). Wrap or cover other areas in a warm blanket. Don't use direct heat, such as a stove, heat lamp, fireplace or heating pad, because these can cause burns.
- *Don't walk on frostbitten feet or toes, if possible.* This will further damage the soft tissues on your feet.
- *If there's any chance the affected areas will freeze again, don't thaw them out.* If they're already thawed out, wrap them up so that they don't become frozen again.
- *Know what to expect as skin thaws.* If the skin turns red and there's a tingling and burning sensation as it warms, circulation is returning. But if numbness or sustained pain remains during warming or if blisters develop, seek medical attention.
- *Apply aloe vera gel or lotion to the affected area several times a day.* This helps reduce inflammation.

✚ Medical Help

Seek medical care if numbness remains during rewarming, you experience increased pain or discharge, you develop blisters, or damage to the skin appears severe.

Gas, belching and bloating

Gas, belching and bloating are natural occurrences, typically caused by swallowed air in the gastrointestinal tract or by the normal breakdown of food during the digestive process. You may only occasionally experience these symptoms, or you may have to deal with them frequently or repeatedly in a single day.

Passing gas (flatulence)

Most intestinal gas (flatus) is produced in the colon. Gas buildup is typically caused by the fermentation of undigested food, such as plant fiber. Gas can also form when your digestive system doesn't completely break down certain components in food, such as gluten or sugar. Other sources of gas may include changes in intestinal bacteria due to medications, as well as swallowed air and constipation.

Belching

Belching, or burping, is your body's way of getting rid of excess air from your stomach. You may swallow too much air if you eat or drink too fast, talk while you eat, drink carbonated beverages, or drink through a straw. Some people swallow air as a nervous habit. Indigestion and heartburn may be relieved by belching.

Bloating and gas pains

When gas is not expelled by belching or flatulence, it can build up in the stomach and intestines and lead to bloating. Abdominal pain, either mild and dull or sharp and intense, often occurs with bloating. Passing gas may relieve the pain. Bloating is also related to conditions such as irritable bowel syndrome or lactose intolerance.

In addition to eating fatty and gas-producing foods, such as beans and raw vegetables, bloating and gas pain may also result from stress and anxiety or from smoking.

Continued next page >

🏠 Home Remedies

To reduce excess gas

- Avoid foods that affect you the most. Common gas producers may include: beans, lentils, peas, cabbage, onions, broccoli, cauliflower, bananas, raisins, prunes, whole-wheat bread, bran cereals or muffins, and carbonated drinks. This doesn't mean eliminating all of these foods from your diet, only the worst offenders.
- Temporarily cut back on high-fiber foods. Add them back gradually over weeks.
- Eat fewer fatty foods. They slow digestion, allowing food more time to ferment.
- Eat slowly. Eating when stressed or on the run can interfere with normal digestion.
- Exercise is good for your gut. Take a short walk after meals.
- Try low-lactose or lactose-free products, such as Lactaid or Dairy Ease, if dairy products are a problem. Products with simethicone can break up the bubbles in gas.
- Try Beano. The natural enzyme in this product assists digestion by making certain foods more digestible and helping reduce intestinal gas.

To reduce belching

- Eat and drink slowly. Take your time and avoid gulping. Limit drinking through straws.
- Cut down on carbonated drinks and beer, which release carbon dioxide gas.
- Avoid chewing gum or sucking on hard candy.
- Don't smoke cigarettes, pipes or cigars.
- Manage stress, which may aggravate the nervous habit of swallowing air.
- Check your dentures. A poor fit may cause you to swallow excess air when eating.
- Avoid lying down immediately after you eat and take steps to treat your heartburn.

To reduce bloating

- Eat fewer fatty foods, which delay stomach emptying.
- Eat fewer gas-producing foods, including the ones listed previously. Also avoid chewing gum and hard candy.

➕ Medical Help

Bouts of excess gas, belching and bloating often resolve on their own. Consult your doctor if your symptoms don't improve with changes in your eating habits or if you notice:

- Diarrhea
- Constipation
- Nausea or vomiting
- Weight loss
- Abdominal or rectal pain
- Persistent heartburn
- Blood in stools
- Fever

These symptoms may signal a more serious, underlying digestive condition.

Gout

Gout is a complex form of arthritis characterized by sudden, severe attacks of pain, redness and tenderness in your body's joints. It may affect your feet, ankles, knees, hands and wrists, but most often occurs at the base of your big toe.

Gout develops when there is a high level of uric acid in your blood. As a result, sharp, needle-like urate crystals form in a joint or surrounding tissue that cause the pain and swelling.

An acute attack of gout can wake you up in the middle of the night feeling like your big toe is on fire. The affected joint is hot, swollen and so tender that even the weight of the sheet on it seems intolerable.

Gout can affect anyone. Men are more likely to develop it, but women become increasingly susceptible to gout after they reach menopause.

Risk factors include obesity, excessive alcohol use, medical conditions such as high blood pressure, high cholesterol and diabetes, and having a family history of gout.

🏠 Home Remedies

Gout is treatable, and there are ways to reduce the risk that gout will recur. The American Dietetic Association recommends following these guidelines during a gout attack:

- Drink 8 to 16 cups of fluid each day, with at least half being water.
- Avoid alcohol.
- Eat a moderate amount of protein, preferably from healthy sources, such as low-fat or fat-free dairy, tofu, eggs, and nut butters.
- Limit your daily intake of meat, fish and poultry to 4 to 6 ounces. These high-protein foods increase uric acid in your bloodstream.
- Maintain a healthy weight.

Alternative treatments that may help

Since few alternative treatments have been studied in clinical trials, it's difficult to assess whether they're actually helpful for gout pain. The strategies that have been studied include:

- *Coffee.* Studies have found an association between coffee drinking — both regular and decaffeinated coffee — and lower uric acid levels in your blood, although no study has determined how or why coffee may have this effect.
- *Vitamin C.* Supplements containing vitamin C may reduce the levels of uric acid in your blood. However, vitamin C hasn't been studied specifically as a treatment for gout. Don't assume that if a little vitamin C is good for you, then lots is even better. In fact, megadoses of vitamin C may increase your body's uric acid levels. In place of supplements, you can increase your vitamin C intake by eating more fruits and vegetables, especially oranges.
- *Cherries.* Studies show an association between cherries and lower levels of uric acid in your blood, but it isn't clear if the cherries have any effect on the signs and symptoms. Eating cherries and other dark-colored fruits, such as blackberries, blueberries, raspberries and purple grapes, may be a safe way to supplement gout treatment, but discuss this strategy with your doctor first.

✚ Medical Help

Seek medical care immediately if you develop a fever and the joint becomes hot and inflamed. This can be a sign of infection.

Headache

Headache is pain in any region of the head. It may be focused at one or both sides of the head, radiate across the head from a single point or have a vise-like quality. The pain may be sharp, throbbing or dull. Symptoms may appear gradually or suddenly, and last for less than an hour or for several days.

Headaches are the most commonly reported medical complaint. They may point to an underlying medical condition but that situation is rare. About 90 percent of all headaches have no underlying cause. These so-called primary headaches may be the result of dysfunction or overactivity of the pain-sensitive features in your head — nerves, blood vessels, muscles — or of chemical activity in the brain.

Three well-known types of primary headache are:

Tension-type

This is the most common type of headache, and yet its causes aren't well understood. The pain is generally mild to moderate and diffuse — many people describe feeling as if there's a tight band wrapped around their head. Headaches can last from 30 minutes to a week.

Migraine

Migraines are chronic headaches that can last for hours or even days. The pain is moderate to severe, often with a pulsating or throbbing quality. Symptoms can be so severe that all you can think about is finding a dark, quiet place to lie down.

Some migraines are preceded, or accompanied, by sensory warning signs (auras), such as flashes of light, blind spots or tingling in the arm or leg. The headache is often accompanied by nausea, vomiting and extreme sensitivity to light, odor and sound.

Cluster

A cluster headache is one of the most painful types of headache. Excrutiating pain, generally located in or around the eye, strikes quickly, and usually without warning.

A striking feature of cluster headaches is that attacks occur in cyclical patterns, or clusters — giving the condition its name. Bouts, or cluster periods, may last from weeks to months, followed by long periods of remission.

Rebound headaches

Rebound headaches are caused by the frequent use of headache medication. Pain relievers can offer relief for occasional headaches, but if you take them more than a couple of days a week, you may trigger medication overuse, or rebound, headaches.

How frequently rebound headaches occur depends on the type of overused drug. This happens because your body adapts to the medication.

- *Simple pain relievers.* Common drugs such as aspirin and acetaminophen (Tylenol, others) may contribute to rebound headaches — especially if you exceed the recommended daily dosages. Ibuprofen (Advil, Motrin, others) and naproxen (Aleve, others) are considered low risk for rebound headaches.
- *Combination pain relievers.* Over-the-counter drugs that combine caffeine, aspirin and acetaminophen (Excedrin, others) are common culprits. Prescription medications such as Fioricet, Fiorinal and Esgic-Plus also contain the sedative butalbital. All of these medications are high risk for the development of rebound headaches.
- *Migraine medications.* Migraine drugs linked to rebound headaches include triptans (Imitrex, Zomig, others) and certain ergots, such as ergotamine (Ergomar, others). They have a moderate risk of causing rebound headaches.
- *Opiates.* Painkillers derived from opium or from synthetic opium compounds, including combinations of codeine and acetaminophen (Tylenol with Codeine No. 3 and No. 4, others), are considered high risk for rebound headaches.

To stop rebound headaches, reduce or stop taking pain medication. It's tough in the short term, but your doctor can help you beat rebound headaches for long-term relief.

For tension-type headaches

- Try massage, hot or cold packs, warm shower, rest, or other relaxation techniques.
- Try a low dose of aspirin (adults only), acetaminophen (Tylenol, others), ibuprofen (Advil, Motrin, others) and naproxen (Aleve).
- Moderate exercise may help a tension-type headache.
- Poor posture may lead to tension headaches in some people. When sitting, don't slump your head forward. When standing, hold your shoulders back and your head high.
- Rub peppermint oil on your forehead and temples. Most peppermint oil contains menthol, which may ease pain.

For migraines

- Start treatment as soon as you feel a migraine coming — it's your best chance to stop the headache early. Use acetaminophen, ibuprofen or aspirin (adults only) at the recommended dosage.
- Some people can abort an migraine by going to sleep in a darkened room or by consuming caffeine (coffee or cola).
- Try muscle relaxation exercises, including meditation, yoga and progressive muscle relaxation. Or spend at least a half-hour each day doing something you find relaxing – listening to music, gardening or reading.

For cluster headaches

- Stick to a regular sleep schedule. Cluster periods may be triggered by changes in your normal sleep schedule.
- Avoid alcohol. Consuming alcohol usually triggers a headache when you're in a cluster period.
- Avoid being around volatile substances. Exposure to substances such as solvents, gasoline and oil-based paints may trigger headaches.
- Be cautious in high altitudes. The reduced oxygen levels may trigger headaches.
- Avoid tobacco. If you're prone to cluster headaches, it's best to stop smoking and avoid other tobacco products.
- Avoid nitrates. These compounds may trigger headaches for some people. Foods that contain nitrates include smoked and processed meats. Medications, such as nitroglycerin, also may contain nitrates.

Herbs, vitamins and minerals

- Evidence suggests that the herbs feverfew and butterbur may prevent or reduce the severity of headache symptoms. Don't take these if you're pregnant.
- A high dose of riboflavin (vitamin B-2) may help ease symptoms.
- Magnesium supplements seem to help some people with migraines, especially those with low levels of magnesium.
- Coenzyme Q10 is under study as a potential preventive agent for migraines. Research suggests it can decrease migraine frequency by about 30 percent.

Continued next page >

➕ **Medical Help**

If self-care doesn't help after one or two days, see your doctor. He or she will try to determine the type and cause of your headache and exclude other possible sources of pain with a variety of tests. Seek emergency care if the headache is the worst headache of your life or is associated with weakness, slurred speech or fainting.

Avoiding headache triggers

Some people can eliminate their headaches by avoiding headache triggers — certain foods, beverages, activities or environments that seem to produce a headache.

Headache triggers vary, but here are common examples:

- Red wine or other alcohol
- Caffeine
- Fermented, pickled or marinated food, aged cheese, bananas, citrus fruit, dried fruit, food additives and seasonings (sodium nitrite in hot dogs and luncheon meat, or monosodium glutamate in Chinese foods), nuts, peanut butter and chocolate
- Smoking
- Stress or fatigue
- Depression or anxiety
- Lack of sleep
- Changing sleeping patterns or mealtimes
- Skipping meals
- Eyestrain
- Poor posture
- Weather, altitude or time zone changes
- Oral contraceptive use or hormone replacement therapy
- Strong or flickering lights
- Strong odors, including perfumes, flowers or natural gas
- Polluted air or stuffy rooms
- Excessive noise

Caffeine and headaches

A morning headache can occur, especially if you regularly consume four or more cups of caffeinated drinks each day. It may be a withdrawal headache, following a night without caffeine.

Caffeine may also help. Some kinds of headaches cause blood vessels to widen. Caffeine temporarily causes them to narrow.

So, for adults, if aspirin or acetaminophen doesn't help, use a medicine that includes caffeine. But don't overdo it. Too much caffeine can cause jitteriness, rapid heart rate, sweating and, yes, withdrawal headaches.

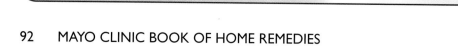

Heartburn

Heartburn is a burning sensation in your chest, just behind your breastbone. Technically called gastroesophageal reflux disease (GERD), heartburn occurs when stomach contents back up into your esophagus. Sour taste and the sensation of food coming back into your mouth may accompany the sensation.

Heartburn usually happens after you've eaten a meal, and it may occur at night. The pain usually worsens when you're lying down or bending over.

Why does food back up into your esophagus? Normally, a strong band of muscle (lower esophageal sphincter) closes off the bottom of the esophagus and opens to allow food and liquid to flow down into your stomach. Then it closes again. If the muscle relaxes abnormally or becomes weakened, stomach contents can wash back up (reflux), irritating the esophagus.

Occasional heartburn is common and no cause for alarm. Most people manage the discomfort on their own. More frequent heartburn that interferes with your daily routine may be a symptom of something more serious that requires assistance from your doctor.

Continued next page >

Most people can manage the discomfort of heartburn with lifestyle changes and over-the-counter medications.

- *Maintain a healthy weight.* The pressure of excess pounds on your abdomen pushes up your stomach, causing acid to back up into your esophagus. If you are overweight or obese, work to slowly lose weight — no more than 1 or 2 pounds a week. Ask your doctor for help in devising a weight-loss strategy.

- *Avoid tightfitting clothing.* Clothes that fit tightly around your waist put pressure on your abdomen, helping force stomach acid to wash back into your esophagus.

- *Avoid foods and drinks that trigger heartburn.* Everyone has specific triggers. These may include: fatty foods, alcohol, caffeinated or carbonated beverages, decaffeinated coffee, peppermint, spearmint, garlic, onion, cinnamon, chocolate, citrus fruits and juices, and tomato products.

- *Avoid big meals.* Avoid overeating by eating smaller, and more frequent meals.

- *Delay lying down after a meal.* Wait at least two to three hours after eating before lying down to rest or take a nap.

- *Don't eat before bed.* Don't eat two to three hours before bedtime at night.

- *Elevate the head of your bed.* An elevation of about 6 to 9 inches at the head of your bed helps gravity work for you against stomach reflux. Place wood or cement blocks under the bedposts at the head of your bed. If it's not possible to elevate the bed frame, insert a wedge between the mattress and box spring that elevates your body from the waist up. Wedges are available at drugstores and medical supply stores.

- *Don't smoke.* Smoking interferes with proper function of the lower esophageal sphincter.

- *Use over-the-counter antacids occasionally.* These products can temporarily neutralize stomach acid and relieve mild heartburn. However, prolonged or excessive use of antacids containing magnesium can cause diarrhea. Calcium or aluminum-based products can lead to constipation.

- *Try other medications.* Products such as famotidine (Pepcid), omeprazole (Prilosec), cimetidine (Tagamet) and ranitidine (Zantac) may relieve heartburn symptoms by reducing the production of stomach acid. These medicines are available in both over-the-counter and prescription strengths.

✚ Medical Help

Most problems with heartburn are occasional and mild. If you have severe or daily discomfort, don't ignore the symptoms. Left untreated, chronic heartburn can scar the lower esophagus and make swallowing difficult. In rare cases, severe heartburn leads to Barrett's esophagus, which may increase your risk of esophageal cancer.

Seek immediate medical attention if you experience chest pain, especially when accompanied by other signs and symptoms, such as shortness of breath or pain in the jaw or arm. These may be signs and symptoms of a heart attack.

Heat exhaustion

Under normal conditions, the natural mechanisms that control your body temperature adjust well to the outside environment. Working hard in hot or humid conditions for prolonged periods, however, may overstress the systems, causing an excessive increase in body temperature.

Heat exhaustion may come on suddenly or may develop after days of heat exposure. Signs and symptoms include: cool, moist skin with goose bumps when in the heat, heavy sweating, faintness, dizziness, fatigue, weak rapid pulse, muscle cramps, nausea, and headache.

What's heatstroke?

Heatstroke is a life-threatening condition that occurs when your body temperature reaches 104 F (40 C) or higher. It's an escalation of two other heat-related health problems: heat cramps and heat exhaustion. With heat stroke, you stop sweating and your skin becomes hot, flushed and dry. You may feel confused and disoriented. Other signs and symptoms include rapid, shallow breathing, rapid heartbeat, headache and muscle cramps or weakness.

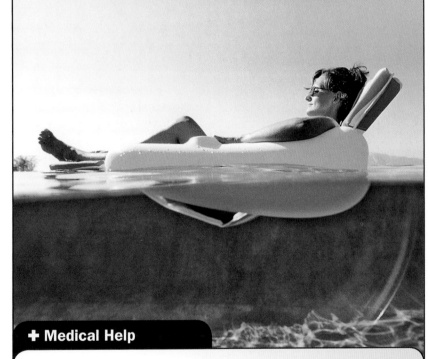

🏠 Home Remedies

To avoid heat-related conditions:
- Avoid being outside during the hottest part of the day, which is generally from noon to 4 p.m. Reserve vigorous exercise or activity for early morning or evening. If possible, exercise in the shade.
- Drink plenty of fluids, especially water and sports drinks. Avoid alcohol and caffeine, which can contribute to fluid loss.
- Wear loosefitting, lightweight, light-colored clothing.
- Avoid hot and heavy meals.
- Pace yourself. Let your body acclimate to the heat.
- At the first sign of heat exhaustion, get out of the sun and rest in the shade or in an air-conditioned building.
- Apply cool water to your skin. If possible, take a cool shower or soak in a cool bath. Don't use alcohol on your skin.

➕ Medical Help

Untreated, heat exhaustion can progress to heatstroke. If you don't begin to feel better within 60 minutes, seek prompt medical attention. If you suspect heatstroke, call 911 or emergency medical help immediately.

Heel pain

Your heels take a lot of punishment — every mile you walk puts heavy stress on each foot. Too much physical activity, poorly fitting shoes and excess weight can cause pain and inflammation.

The pain usually develops directly under your heel (plantar fasciitis). This is an inflammation of the plantar fascia, the fibrous tissue along the bottom of your foot that connects to your heel bone. Pain can also occur just behind the heel, where the Achilles tendon attaches to the heel bone (Achilles tendinitis). Although the cause often isn't serious, heel pain can be severe and occasionally disabling.

Heel pain usually develops gradually, but can also occur suddenly and severely. Although both feet may be affected, it usually occurs in only one foot.

Pain tends to be worse when you get out of bed in the morning, and generally goes away as your foot limbers up. It can recur if you stand for a long time, get up from a sitting or lying position, climb stairs, or stand on tiptoes. A bone spur (usually painless) may form due to the tension on your heel bone.

Treatment generally involves relieving pain and inflammation. However, don't expect a quick cure. Relief may take six months or longer.

⌂ Home Remedies

To relieve heel pain:

- *Cut back on exercises such as jogging or walking, which impact the heel.* Substitute exercises that put less weight on your heel, such as swimming or bicycling.
- *Apply ice to the painful area.* Do this for up to 20 minutes after an activity to reduce inflammation.
- *Stretch your heel.* Stretching increases your flexibility. Stretching in the morning before you get out of bed helps reverse the tightening that occurs overnight. Reach for your toes and gently flex your feet. Pull the top of the foot forward toward the front of the leg. Stretch your heel after exercise, such as walking or running. See the stretches on page 97.
- *Wear the right shoes.* Buy shoes with a low to moderate heel (1 to 2 inches), good support and shock absorbency.
- *Try heel pads or cups that cushion and support your heel.*
- *Don't walk barefoot, especially on hard surfaces.* Going shoeless can aggravate heel pain.
- *Try nonprescription pain relievers.*
- *If you're overweight, lose weight to reduce stress on your heel.*

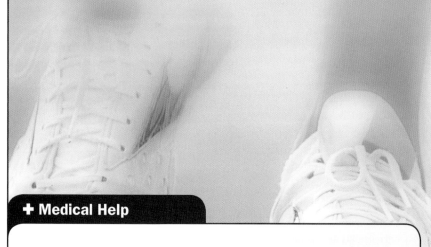

✚ Medical Help

If self-care measures aren't effective, or if you believe your condition may be caused by a foot abnormality, see your doctor.

Heel exercises

These exercises stretch or strengthen your plantar fascia, Achilles tendon and calf muscles. The two exercises illustrated at right are best performed while seated. Hold each stretch for 20 or 30 seconds. Do two to three repetitions two or three times a day.

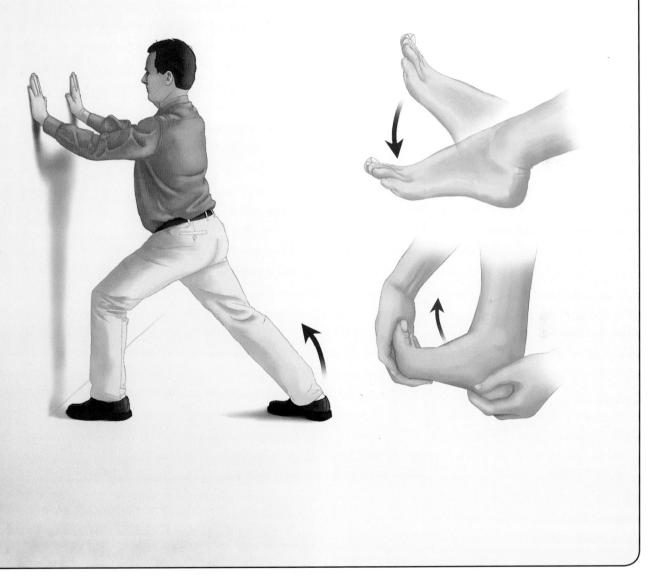

Hemorrhoids

Hemorrhoids are swollen and inflamed veins in your anus and lower rectum. By age 50, about half of adults have experienced the itching, burning and discomfort that signals their presence. You may also notice small amounts of blood on toilet tissue or in the toilet bowl.

Hemorrhoids usually develop due to increased pressure, for example, as you strain to pass hard stools. Lifting heavy objects, obesity, pregnancy, childbirth, stress and diarrhea also can increase the pressure on these veins and lead to hemorrhoids.

There are two common types of hemorrhoid. An internal hemorrhoid develops within the anal canal. You can't see or feel it, and it usually doesn't cause any discomfort. An external hemorrhoid is under the skin around your anus. When irritated, it can itch and bleed.

In addition to hemorrhoids, bleeding from the rectum can occur for other reasons, some of which can be serious. Therefore, it's important not to dismiss all rectal bleeding as hemorrhoids.

🏠 Home Remedies

Although uncomfortable, hemorrhoids are not a serious medical condition. You can temporarily relieve mild pain, swelling and inflammation with the following self-care measures:

- Drink plenty of water each day and eat high-fiber foods such as wheat-bran cereal, whole-wheat bread, fresh fruit and vegetables.
- Bathe or shower daily to gently cleanse the skin around your anus. Regular soaking in a warm bath is best. Soap isn't necessary and may aggravate the irritation.
- Stay active and exercise. If you must sit or stand for long periods, try to take quick walks or frequent breaks.
- Try not to strain during bowel movements or sit on the toilet for long periods of time.
- Apply ice packs or cold compresses to relieve inflammation.
- To relieve mild itching and irritation, apply over-the-counter creams containing hydrocortisone or pads containing witch hazel or a topical numbing agent.
- Taking fiber supplements (Citrucel, Metamucil) can help keep stools soft and regular.

➕ Medical Help

Hemorrhoids become most painful when a clot forms in the enlarged vein. If this happens, your doctor may prescribe a cream or suppository containing hydrocortisone to reduce inflammation. Troublesome internal hemorrhoids may require surgery or other procedures to shrink or eliminate them.

Hiccups

Hiccups involve an involuntary contraction of your diaphragm — the thin muscular partition that separates your chest from your abdomen and plays an important role in breathing. Each involuntary contraction is followed by a sudden closure of your vocal cords, producing the characteristic "hic" sound.

A bout of hiccups usually lasts only a few minutes. Many people have home remedies for hiccups that they swear by. But in some people — about 1 in 100,000 — hiccups may persist for several months, no matter what remedies they may try to stop them.

Many factors may cause hiccups but only rarely are they a sign of an underlying medical condition.

♠ Home Remedies

Although there's no surefire way to stop them, if you have a bout of hiccups that lasts longer than a few minutes, the following home remedies may provide relief:
- Swallow a teaspoon of sugar
- Breathe into a paper bag
- Gargle with ice water
- Hold your breath

Prevention
You may be able to decrease the frequency of hiccups by avoiding common hiccup triggers, such as:
- Eating large meals
- Drinking carbonated beverages or alcohol
- Sudden changes in temperature
- Excitement or emotional stress

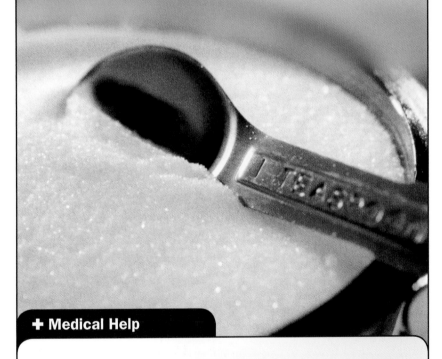

✚ Medical Help

Make an appointment to see your doctor if your hiccups last more than 48 hours or if they are so severe that they cause problems with eating or breathing.

High blood pressure

Most people with high blood pressure (hypertension) don't experience any signs or symptoms, even if their blood pressure reaches dangerously high levels. That's why it's called a silent killer. Uncontrolled blood pressure can damage your arteries, heart, brain, kidneys and eyes. It increases your risk of serious health problems, including heart attack and stroke.

Blood pressure basics

Blood pressure is determined by the amount of blood your heart pumps and the amount of resistance to blood flow in your arteries. The more blood your heart pumps and the narrower your arteries, the higher your blood pressure.

Blood pressure is highest when your heart muscle contracts and pumps out blood — that's your systolic blood pressure. Between each contraction, your heart rests, lowering your blood pressure — that's your diastolic blood pressure. Your blood pressure readings have two numbers: the systolic pressure (top number) and diastolic pressure (bottom number).

Know your numbers

Top number (systolic)	Bottom number (diastolic)	What it means	What to do
Below 120	and Below 80	*Normal*	*Maintain or adopt a healthy lifestyle*
120-139	or 80-89	*Prehypertension*	*Adopt a healthy lifestyle**
140-159	or 90-99	*Stage 1 hypertension*	*Lifestyle changes plus a medication†*
160 or higher	or 100 or higher	*Stage 2 hypertension*	*Lifestyle changes plus more than one medication*

* These recommendations address high blood pressure as a single health condition. If you also have heart disease, diabetes, chronic kidney disease or certain other conditions, you'll need to treat your blood pressure more aggressively.
† If your blood pressure isn't normal, a healthy lifestyle — often times along with medication — can help bring it under control and reduce your risk of life-threatening complications.

Note: This chart applies to adults 18 and older. Numbers are in millimeters of mercury (mm Hg). Diagnosis is based on the average of two or more readings taken at two different visits, after the initial screening. If your readings fall into two different categories, your result is the higher category.

Lifestyle changes can help you prevent or control high blood pressure – even if you're taking blood pressure medication. Here's what you can do:

Eat healthy foods

Try the Dietary Approaches to Stop Hypertension (DASH) diet, which emphasizes fruits, vegetables, whole grains and low-fat dairy products. Get plenty of potassium, which can help control high blood pressure. Eat less saturated fat and total fat.

Limit salt

Salt causes the body to retain fluids and so, in many people, can raise blood pressure. Don't add salt to food. Avoid foods that include a lot of salt in processing, such as cured meats, snack foods, and many canned or frozen foods.

Maintain a healthy weight

If you're overweight, losing even 5 pounds may lower your blood pressure. In some people, weight loss alone is sufficient to avoid the need to take blood pressure medications.

Increase physical activity

Regular physical activity can help lower your blood pressure and keep your weight under control. Try to get at least 30 minutes of physical activity every day. Don't think you've got to run a marathon or join a gym. Consider moderate aerobic activity, such as walking or bicycling.

Don't smoke

Smoking tobacco products injures blood vessel walls and makes them less flexible (hardening of the arteries). If you smoke, ask your doctor to help you quit.

Limit alcohol

Even if you're healthy, alcohol can raise your blood pressure. If you choose to drink alcohol, do so in moderation — no more than one drink a day for women and anyone over age 65, and a limit of two drinks a day for men.

Manage stress

Reduce daily stress as much as possible. Get plenty of sleep. Practice healthy coping techniques, such as deep breathing.

Monitor your blood pressure

Home blood pressure monitoring can help you keep closer tabs on your blood pressure, indicate if your medication is working, and even alert you and your doctor to potential complications.

Eat dark chocolate

Certain compounds in dark chocolate can lower blood pressure slightly. Milk chocolate does not have the same effect.

Try paced respiration

Paced respiration refers to slow, deep breathing. In various clinical trials, regular use of a nonprescription device (Resperate) that helps analyze and guide your breathing patterns was found to help lower blood pressure. However, some researchers have questioned whether this benefit is due to the device or simply a result of taking 15 minutes to relax.

➕ Medical Help

High blood pressure requires medical attention. See a doctor if you think you have high blood pressure. The doctor can determine if you need medication and, if so , which type may work best for you.

High cholesterol

Cholesterol is a waxy substance that's found in the fats (lipids) in your blood and used by your body to build healthy cells. There are different types of cholesterol, including low-density lipoprotein (LDL, or "bad") cholesterol and high-density lipoprotein (HDL, or "good") cholesterol.

Problems occur when you regularly carry undesirable levels of cholesterol in your bloodstream: too much of one type, not enough of another type, or both. High levels of LDL cholesterol can cause fatty deposits to build up in your blood vessels. Eventually, these deposits restrict bloodflow through your arteries. The lack of oxygen-rich blood to your heart increases the risk of heart attack. Decreased blood flow to your brain can cause a stroke.

What about triglycerides?

Triglycerides are a type of fat associated with blood cholesterol. When you eat, your body converts any calories it doesn't need into triglycerides. The triglycerides are stored in your fat cells, and later released as a source of energy between meals.

High triglyceride levels may be caused by excess weight and inactivity. People with high triglyceride levels often have high levels of LDL cholesterol as well. High triglyceride levels increase your risk of heart disease and stroke.

Know your numbers

Cholesterol and triglycerides are fats that circulate in your blood. These cholesterol goals are appropriate for most people. But your goals may differ — talk with your doctor, especially if you have heart or blood vessel disease.

Type of blood fat	Typical goals
Total cholesterol	Below 200
LDL* ("bad") cholesterol	Below 100 (Below 70 if you're at very high risk of a heart attack)
HDL* ("good") cholesterol	Men: 40 or higher Women: 50 or higher
Triglycerides	Below 150†

Numbers are in milligrams per deciliter of blood (mg/dL).
*LDL means low-density lipoprotein. HDL means high-density lipoprotein.
†Emerging data indicates that below 100 is ideal.
Adapted from American Heart Association, 2007

Lifestyle changes are essential to improving your cholesterol level:

Lose excess pounds

Excess weight contributes to high cholesterol. Losing even 5 to 10 pounds of excess weight can help lower total cholesterol levels. Take an honest look at your diet and daily routines. Consider ways to overcome your challenges.

Eat heart-healthy foods

What you eat has a direct impact on your cholesterol level. In fact, researchers say that a diet rich in fiber and other cholesterol-lowering foods may help lower cholesterol as much as prescription medications will for some people.

Choose healthy fats

Fats come in different forms, and some fats are healthier than others. Select more foods made with unsaturated fats (polyunsaturated and monounsaturated). This would include products made with olive oil, vegetable oils, avocado, nuts and nut butters, and oils that come from nuts.

Eliminate trans fats

Trans fats are often found in margarines and commercially baked cookies, crackers and snack cakes. Trans fats are double trouble for heart health, raising LDL ("bad") cholesterol levels and lowering HDL ("good") cholesterol levels.

Select whole grains

Whole grains are packed with essential vitamins, minerals and fiber that promote heart health. Choose whole-grain breads, pasta, and flour. Brown rice, oatmeal and oat bran are other good choices.

Eat fruits and vegetables

Fruits and vegetables are the foundation of a healthy diet and successful weight loss. Explore different types and varieties for appealing tastes and textures.

Eat heart-healthy fish

Fish such as cod, tuna and halibut have less total fat and cholesterol than do meat and poultry. Salmon, mackerel and herring are rich in omega-3 fatty acids, which help promote heart health.

Drink alcohol in moderation

In some studies, moderate use of alcohol has been linked with higher levels of HDL cholesterol — but this benefit isn't strong enough to recommend alcohol for anyone who doesn't drink already.

Exercise regularly

Regular exercise can help improve cholesterol levels. Try to include 30 to 60 minutes of exercise daily. Take a brisk walk. Ride your bike. Swim laps. If you can't fit a single session into your schedule, you can get similar benefits from several 10-minute workouts. See your doctor before beginning any type of vigorous exercise program.

Don't smoke

Stopping smoking can improve your HDL cholesterol level. And the benefits don't end there. Within one year, your risk of getting heart disease is half that of a smoker's. Within 15 years, your risk is similar to that of someone who's never smoked at all.

Continued next page >

✚ Medical Help

Ask your doctor for a baseline cholesterol test at age 20 and then have your cholesterol retested at least every five years. If your test results aren't within desirable ranges, your doctor may recommend more frequent measurements.

Experiment with natural products

Although few natural products have been proven to reduce cholesterol, some may be helpful. You might consider trying these cholesterol-lowering supplements and products:

- Artichoke
- Barley
- Blond psyllium (found in seed husk and products such as Metamucil)
- Flaxseed
- Garlic
- Oat bran (found in oatmeal and whole oats)
- Plant sterols and stanols. These compounds include beta-sitosterol (found in oral supplements and some margarines, such as Promise Activ) and sitostanol (found in oral supplements and some margarines, such as Benecol). They help block the absorption of cholesterol and can lower LDL ("bad") cholesterol.

Beware of red yeast rice

You may have heard of a supplement for reducing cholesterol called red yeast rice. The Food and Drug Administration has released a warning regarding three brands of red yeast rice because they were found to contain lovastatin, the active ingredient in the drug Mevacor. This can be unsafe, since there's no way to determine the quantity or quality of the lovastatin in the red yeast supplements.

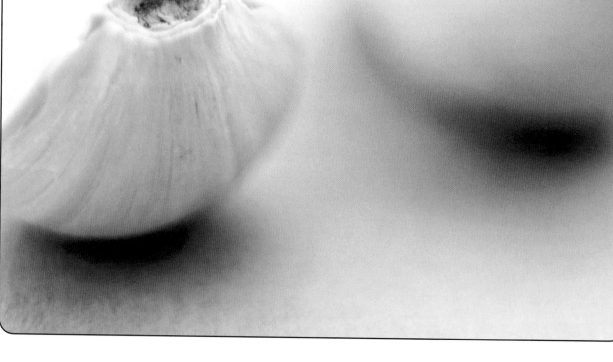

Hives

Hives are raised, red, often itchy welts of various sizes that appear and disappear on your skin. They tend to occur in batches and last anywhere from a few minutes to several days. Hives are more common on areas of the body where clothes rub the skin.

Angioedema, a similar kind of swelling, causes large welts just below your skin, especially near your eyes and lips, but also on your hands and feet and inside your throat.

Hives and angioedema are a result of your body releasing a natural chemical called histamine in your skin. Allergies to foods, drugs, insect bites, infections, illness, pollen, cold and heat, and emotional distress may trigger this reaction.

In most cases, hives and angioedema are harmless and leave no lasting marks. However, serious angioedema may cause swelling in your throat or tongue that blocks your airway and causes loss of consciousness.

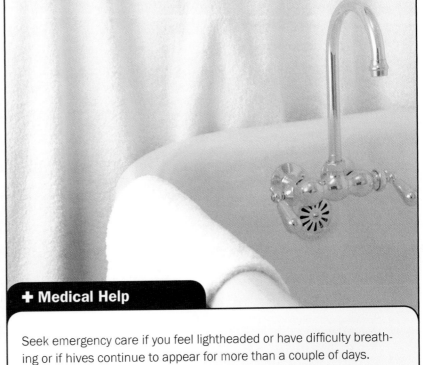

🏠 Home Remedies

If you're experiencing mild hives or angioedema, these tips may help relieve your symptoms:

- *Look for triggers.* Try to identify and avoid substances that irritate your skin or that cause an allergic reaction. These may include foods, medications, pollen, pet dander, latex and insect stings.
- *Use over-the-counter antihistamine.* A nonprescription oral antihistamine, such as diphenhydramine (Benadryl, others) or loratadine (Claritin) may help relieve itching.
- *Apply cool, wet compresses.* Covering the affected area with bandages and dressings can help soothe the skin and prevent scratching.
- *Take a comfortably cool bath.* To relieve itching, sprinkle the bath water with baking soda, uncooked oatmeal or colloidal oatmeal – a finely ground oatmeal made for bathing (Aveeno, others).
- *Wear loose, smooth-textured cotton clothing.* Avoid clothing that's rough, tight, scratchy or made from wool, to reduce irritation.
- *Keep a diary.* If you suspect foods are causing the problem, keep a food diary. Be aware that food labels may list some ingredients under less common names.

➕ Medical Help

Seek emergency care if you feel lightheaded or have difficulty breathing or if hives continue to appear for more than a couple of days.

Hoarse voice

You've likely had days when your voice sounds excessively husky, raspy or weak. You may have even lost your voice for a short time (laryngitis). This occurs when your vocal cords become swollen or inflamed and are no longer able to vibrate normally. They produce unnatural sounds, or possibly no sound at all.

In addition to difficulty speaking, you may feel some pain or have a raw, scratchy throat. Your voice may change pitch, sounding higher or lower than normal.

A common cause of hoarseness is infection, especially a viral infection of the upper respiratory system, such as a cold or flu. You can also become hoarse from vocal strain caused by yelling or overusing your voice. Other causes include allergies, smoking, and the chronic reflux of stomach acid into your esophagus.

Hoarseness and laryngitis may be short-lived (acute) or long lasting (chronic). Most acute cases are not serious, but persistent hoarseness may signal a serious underlying condition.

♠ Home Remedies

The following steps may reduce strain on your voice and relieve the symptoms of hoarseness and laryngitis:

- *Rest your voice.* Limit how much talking you do. Whispering puts even more strain on your vocal cords than does normal speech.
- *Drink lots of warm, noncaffeinated fluids.* Fluids help keep your throat moist. Also try sucking on lozenges, gargling with salt water or chewing a piece of gum.
- *Inhale steam.* Breathe in steam from a bowl filled with hot water. (Never inhale steam directly from water as it boils.) Lean over the container with a towel draped over your head to help catch the steam. Breathing deeply during a hot shower also may help.
- *Use a humidifier to moisturize the air.* Follow the manufacturer's instructions to clean the humidifier and prevent bacterial buildup.
- *Avoid clearing your throat.* This action irritates your vocal cords.
- *Stop drinking alcohol and smoking, and avoid exposure to smoke.* Alcohol and smoke dry your throat and irritates your vocal cords.
- *Avoid decongestants.* These medications can dry out the throat.

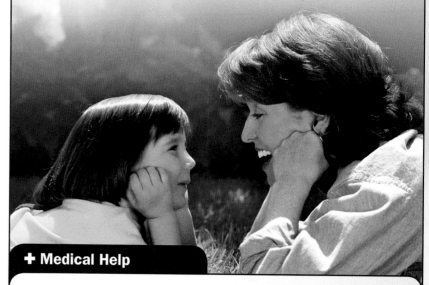

✚ Medical Help

If hoarseness lasts for more than two weeks, seek medical help. Seek immediate medical attention if your child makes noisy, high-pitched breathing sounds when inhaling, drools more than usual, has trouble swallowing and has a fever higher than 103 F. These signs and symptoms may indicate epiglottitis, which requires medical attention.

Impetigo

Impetigo is a highly contagious skin infection that usually appears on the face. The infection begins when common bacteria penetrate your skin through a cut, scratch or insect bite. Although a much less common occurrence, it may also develop in healthy skin.

The infection appears as red sores that blister briefly, ooze for several days and then form a sticky, yellowish-brown crust. Scratching or touching the sores can spread the infection on your body or to other people.

Other signs and symptoms of impetigo include:

- Itching
- Painless, fluid-filled blisters
- In a more serious form, painful fluid- or pus-filled sores that turn into deep ulcers

Impetigo is more common among young children. In adults, it develops mostly as a complication of other skin problems, such as dermatitis. There's a small chance of kidney damage or rheumatic fever following the infection.

★ Home Remedies

Good hygiene is essential for preventing impetigo and limiting its spread. For minor infections that haven't spread to other parts of your body, try the following:

- *Soak the affected areas of skin with a vinegar solution.* Combine 1 tablespoon of white vinegar with 1 pint of water. Soak the areas for 20 minutes. This makes it easier to gently remove the scabs.
- *After washing the area, apply over-the-counter antibiotic ointment three or four times daily.* Wash the skin before each application, and pat it dry. Keep the sores and skin around them clean.
- *Avoid scratching or touching the sores as much as possible until they heal.* Apply a nonstick dressing to the infected area to help keep impetigo from spreading. Children's fingernails should be trimmed to help reduce damage from scratching.
- *Don't share towels, clothing or razors with others.* Change your bathroom linens daily.

+ Medical Help

See your doctor if the infection doesn't appear to be improving. Antibiotics are often prescribed that may speed healing of the sores and limit the spread of infection.

Incontinence

Urinary incontinence means a loss of bladder control, resulting in accidental and untimely leakage. It's a common problem that may be caused by everyday behaviors, underlying medical conditions or physical problems.

Your concerns may range from occasional minor leaks or dribbles, to sudden, strong urges to urinate. Types of incontinence include:

- *Stress incontinence.* This is a loss of urine when you exert pressure on your bladder from coughing, sneezing, laughing, exercising or lifting.
- *Urge incontinence.* This is a sudden, strong urge to urinate, often with only seconds or minutes to reach a toilet.
- *Overflow incontinence.* An inability to empty your bladder results in frequent and constant dribbling of urine.
- *Functional incontinence.* Some people have a physical or mental impairment, for example, arthritis or dementia, that prevents them from getting to the toilet on time.

Other causes of incontinence include overhydration or dehydration, drinking alcohol or caffeine, taking certain medications, and consuming substances that irritate the bladder.

♠ Home Remedies

Lifestyle changes work well for treating certain types of urinary incontinence:

Bladder training
This involves learning to delay urination every time you get the urge to go. You may start by trying to hold off for 10 minutes. The goal is to lengthen the time between toilet trips until you're urinating every two to four hours. Bladder training may also involve double voiding — urinating, then waiting a few minutes and trying again to empty your bladder more completely.

Scheduled toilet trips
The idea here is timed urination — going to the toilet according to the clock rather than waiting for the need to go. Try to go every two to four hours.

Fluid and diet management
You may be able to simply modify your daily habits to regain control of your bladder. You may need to cut back on or avoid alcohol, caffeine or acidic foods.

Pelvic floor muscle exercises
These exercises, called Kegels, strengthen the abdominal muscles that help control urination. Imagine that you're trying to stop the flow of urine. If you're using the right muscles, you'll feel a pulling sensation. Pull in your pelvic muscles and hold for a count of three. Relax for a count of three. Work up to 10 to 15 repetitions each time you exercise. Do Kegel exercises at least three times a day. It may take up to 12 weeks before you notice an improvement in bladder control.

✚ Medical Help

You may feel uncomfortable discussing incontinence. But if incontinence is frequent or is affecting your quality of life, don't hesitate to discuss your concerns with your doctor.

Indigestion

Indigestion, also called upset stomach, is a general term that describes discomfort in your upper abdomen. Indigestion isn't a disease but rather a collection of signs and symptoms, such as bloating, belching, nausea and feeling uncomfortably full after eating a meal.

There are many possible causes of indigestion. Some are related to your lifestyle and others to what you eat and drink. Anxiety, smoking, emotional trauma, mealtime habits (such as eating too quickly) and digestive conditions, such as ulcers or gallstones, also may cause indigestion.

Sometimes people with indigestion also experience heartburn, but heartburn and indigestion are two separate conditions. Heartburn is a pain or burning feeling in the center of your chest (see pages 93-94).

Although the condition is common, how you experience indigestion may differ from how others do. Fortunately, you may be able to prevent or treat symptoms with self-care.

🏠 Home Remedies

Healthy lifestyle choices may help prevent mild indigestion.

- *Eat smaller, more frequent meals.* Choose mostly fresh vegetables, fruits and whole grains. Chew your food slowly and thoroughly.
- *Avoid triggers.* Common triggers of indigestion include fatty and spicy foods, carbonated beverages, caffeine, alcohol and smoking.
- *Maintain a healthy weight.* Extra pounds put pressure on your abdomen and may cause stomach acid to back up into your esophagus.
- *Exercise regularly.* Exercise helps you keep off extra weight and promotes better digestion. With your doctor's OK, aim for 30 to 60 minutes of physical activity on most days of the week.
- *Manage stress.* Get plenty of sleep. Spend time doing things you enjoy. Practice relaxation techniques such as meditation or yoga.
- *Reconsider your medications.* With your doctor's approval, stop or cut back on aspirin or other anti-inflammatory drugs that can irritate your stomach lining. If that's not an option, be sure to take these medications with food.
- *Drink herbal tea with peppermint.* Some people find relief from indigestion with peppermint, although more research is needed to determine its effectiveness.

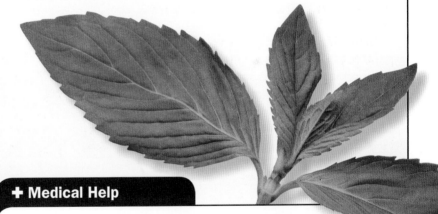

➕ Medical Help

Mild indigestion is usually nothing to worry about. Consult your doctor if discomfort persists for more than two weeks. Contact your doctor right away if indigestion is severe or accompanied by:

- Weight loss or loss of appetite
- Vomiting
- Black, tarry stools
- Jaundice, or yellow coloring in the skin and eyes

Ingrown hairs

An ingrown hair occurs when the tip of a hair curls back and grows into the skin, causing inflammation and irritation. This is more likely to happen after hair has been cut close to the skin, for example, by shaving or tweezing. The sharp tip of hair that's formed by these actions can penetrate the skin more easily than can uncut hair.

Ingrown hairs most commonly appear in the beard area of males, including the chin, cheeks and, especially, the neck. In females, the most common areas are the armpits, pubic area and legs. Signs and symptoms may include:

- Localized pain
- Areas of small, dry, rounded bumps
- Small, pus-filled, blister-like lesions
- Skin darkening
- Itching

Ingrown hairs are most likely to occur in black males, ages 14 to 25. But an ingrown hair can develop in anyone who shaves, tweezes, waxes or uses electrolysis to remove hair.

🏠 Home Remedies

To release ingrown hairs:
- Wash the affected area using a washcloth or soft-bristled toothbrush — using a circular motion — for several minutes before shaving and at bedtime
- Use a sterile needle, inserting it under hair loops, to gently lift hair tips that are embedded in your skin

Prevention
Of course, not removing hair is one way to avoid an ingrown hair. If that's not an option, there are hair-removal methods that make ingrown hairs less likely. If you shave:
- Wet the hair or whiskers to be removed with warm water
- Avoid close shaves
- Use a lubricating shave gel
- Use a single-blade razor
- Use a sharp blade
- Don't pull your skin taut while shaving
- Shave in the direction of hair growth
- Rinse the blade after each stroke
- Apply cool compresses to the shaved area when you're finished

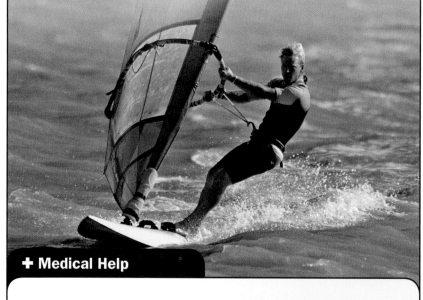

➕ Medical Help

See your doctor if ingrown hairs are a chronic problem.

Ingrown toenails

An ingrown toenail is a common condition in which the corner or side of one of your toenails grows into the soft flesh of the toe. The result is pain, redness, swelling around a nail and, sometimes, an infection. An ingrown toenail usually develops on your big toe.

Common causes include wearing shoes that crowd your toenails, cutting your toenails too short or not straight across, injuring your toenail, or having unusually curved toenails.

Usually, an ingrown toenail is taken care of before any serious problems can develop. But, if left untreated, tissue surrounding the toe and the underlying bone can become infected.

🏠 Home Remedies

You can treat most ingrown toenails at home. Here's how:

- *Soak your feet in warm salt water.* For every pint of water, add 1 teaspoon of salt. Soak your feet for 15 to 20 minutes three times a day. Soaking reduces swelling and relieves tenderness.
- *Place cotton under your toenail.* Put fresh bits of cotton or dental floss under the ingrown edge after each soaking. This will help the nail eventually grow above the skin edge. Change the cotton or floss daily until the pain and redness subside.
- *Use a topical antibiotic.* Apply an antibiotic ointment and bandage to the tender area.
- *Choose sensible footwear.* Consider wearing open-toed shoes or sandals until your toe feels better.
- *Check your feet.* If you have diabetes, check your feet daily for signs of ingrown toenails or other foot problems.
- *Take pain relievers.* If the pain is severe, take over-the-counter pain relievers, such as ibuprofen (Advil, Motrin, others), naproxen (Aleve) and acetaminophen (Tylenol, others), to relieve the pain until you can make an appointment with your doctor.

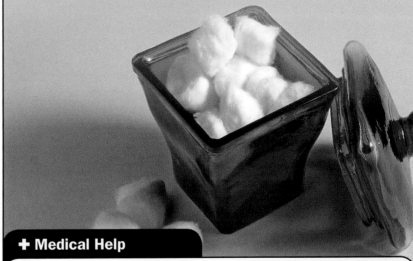

➕ Medical Help

If the pain of an ingrown toenail is severe or spreading, your doctor can take steps to relieve discomfort and help you avoid complications. Also seek medical attention if you experience areas of pus or redness on the toe that appears to be spreading or if you have diabetes or poor blood circulation.

Insect bites and stings

Signs and symptoms of an insect bite are caused by the injection of venom or other substances into your skin. The venom sometimes triggers an allergic reaction. The severity of your reaction depends on how sensitive you are to the venom and whether you've been bitten or stung more than once.

Most reactions are mild, causing a slight itching or stinging sensation and mild swelling that disappear within a day or so. A delayed reaction, which can happen hours or even days later, may cause fever, hives, painful joints and swollen glands.

Only a small percentage of people develop severe reactions to insect venom. For information on severe allergic reactions, see page 186. Signs and symptoms may include:

- Nausea
- Facial swelling
- Difficulty breathing
- Abdominal pain
- Deterioration of blood pressure and circulation

Bites from bees, hornets, wasps, yellow jackets and fire ants are typically the most troublesome. Bites from mosquitoes, ticks, biting flies and some spiders also can cause reactions, but these are generally milder.

Mosquito bites

There's no denying that mosquito bites are annoying. You're most likely to be bitten at dawn or dusk, when the insects are most active. You can take steps to keep mosquitoes at bay, but no method is foolproof. Telltale signs and symptoms — redness, swelling and itching — may not appear for up to two days after the bite.

Mosquito bites may sometimes transmit serious diseases, such as West Nile virus, malaria and dengue fever. Signs and symptoms of more serious infection include fever, severe headache, body aches, lethargy, confusion and sensitivity to light. Such signs and symptoms require prompt medical attention.

Spider bites

Most spider bites produce harmless itching or stinging that goes away in a day or two. Only a few spiders are dangerous to humans, including the black widow — known for the red hourglass marking on its belly — and the brown recluse — with its violin-shaped marking on its top.

These two spiders prefer warm climates and dark, dry places, such as closets, woodpiles and outdoor toilets. Symptoms of a black widow bite start with slight swelling and redness at the bite. Within hours, however, you may experience intense pain, stiffness, chills, fever, nausea and severe abdominal pain.

If bitten by either of these spiders, seek emergency care immediately.

Tick bites

Some ticks carry infections and their bite can transmit bacteria that cause illness. For information on tick bites, see page 173.

Most insect bites and stings feel unpleasant but are generally harmless and easily treated at home. The following steps may help relieve discomfort:

- In the case of a sting, brush off the stinger from the skin with a straight-edged object. Don't pull out the stinger. This may release more venom.
- Wash the bite or sting area with soap and water.
- Apply a cold pack or cloth filled with ice to reduce the pain and swelling.
- Apply 0.5 or 1 percent hydrocortisone cream, calamine lotion, aloe vera, or a paste of baking soda and water to the bite or sting several times daily until your symptoms go away. A baking soda paste can be made with a ratio of 3 teaspoons baking soda to 1 teaspoon water.
- Take an antihistamine (Benadryl, Chlor-Trimeton, others) to reduce itching.

Mosquito bites

The preceding steps can help relieve itching. To reduce your risk of getting bit by mosquitoes:

- Avoid unnecessary outdoor activity when mosquitoes are most active, at dawn, dusk and early evening.
- Wear light-colored, long-sleeved shirts and long pants outdoors.
- Use mosquito repellent that contains DEET. Don't apply DEET on the hands of young children and don't use DEET on infants under 2 months of age.

- Apply permethrin-containing mosquito repellent to your clothing or buy clothing with permethrin in it.

Spider bites

If bitten by a black widow or brown recluse spider:

- Use soap and water to clean the wound and skin around the spider bite.
- Slow the venom's spread. If the spider bite is on an arm or leg, tie a snug bandage above the bite and elevate the limb to help slow or halt the venom's spread. Ensure that the bandage is not so tight that it cuts off circulation in your arm or leg.
- Use a cold cloth at the spider bite location. Apply a cloth dampened with cold water or filled with ice.
- Seek immediate medical attention. Treatment may require anti-venom medication.

➕ Medical Help

If you have any breathing problems, swelling of the lips, tongue or throat, faintness, confusion, rapid heartbeat or hives after a sting, seek emergency care. Less severe allergic reactions include nausea, intestinal cramps, diarrhea or swelling larger than 2 inches wide at the site. See your doctor promptly if you have any of these symptoms.

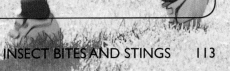

Insomnia

Insomnia is the most common kind of sleep disorder (and there are more than 60 different kinds of sleep disorder). Insomnia includes difficulty falling asleep or staying asleep. More than one-third of adults have had insomnia at some time in their lives, while 10 to 15 percent report long-term (chronic) insomnia.

With insomnia, you typically awaken in the morning feeling tired and unrefreshed. This status takes a heavy toll on your ability to function during the day. It saps your energy and mood, as well as your health and quality of life.

Insomnia mostly stems from some other problem. It may be a symptom of another disorder or it may be from the use of substances that interfere with sleep. Common causes include:

- Stress, anxiety and depression
- Caffeine, nicotine and alcohol
- Some prescription medications for conditions such as depression, heart disease, high blood pressure and allergies
- Some over-the-counter drugs for health concerns such as congestion and pain
- Certain medical conditions linked to insomnia, such as arthritis, cancer, congestive heart failure, diabetes, lung disease and stroke
- Eating too much late in the evening
- Change in environment or work schedule
- Long-term use of sleep medications
- Poor sleep habits
- "Learned" insomnia, from worrying excessively about sleep and trying too hard to fall asleep

Insomnia and aging

Insomnia may become more prevalent as you get older. You may experience:

- *Change in sleep patterns.* Sleep often becomes less restful with age. Because you're sleeping lightly, you're also more likely to awaken.
- *Change in activity.* You may become less physically and socially active. Activity helps promote a good night's sleep. You're also more likely to take daily naps, which can interfere with sleep at night.
- *Change in health.* Chronic pain, depression, anxiety and stress can interfere with sleep. Men often develop an enlarged prostate gland, which can increase the need to urinate and interrupt sleep.
- *Increased use of medications.* Older adults use more medications than younger people do, which increases the chance of insomnia caused by a drug.

How much sleep is enough?

The answer to this question will differ from one person to the next. Most adults seem to need around seven to eight hours a night. However, some people do just fine on less sleep and are able to function during the day.

To nap, or not?

Don't nap during the day if sleeping at night is a problem. Otherwise, if a nap refreshes you:

- *Keep it short.* Limit your nap to 20 or 30 minutes. Longer naps are more likely to interfere with nighttime sleep.
- *Just rest if you can't nap.* Lie down for a short time and focus your mind on calming thoughts.
- *Don't rely on naps to keep you going.* It's important to depend on getting enough sleep at night to build energy reserves and avoid a sleep deficit.

You don't have to put up with sleepless nights. Simple lifestyle changes can resolve insomnia and restore your needed rest:

- *Get on schedule.* Keep bedtimes and wake times consistent, including on weekends.
- *Exercise regularly.* Get at least 30 minutes of exercise on most days of the week. Allow at least five to six hours between the end of exercise and bedtime.
- *Don't take work to bed.* Avoid taking work materials into the bedroom or using the Internet right before bedtime.
- *Take a warm bath.* Bathing one to two hours before bedtime can be soothing.
- *Avoid or limit caffeine, alcohol and nicotine.* Drinking caffeine after lunchtime and using nicotine can prevent you from falling asleep at night. Alcohol can cause unrestful sleep and frequent awakenings.
- *Avoid large meals before bedtime.* Light snacks are fine, but eating too much late in the evening can interfere with sleep at night.
- *Drink fewer fluids before bedtime.* Drinking less will help reduce the need to urinate in the middle of the night.
- *Create a quiet, dark, cool sleeping environment.* If necessary, use eye covers and earplugs. Try adding subtle background noise, such as from a fan.
- *Hide your bedroom clocks.* Set your alarm but then hide all clocks in your bedroom. Watching the time makes it more difficult to fall asleep.
- *Check your medications.* Check the labels and ask the doctor if your medications contain caffeine or other stimulants that may interfere with sleep.
- *Don't try to sleep.* The harder you try, the more awake you become. If you don't fall asleep after 20 minutes, get out of bed. Do a quiet activity, such as reading or listening to music. Stay up until you feel drowsy, and then return to bed.

Remedies to try

These may improve your sleep:

- *Valerian.* This herb may help improve sleep quality. It's generally considered safe when taken in recommended doses. Some people may experience mild side effects, and valerian may increase sedation from alcohol or the anxiety drug lorazepam (Ativan). Also, don't use it if you're pregnant.
- *Melatonin.* Melatonin is a hormone that controls your body's internal system that regulates sleep. It's generally considered safe for use at recommended doses and may be used occasionally to overcome jet lag. Melatonin may cause clotting problems in people taking the anticoagulant warfarin (Coumadin). Also don't use it if you're pregnant.
- *Lavender.* A study of female college students found that lavender fragrance was effective for helping the participants fall asleep.

Continued next page >

➕ Medical Help

If, after a week or two, you still have trouble sleeping, see your doctor. Doctors generally don't recommend taking sleeping pills for more than a few days. However, they may recommend sleeping pills as temporary help until other treatments begin to work. If your doctor thinks you may have a sleep disorder other than insomnia, you may be referred to a sleep center for special testing.

What about nonprescription sleeping pills?

Most nonprescription sleep aids in any drugstore or pharmacy contain antihistamines, which can cause drowsiness. Commonly available store-brand sleep aids have the same active ingredients (and carry the same risks and benefits) as their brand-name counterparts, but often can be purchased at a more reasonable cost.

Before taking the aid, inform your doctor if you're taking a type of antidepressant called monoamine oxidase inhibitor (MAOI), such as phenelzine (Nardil) or tranylcypromine (Parnate), either currently or as recently as two weeks ago.

Also check with your doctor if you take any other drugs for depression, any psychiatric or emotional condition, or Parkinson's disease.

Although antihistamine-based medications may improve mild symptoms of insomnia for a short time, they aren't likely to help for longer than a couple of weeks.

Some common nonprescription sleep aids include:

- *Diphenhydramine (Benadryl, Sominex, others).* These products may cause dry mouth, dizziness, prolonged drowsiness and memory problems. They're not recommended if you're pregnant or breast-feeding or you have a history of glaucoma, heart problems or an enlarged prostate.
- *Doxylamine (Unisom).* This medication may cause periods of prolonged drowsiness. It may not be safe if you're pregnant or breast-feeding, or if you have a history of asthma, bronchitis, glaucoma, peptic ulcers or an enlarged prostate gland. While taking this type of medication, don't drive or attempt other activities that require alertness.

What about antihistamines?

Antihistamines may help you fall asleep for a few nights — but routine use of antihistamines for insomnia isn't recommended.

Antihistamines induce drowsiness by counteracting histamine, a chemical produced by the central nervous system. In fact, most over-the-counter sleep aids contain antihistamines. These products are intended to be used for only two to three nights at a time, such as when stress, travel or other disruptions prevent you from falling asleep. You can quickly develop a tolerance to the sedative effects of antihistamines — so the longer you take them, the less likely they are to make you sleepy.

Irritable bowel syndrome

Irritable bowel syndrome (IBS) is a common disorder of the gastrointestinal tract. IBS can be worrisome, painful and at times embarrassing, but it's not life-threatening.

It's not known what causes IBS, but the condition involves abnormal muscle spasms in the walls of your stomach or intestines. The muscular walls regularly contract and relax to move food through the gastrointestinal tract. If you have IBS, the contractions are much stronger and longer lasting, forcing food through the tract more rapidly.

You're more likely to have IBS if you are young, female and have a family history of IBS. Researchers are studying whether this family history relates to a genetic inheritance, to a shared environment or to a combination of both.

Fortunately, irritable bowel syndrome doesn't cause inflammation or tissue changes, nor does it increase your risk of colorectal cancer. Most people discover that signs and symptoms improve as they learn to control the condition through the proper management of diet, lifestyle and stress.

Signs and symptoms

Signs and symptoms of IBS vary widely, and often resemble those of other diseases. The most common signs and symptoms include abdominal pain or cramping, diarrhea or constipation (sometimes occurring in alternating bouts), bloating, indigestion, gas and mucus in the stool.

Although bowel movements temporarily relieve pain, you may feel as though you can't empty your bowels completely. Your stools become thin and ribbon-like, laced with mucus or hard, dry pellets.

Like many people, you may experience only mild signs and symptoms, but for some, these problems are disabling. IBS is generally a chronic condition, although there are times when the signs and symptoms are worse and other times when they improve or disappear completely.

Triggers

For reasons that aren't clear, if you have IBS you may be reacting strongly to certain stimuli that may have little effect on other people. Common triggers for IBS may include:

• *Foods.* Symptoms may worsen when you eat certain foods, including chocolate, milk and alcohol. Be aware that if you experience cramping and bloating after eating dairy products, food with caffeine or sugar-free candy, the problem may be an intolerance to sugar (lactose), caffeine or the artificial sweetener sorbitol.

• *Stress.* Many people with IBS find their symptoms worsen or become more frequent during stressful events, such as changes in the daily routine or during family arguments. However, while stress may aggravate the symptoms, it doesn't cause them.

• *Hormones.* Because women are twice as likely to have IBS, researchers believe that hormonal changes play a role in this condition. Many women find their symptoms are worse during or around their menstrual periods.

• *Other illnesses.* Sometimes other illnesses, such as an acute episode of infectious diarrhea (gastroenteritis), can trigger IBS.

Continued next page >

♠ Home Remedies

Simple lifestyle changes may provide some relief from irritable bowel syndrome (IBS):

- *Experiment with fiber.* Fiber can be a mixed blessing. Although it helps reduce constipation, it can also make gas and cramping worse. The best approach is to gradually increase the fiber in your diet over a period of weeks. Examples of foods that contain fiber are whole grains, fruits, vegetables and beans. Some people do better taking a fiber supplement, such as Metamucil or Citrucel, which causes less gas and bloating. Be sure to introduce a supplement gradually and drink plenty of water every day.
- *Avoid problem foods.* If certain foods make your signs and symptoms worse, don't eat them. Common culprits include alcohol, chocolate, caffeinated beverages such as coffee and sodas, medications that contain caffeine, dairy products, and sugar-free sweeteners such as sorbitol or mannitol. If gas is a problem, foods that may trigger symptoms include beans, cauliflower, cabbage and broccoli. Fatty foods also may be a problem.
- *Take care with dairy products.* If you're lactose intolerant, try substituting yogurt for milk, or using an enzyme product that breaks down lactose. Consuming milk products in small amounts or combining them with other foods also may help. Some people may need to eliminate dairy completely.
- *Eat at regular times.* Not skipping meals and eating at about the same time each day helps you stay regular. If you have diarrhea, eating small, frequent meals may help ease bouts. If you're constipated, eating high-fiber foods may help move food through your intestines.
- *Drink plenty of liquids.* Water is best. Caffeinated or carbonated drinks may make symptoms worse.
- *Exercise regularly.* Exercise stimulates normal intestinal contractions and helps relieve stress. If you've been inactive, start slowly and gradually. If you have medical concerns, check with your doctor before starting an exercise program.
- *Try peppermint.* In some studies, symptoms of IBS improved significantly among people taking peppermint capsules. In other studies, there was no benefit. Peppermint contains menthol, which is thought to relax stomach muscles and speed passage of food through the stomach.
- *Eat yogurt and other probiotics.* Probiotics are foods containing "good," bacteria similar to those normally found in your body. Good bacteria help maintain a microorganic balance in your intestinal tract. Probiotics include yogurt, miso, tempeh, and some juices and soy drinks. They're available in supplement form.

✚ Medical Help

Because symptoms of IBS may mimic those of more serious medical problems, such as cancer, gallbladder disease and ulcers, see your doctor if self-care measures don't help within a couple of weeks. You may need testing if the following occurs: new onset after age 50, weight loss, rectal bleeding, fever, nausea or recurrent vomiting, abdominal pain (especially if it's not completely relieved by bowel movement), and persistent diarrhea.

Jammed finger

A jammed finger is typically a sprain to the joint, or knuckle, of the finger. There may also be a small fracture or dislocation of the joint. The injury can be extremely painful, and the joint usually becomes swollen.

A jammed finger is a common sports injury. For example, your fingertip receives the full impact of a hard-hit baseball, basketball rebound or volleyball spike. A jammed finger may also result for other reasons. You reach out your arm to break a fall, and your finger jabs into the ground. The result is often a jammed finger.

This type of injury usually heals quickly if there is no fracture, although the pain may linger for months when direct pressure is applied to the finger.

🏠 Home Remedies

To treat a jammed finger:
- Ice the finger with a cold pack for 15 minutes. Placing your finger in ice water works, too.
- Elevate your hand to reduce swelling.

To protect the finger during use:
- "Buddy tape" the injured finger to an adjacent finger. Use a self-adhesive wrap to tape above and below the finger joint — for example, index finger to middle finger or ring finger to small finger.

➕ Medical Help

Seek medical care if:
- Your finger appears deformed
- You cannot straighten your finger
- The area becomes hot and inflamed and you develop a fever
- Swelling and pain becomes significant or persistent
- The finger becomes numb, and turns white or pale (less pink)

Children require medical care because damage to the growth plate of a finger bone can lead to long-term deformity.

Jet lag

If you've traveled by air to another location in a different time zone, you're probably familiar with that dragged-out feeling called jet lag. The sleep disorder is caused by a disruption of your body's internal clock or circadian rhythm — which signals when it's time to be awake and when it's time to sleep. The more time zones you cross, the more likely you are to have jet lag.

Symptoms of jet lag may vary but can include:
- Disturbed sleep
- Daytime fatigue
- Difficulty concentrating
- Stomach problems
- Not feeling well
- Muscle soreness

Your body will readjust at the rate of about an hour a day. Thus, if you change four time zones, your body may require about four days to get back into its usual rhythm. Flying eastward — and resetting your body clock forward — is often more difficult than flying westward and adding hours to your day.

♠ Home Remedies

To reduce or prevent jet lag:
- *Reset your body's clock.* Several days in advance of your departure, adopt a waking-sleeping cycle that's closer to what you'll have at your destination.
- *Drink plenty of fluids and eat lightly.* Drink extra liquids during your flight to avoid dehydration, but limit beverages with alcohol and caffeine. They increase dehydration and may disrupt your sleep.
- *Avoid taking a sleeping pill on the flight over.* However, taking an over-the-counter sleep aid for the first three nights after reaching your destination may help you to adjust.
- *Switch immediately to local time.* On arrival at your destination, reset your watch to local time. If possible, don't plan a hectic schedule on the first day. Consider arriving at your destination in the evening, if traveling eastward.
- *Try melatonin.* The use of melatonin has its pros and cons. The latest research suggests that melatonin does indeed aid sleep during times when you wouldn't normally be resting, making it of particular benefit for people with jet lag. Small doses — as little as 0.5 milligram — seem just as effective as larger doses. Take melatonin 30 minutes before you plan to sleep or ask your doctor about the proper timing. Avoid alcohol when taking melatonin. Side effects are uncommon but may include dizziness, headache and loss of appetite, and possibly nausea and disorientation.

✚ Medical Help

Jet lag is a temporary condition. But if you are a frequent traveler and struggle with jet leg, you may benefit from seeing a sleep specialist.

Kidney stones

Kidney stones are small, hard deposits that form inside your kidneys. The stones are made of mineral and acid salts. Kidney stones have many causes. For example, they can form when your urine becomes concentrated, allowing minerals to crystallize and stick together.

Passing a stone through the urinary tract can be painful. The pain typically starts in your side or back, just below your ribs, and moves to your lower abdomen and groin. The location of pain may change as the stone moves through your tract.

Factors that increase your risk of kidney stones include:

- Family or personal history of kidney stones
- Being adult
- Being male
- Dehydration
- Eating a high-protein, high-sodium and high-sugar diet
- Obesity
- Digestive diseases and surgery that can cause changes in the digestive process
- Other medical conditions, including gout, hyperparathyroidism and certain urinary tract infections

♠ Home Remedies

One of the most effective ways to reduce your risk of kidney stones is to drink more fluids — ideally water — to increase your urine output to about 2.5 liters in a 24-hour period. Aim to drink enough fluid that your urine is nearly clear or has only a light yellow tinge. Other measures that may help prevent kidney stones include:

- Avoid foods and beverages that contain high-fructose corn syrup.
- Reduce your daily salt intake.
- Avoid calcium-containing antacids.
- Limit intake of beef, pork and poultry to less than 4 to 6 ounces a day.
- Eat moderate amounts of dairy products — between one and three servings — each day.
- Eat fewer oxalate-rich foods. If you tend to form calcium oxalate stones, your doctor may recommend restricting foods rich in oxalates. These include rhubarb, beets, okra, spinach, Swiss chard, sweet potatoes, tea, chocolate and soy products.
- Drink tea. Drinking a cup of black tea or green tea each day could reduce your risk of kidney stones. One study found that a group of women who drank the most black tea had a slightly lower risk of kidney stones. Although this study was not a rigorous one, if you currently enjoy tea, there's a chance that continuing to drink it may help reduce your risk of kidney stones.
- Drink lemon juice and orange juice. The citric acid levels in lemon juice and orange juice may reduce calcium levels in your urine, leading to fewer kidney stones, even though no studies have proved this theory. If you enjoy drinking water flavored with lemon or drinking orange juice every morning, you may actually be helping to reduce your risk.

✚ Medical Help

Make an appointment with your doctor if you have any signs or symptoms that worry you. Seek immediate medical attention if you experience:

- Pain so severe that you can't sit still or find a comfortable position
- Pain accompanied by nausea and vomiting
- Pain accompanied by fever and chills
- Blood in your urine

Knee pain

Knee injuries are often complex. A knee bears a lot of weight and isn't designed to handle sideways stress. The injury may affect any of the ligaments, tendons, or fluid-filled sacs (bursae) that surround your knee as well as the bones, cartilage and ligaments that form the joint itself. The signs and symptoms vary widely. Pain may be the result of:

- Trauma or blow to the knee
- Repeated stress or overuse
- Sudden turning, pivoting, stopping and cutting from side to side
- Awkward landings from a fall or from jumping
- Rapidly growing bones
- Degeneration from aging

Many knee injuries are sports related. Relatively minor knee pain usually responds well to self-care measures. More serious injuries, such as ruptured ligaments or tendons, may require surgical repair.

🏠 Home Remedies

The key to treating knee pain is to break the cycle of inflammation that begins right after the injury, decreasing the swelling and pain. Simple self-care measures can be remarkably effective in ending this cycle:

- *Follow the instructions for R.I.C.E..* See page 157.
- *Take an anti-inflammatory medication.* Nonsteroidal anti-inflammatory medications such as ibuprofen (Advil, Motrin, others) and naproxen (Aleve) help relieve inflammation.
- *Flex and straighten your leg gently every day.* If it's difficult to move your knee, have someone help you at first. Try to straighten it and keep it straight.
- *Avoid strenuous activity until your knee heals.* Start nonimpact exercises slowly.
- *Avoid squatting, kneeling or walking up and down hills.* Stress of this kind may aggravate your knee injury.

Prevention

Regular exercise strengthens your knee muscles and helps prevent knee pain. Bend your knee only to a 90-degree angle during exercise. Don't do deep knee bends.

✚ Medical Help

Seek medical care immediately if the injury produces intense pain and the knee doesn't function properly, or if the pain follows a popping sound or a snapping or locking feeling. Also, seek care if the knee locks in one position or seems unusually loose or unstable.

Lactose intolerance

Lactose intolerance means that you aren't able to fully digest lactose, a natural sugar in milk and other dairy products. The condition usually is not dangerous, but its symptoms can be uncomfortable.

The problem behind lactose intolerance is your body's deficiency of lactase — an enzyme that breaks down lactose during the digestive process. In fact, many people have low levels of lactase, but only a segment of this larger group have associated signs and symptoms. These are the individuals who have, by definition, lactose intolerance.

Signs and symptoms of lactose intolerance usually begin 30 minutes to two hours after eating or drinking foods that contain lactose. Common signs and symptoms include:

- Diarrhea
- Nausea
- Abdominal cramps
- Bloating and gas

Symptoms of lactose intolerance are usually mild, but they may sometimes be severe. It may not be necessary to completely avoid all dairy foods. Most people with lactose intolerance can enjoy some milk products without symptoms — they just choose what to eat with caution.

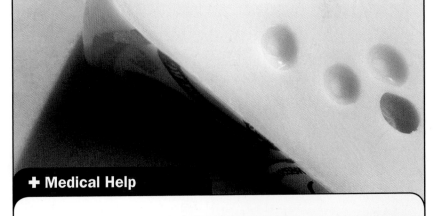

⌂ Home Remedies

People with lactose intolerance can reduce signs and symptoms by carefully selecting and limiting dairy products. Simple ways to adjust your diet include:

- *Choosing smaller servings of dairy.* Sip small servings of milk — up to 4 ounces at a time. The smaller the serving, the less likely it is to cause gastrointestinal problems.
- *Experimenting with an assortment of dairy products.* Not all dairy products have the same amount of lactose. For example, hard cheeses, such as Swiss or cheddar, have small amounts of lactose and generally cause no symptoms. You may be able to tolerate products such as yogurt, because bacteria used in the culturing process naturally produce the enzyme lactase.
- *Buying lactose-reduced or lactose-free products.* You can find these products at most supermarkets in the refrigerated dairy section.
- *Using lactase enzyme products.* Over-the-counter tablets or drops containing the lactase enzyme may help you digest dairy products.
- *Eating foods containing probiotics.* Probiotics are foods or supplements containing beneficial, or "good," bacteria that inhibit harmful, disease-causing bacteria, to help maintain a proper microorganic balance in your intestinal tract. Probiotics come from food sources, such as yogurt, miso, tempeh, and some juices and soy drinks. They're also available as capsules, tablets, suppositories and powders.

✚ Medical Help

There's currently no way to boost your body's production of the lactase enzyme. However, make an appointment with your doctor if you or your child has any signs or symptoms that worry you.

Leg swelling

Swelling can occur in any part of your legs, including feet, ankles, calves or thighs. The swelling may result from fluid buildup or from inflammation in injured or diseased tissues or joints.

Many causes of leg swelling are relatively harmless in the long term, but sometimes, the swelling may be a sign of a more serious disorder, such as heart disease or a blood clot.

Some generalizations that may help you determine the cause of leg swelling include:

- Swelling in only one leg is more likely related to a condition in that leg alone.
- Swelling in both legs is more likely caused by a condition not directly related to the legs, such as prolonged standing or sitting.
- Leg swelling usually isn't the only sign of a serious disorder. For example, leg swelling related to heart disease is likely to occur along with shortness of breath or chest pain.
- Leg swelling from a blood clot usually appears suddenly and for no obvious reason. The clots often cause an aching pain deep in the calf or inner thigh. The leg may also be cool and pale.

⌂ Home Remedies

To help prevent or remedy occasional leg swelling:

- Lose weight and limit your salt intake.
- Elevate your legs to a level above your heart for 15 to 20 minutes every few hours to let gravity help move fluid toward your heart.
- During periods of prolonged sitting and travel, try to walk around frequently and stretch your legs.
- Consider using compression stockings, especially when you're on your feet for long periods of time or while traveling on an airplane.

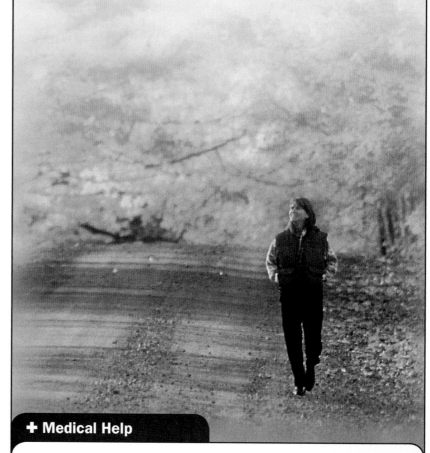

✚ Medical Help

Swelling in your legs can be a sign of a more serious condition. Seek medical care immediately if you have unexplained, painful swelling in your legs or if a swollen leg becomes warm, red and inflamed. Also see your doctor if the swelling remains despite self-care.

Lice

Lice are tiny parasitic insects that feed on your blood. They are easily spread through personal contact, and by sharing belongings such as combs, clothing and bedding.

Several types of lice exist, named for the areas of the body where they prefer to feed: head lice, body lice and pubic lice, commonly called crabs. Lice live only three days off the body. Eggs (nits) hatch in about one week.

Signs and symptoms include intense itching, tickling sensations, and small, red bumps on the scalp, neck and shoulders. The eggs, resembling tiny pussy willow buds, can be found on hair shafts. With body lice, some people develop hives while others have abrasions from scratching.

Head lice are easiest to see at the nape of the neck and over the ears. Body lice are difficult to find because they burrow into the skin, but may be detected in the seams of underwear.

Scabies

Other unwelcome visitors may be tiny burrowing mites that cause an itchy condition called scabies, marked by thin, irregular burrow tracks on your skin made up of tiny blisters or bumps. Scabies is highly contagious and can spread quickly through physical contact. Medicated cream applied to your skin can kill the mites, although you may experience some itching for several more weeks.

🏠 Home Remedies

These steps may help you eliminate lice infestations:

- *Use lotions and shampoos.* Several over-the-counter lotions and shampoos (Nix, Rid, others) are designed to kill lice. Apply the product according to package instructions. You may need to repeat the treatment in seven to 10 days. These lotions and shampoos typically aren't recommended for children under age 2.
- *After shampoo treatment, rinse your hair with vinegar.* Grasp a lock of hair with a cloth saturated with vinegar and strip the lock downward to remove nits. Repeat until you've treated all the hair in this way. Or soak hair with vinegar and leave it on for a few minutes before combing. Then towel-dry the hair.
- *Comb wet hair.* Use a fine-toothed or nit comb to physically remove the lice from wet hair. Repeat every three to four days for at least two weeks. This method may be used in combination with other treatments and is usually recommended as the first line of treatment for children under age 2.
- *Wash contaminated items.* Wash bedding, stuffed animals, clothing and hats with hot, soapy water — at least 130 F — and dry them at high heat for at least 20 minutes.
- *Seal unwashable items.* Place in an airtight bag for two weeks.
- *Vacuum.* Give the floor and furniture a good vacuuming.
- *Cover furniture.* Use a plastic painter's dropcloth to cover furniture for two weeks to prevent acquiring another case of lice. Don't do this if you have a toddler who may become tangled in the plastic.
- *Wash combs and brushes.* Use hot, soapy water — at least 130 F — or soak combs and brushes in rubbing alcohol for an hour.

➕ Medical Help

Consult your doctor before using products on a child younger than 2 months or if you're pregnant. The Food and Drug Administration (FDA) cautions that products containing lindane can cause serious side effects, even when used as directed.

Menopause

Menopause is the permanent end of menstruation and fertility, defined as occurring 12 months after your last menstrual period. Some women reach menopause in their 30s or 40s, while others do so in their 50s or 60s. The average age for women in the United States is 51.

Menopause is a natural biological process, not a medical illness. Even so, the physical and emotional symptoms of menopause may disrupt your sleep, sap your energy and trigger feelings of sadness and loss.

Hormonal changes cause the physical symptoms, but mistaken beliefs are partly to blame for many emotional ones. First, menopause doesn't mean the end is near — you've still got as much as half your life to go.

Second, menopause will not snuff out your femininity and sexuality. In fact, you may be one of many women who find it liberating to enjoy intimacy without having to worry about pregnancy and periods.

Most important, even though menopause is not an illness, you shouldn't hesitate to get treatment for severe symptoms.

Signs and symptoms often appear long before you "hit" menopause. They include:
- Irregular periods
- Decreased fertility
- Vaginal dryness
- Hot flashes
- Sleep disturbances
- Mood swings
- Increased abdominal fat
- Thinning hair
- Loss of breast fullness

Stages of menopause

Because the transition occurs over months and years, menopause is commonly divided into these stages:
- *Perimenopause.* You begin to experience menopausal signs and symptoms, even though you still menstruate. Your hormone levels rise and fall unevenly, and you may have hot flashes and other symptoms. This may last four to five years or longer. During this time, it's still possible to get pregnant, but not likely.
- *Postmenopause.* Once 12 months have passed since your last period, you've reached menopause. In the postmenopausal years that follow, your ovaries produce less of the sex hormones and don't release eggs.

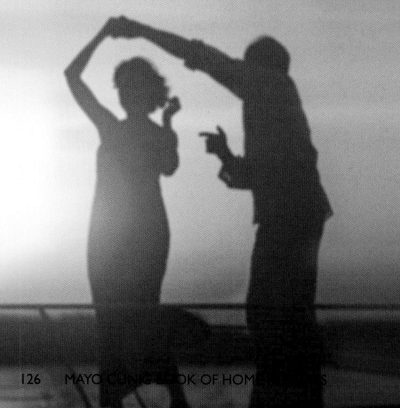

Fortunately, many signs and symptoms of menopause are temporary. The following steps may help reduce or prevent their effects.

Eat well
Eat a balanced diet that includes a variety of fruits, vegetables and whole grains and that limits saturated fats, oils and sugars. Include 1,200 to 1,500 milligrams of calcium and 800 international units of vitamin D a day.

Optimize your sleep
If you have trouble sleeping, avoid caffeinated beverages and don't exercise right before bedtime.

Exercise regularly
Get at least 30 minutes of moderately intense physical activity on most days to help protect against many conditions associated with aging. More vigorous exercise for longer periods may provide further benefit and is particularly important if you're trying to lose weight and reduce stress.

Decrease vaginal discomfort
For vaginal dryness or discomfort with intercourse, use over-the-counter water-based vaginal lubricants (Astroglide, K-Y Jelly), moisturizers (Replens, Vagisil) or vaginal estrogen. Staying sexually active also helps.

Cool hot flashes
To cope with hot flashes, get regular exercise, dress in layers and try to pinpoint what triggers your hot flashes. Triggers may include hot beverages, spicy foods, alcohol, hot weather and even a warm room. Other remedies you might try include:

- *Black cohosh.* Studies show mixed results for black cohosh reducing menopausal symptoms, such as hot flashes. When taken short term, it appears to have a low risk of side effects. Don't take it for more than six months.
- *Isoflavones.* Soy is a common source of isoflavones, compounds with weak estrogen-like effects. These compounds may help with hot flashes. Study results regarding their safety and effectiveness are mixed. If you've had breast cancer, talk to your doctor before taking soy supplements.
- *Flaxseed.* Flaxseed is a source of phytoestrogens as well as omega-3 fatty acids. Some research suggests daily consumption of flaxseed improves mild menopause symptoms, such as hot flashes. Flaxseed is a healthy alternative to other fats and it's safe. However, it shouldn't be taken in large amounts by people who take warfarin (Coumadin).

Practice relaxation techniques
Techniques such as deep breathing, guided imagery, yoga and meditation don't directly target the hormonal fluctuations of menopause, but they may help you cope with mood swings, stress and sleep disturbances.

Vaginal bleeding after menopause is not normal and should be promptly evaluated by your doctor. The cause of bleeding may be entirely harmless, but postmenopausal bleeding has a number of serious causes, including cancer.

Menstrual cramps

If you're a woman, chances are you have dealt with menstrual cramps – even if you've never heard of the medical term for them: dysmenorrhea. Dull, throbbing or cramping pains develop in your lower abdomen and may extend to the lower back and thighs. Some women also have nausea, vomiting, diarrhea, sweating or dizziness.

Many women experience painful cramps just before or during their menstrual period. The discomfort may be merely annoying. But for some women, the pain they live with for a few days every month is severe enough to affect their mood and disrupt activities.

Many experts believe that cramping is a result of severe contractions of the uterus, which constrict blood vessels feeding the uterus. Menstrual cramps may also be caused by gynecologic conditions such as endometriosis and uterine fibroids.

Menstrual cramps tend to lessen with age and often disappear following childbirth.

🏠 Home Remedies

To relieve or prevent menstrual cramps, try the following:
- *Pain relievers.* Nonsteroidal anti-inflammatory drugs, such as aspirin, ibuprofen (Advil, Motrin, others), naproxen (Aleve) and acetaminophen (Tylenol, others), taken as directed from the start of cramps until the cramps go away will relieve pain in most women. Girls under age 18 should not use aspirin.
- *Heat.* Try soaking in a warm tub or applying a heating pad on your lower abdomen.
- *Exercise.* Many women find that exercise helps lessen the symptoms of menstrual cramps.
- *Dietary supplements.* Some studies have indicated that vitamin E, thiamin and omega-3 supplements may help reduce the symptoms of menstrual cramps.

➕ Medical Help

Talk to your doctor if the cramping pain is severe or associated with a fever, or if the pain lasts several days a month and disrupts your life. Also see your doctor if you have nausea and vomiting or unusual vaginal discharge or odor.

Morning sickness

Morning sickness refers to nausea that occurs during pregnancy. The name is a misnomer, however, because morning sickness can strike at any time of the day (or even at night).

Morning sickness affects an estimated 50 to 90 percent of pregnant women. It's most common during the first trimester, but for some women morning sickness lingers throughout the pregnancy.

The condition is distressful and uncomfortable but is generally harmless. Medical treatment isn't usually necessary, although various home remedies often help relieve the nausea.

♠ Home Remedies

To help relieve morning sickness:

- *Choose foods carefully.* Opt for foods that are high in carbohydrates, low in fat and easy to digest. Salty foods are sometimes helpful, as are foods that contain ginger – such as ginger lollipops. Avoid greasy, spicy and fatty foods.
- *Snack often.* Before getting out of bed in the morning, eat a few soda crackers or a piece of dry toast. Nibble throughout the day, rather than eating three large meals. An empty stomach may aggravate nausea.
- *Drink plenty of fluids.* Sip water or ginger ale. It may also help to suck on hard candy, ice chips or ice pops.
- *Pay attention to situations that trigger nausea.* Avoid foods or smells or environments that seem to make your nausea worse.
- *Get plenty of fresh air.* Weather permitting, open the windows in your home or workplace. Take a daily walk outdoors.
- *Take care with prenatal vitamins.* If you feel queasy after taking prenatal vitamins, take the vitamins at night or with a snack. It may also help to chew gum or suck on hard candy after taking your vitamin. If these steps don't help, ask your doctor about switching to a type of prenatal vitamin that doesn't contain iron.
- *Try ginger.* A few studies suggest that ginger may help ease nausea from pregnancy. Ginger supplements are generally considered safe when taken in small amounts for a short time. However, it takes a few days for the ginger to work. Before taking the supplement, it may be best to talk with your doctor.

✚ Medical Help

Contact your doctor if, during periods of morning sickness:

- Nausea or vomiting is severe
- You pass only a small amount of urine or it's dark in color
- You can't keep down liquids
- You feel dizzy or faint when you stand up
- Your heart races
- You vomit blood

Motion sickness

Any type of transportation can cause motion sickness — boat, plane, train or automobile. Symptoms may strike suddenly, building from a feeling of unease to a cold sweat, dizziness and then vomiting.

Typically, you start feeling better as soon as the motion stops. The more you travel, the more easily you'll adjust to the motion.

You may be able to escape motion sickness by planning ahead. When you travel, reserve seats where motion is felt least:

- *By ship.* Request a cabin in the front or middle of the ship, or on the upper deck.
- *By plane.* Ask for a seat over the front edge of a wing. Once aboard, direct the air vent flow to your face.
- *By train.* Take a seat near the front and next to a window. Face forward.
- *By automobile.* Drive or sit in the front passenger's seat.

♠ Home Remedies

If you're susceptible to motion sickness:

- Focus on the horizon or on a distant, stationary object. Don't read.
- Keep your head still, while resting against a seat back.
- Don't smoke or sit near smokers.
- Breathe plenty of fresh air.
- Avoid spicy or greasy foods and alcohol. Don't overeat.
- Take an over-the-counter motion sickness drug such as meclizine (Bonine, Dramamine Less Drowsy Formula) or dimenhydrinate (Dramamine) before your outing.
- Consider scopolamine (Transderm Scōp), available in a prescription adhesive patch. Several hours before you plan to travel, apply the patch behind your ear for 72-hour protection. Talk to your doctor before using the medication if you have health problems such as asthma, glaucoma or urine retention.
- Eat dry crackers or drink a carbonated beverage to help settle your stomach if you become ill.

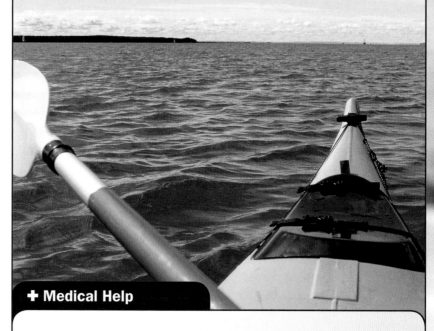

✚ Medical Help

If you're prone to severe motion sickness, talk with your doctor about prescription medications such as scopolamine (Transderm Scōp) before traveling. The drug offers 72-hour protection from motion sickness, although it can cause dry mouth and other side effects.

Muscle strain

A muscle can become strained or pulled — or even torn — when it is stretched unusually far or abruptly. This type of injury may also happen when muscles suddenly and powerfully contract.

Muscle strains often occur in the lower back or in the hamstring muscle in the back of your thigh. A slip on the ice or lifting from an awkward position may cause the muscle strain. Strains can vary in their severity:

- *Mild.* Causes pain and stiffness when you move. Symptoms will last a few days.
- *Moderate.* Causes small muscle tears and more extensive pain, swelling and bruising. Pain may last one to three weeks.
- *Severe.* Muscle is torn or ruptured completely. You may have significant internal bleeding, swelling and bruising around the muscle. The muscle may not function at all. Seek immediate medical attention.

⌂ Home Remedies

To relieve symptoms of muscle strain:

- Follow the instructions for R.I.C.E. (see page 157). The earlier the treatment, the speedier and more complete your recovery.
- For extensive swelling, use cold packs several times each day throughout your recovery.
- Don't apply heat when the area is still swollen.
- Avoid the activity that caused the strain while the muscle heals.
- Use over-the-counter pain medications as needed, such as ibuprofen (Advil, Motrin, others), naproxen (Aleve) and acetaminophen (Tylenol, others). Avoid using aspirin in the first few hours after the strain because aspirin may make bleeding more extensive. Don't give aspirin to children.

✚ Medical Help

Seek medical help immediately if the area quickly becomes swollen and is intensely painful. Call your doctor if the pain, swelling and stiffness don't improve in two to three days or if you suspect a ruptured muscle or broken bone.

Nausea and vomiting

Nausea is a queasy feeling in your stomach that can be caused by many things, including viral infection, headache, gallstones, food poisoning, motion sickness, radiation therapy, general anesthesia, pregnancy, dizziness, fear and anxiety, overeating, and exposure to strong odors. The list of potential causes goes on and on.

Nausea often, but not always, leads to vomiting — a violent, forceful ejection of stomach contents through your mouth. With vomiting, there's always an added risk of dehydration.

Nausea and vomiting are common and uncomfortable but generally not serious. A viral infection called gastroenteritis, often mistakenly called "stomach flu," is a common cause of nausea and vomiting (see pages 158-159). Diarrhea, abdominal cramps, bloating and fever may accompany this condition.

🏠 Home Remedies

If a viral infection is the culprit, nausea and vomiting may last from a few hours to two or three days. Diarrhea and mild abdominal cramping also are common. To stay comfortable and prevent dehydration while you recover, try the following:

- Don't eat or drink anything for a few hours until your stomach has had time to settle.
- Try ice chips or small sips of weak tea, broths, clear soda (such as 7Up or Sprite) or noncaffeinated clear sports drinks to prevent dehydration. Consume 2 to 4 quarts (eight to 16 glasses) of liquid for 24 hours, taking frequent, small sips.
- Try adding semisolid and low-fiber foods gradually — but stop eating if the vomiting returns. Try soda crackers, gelatin, plain toast, eggs, rice or chicken.
- Avoid dairy products, caffeine, alcohol, nicotine, and fatty or highly seasoned foods for a few days.

Infant care

Most babies spit up food at least occasionally. Vomiting is a more forceful and disturbing action to your baby. It may lead to dehydration and weight loss if it's persistent.

To prevent dehydration, let the baby's stomach rest for 30 to 60 minutes and then offer small amounts of liquid. If you're breast-feeding, let your baby nurse smaller amounts more frequently. Offer bottle-fed babies a small amount of formula or an oral electrolyte solution such as Pedialyte.

If the vomiting doesn't recur, continue to offer small sips of liquid or the breast every 15 to 30 minutes.

➕ Medical Help

Contact your doctor if you're unable to drink anything for 24 hours, if vomiting persists beyond two or three days, if you become dehydrated or if you vomit blood. Signs of dehydration include excessive thirst, dry mouth, little or no urination, severe weakness, dizziness or lightheadedness. Vomiting may be a warning of more serious underlying problems such as concussion, gallbladder disease, ulcers, bowel obstruction or meningitis.

Neck pain

Neck pain may involve muscles and nerves as well as cervical vertebrae and the disks that cushion them. Fortunately, most causes of neck pain aren't serious and can be treated with self-care.

Poor posture
Whether leaning over a computer or hunched over a workbench, poor posture can strain muscles.

Muscle strain
Overuse, such as twisting and turning your head, can trigger muscle strains. Even gritting your teeth can strain neck muscles.

Worn joints
Your neck joints tend to experience wear and tear with age, which can cause osteoarthritis.

Nerve compression
A so-called "pinched nerve" can occur when the space around your neck's vertebrae is reduced.

Injury
Whiplash injuries, when the head is jerked sharply back and forth, stretches the soft tissues of the neck beyond their typical range of motion.

Disease
Neck pain may be a symptom of disease, such as rheumatoid arthritis or meningitis.

♠ Home Remedies

Self-care measures to relieve neck pain include:

- *Pain relievers.* Try over-the-counter pain relievers, such as aspirin, ibuprofen (Advil, Motrin, others), naproxen (Aleve) and acetaminophen (Tylenol, others).
- *Alternate heat and cold.* Reduce inflammation by applying an ice pack or ice wrapped in a towel for up to 20 minutes several times a day. Or alternate the cold treatment with heat. Try taking a warm shower or using a heating pad on a low setting. Heat can help relax sore muscles, but it sometimes aggravates inflammation, so use it with caution.
- *Rest.* Lie down from time to time to give your neck a rest from holding up your head. Avoid prolonged rest, since too much inactivity can increase stiffness in the neck muscles.
- *Do gentle stretching.* Gently move your neck to one side and hold it for 30 seconds. Stretch your neck in as many directions as the pain allows. This may help alleviate some of the pain.
- *Take frequent breaks.* This is especially helpful if you drive long distances or work long hours at your computer. Keep your head back, over your spine, to reduce strain. Avoid gritting your teeth.
- *Adjust your computer.* Make sure your desk, chair and computer are aligned so the computer monitor is at eye level. When you sit, your knees should be slightly lower than hips. Use your chair's armrests.
- *Be wise with your phone.* Avoid tucking the phone between your ear and shoulder as you talk. If you use the phone a lot, get a headset.
- *Avoid sleeping on your stomach.* This position puts stress on your neck. Choose a pillow that supports the natural curve of your neck.

✚ Medical Help

Sometimes neck pain can signify something more serious. Seek immediate medical care if you experience:
- Shooting pain into your shoulder or down your arm
- Numbness or loss of strength in your arms or hands
- Change in bladder or bowel habits
- Inability to touch your chin to your chest

Nosebleeds

The lining of your nose contains tiny blood vessels that lie close to the surface and are easily damaged, which may cause bleeding. Most often, nosebleeds are a nuisance and not a true medical problem.

The two most common causes of nosebleeds are:

- Dry air — when your nasal membranes are dry, they're more susceptible to bleeding
- Nose picking

Other causes of nosebleeds include sinusitis, allergies, common cold, foreign body in the nose, trauma, exposure to chemical irritants, such as ammonia, and taking blood thinners, such as warfarin (Coumadin) and heparin.

Rarely, frequent nosebleeds may indicate a serious condition such as a bleeding disorder or leukemia. See your doctor to rule out these conditions if you experience frequent nosebleeds along with easy bruising and bleeding elsewhere in your body.

🏠 Home Remedies

To treat a nosebleed:

- Sit upright and lean forward. By remaining upright, you reduce blood pressure in the veins of your nose. This discourages further bleeding. Sitting forward will help you avoid swallowing blood, which can irritate your stomach.
- Pinch your nose with your thumb and index finger and breathe through your mouth. Continue to pinch for five to 10 minutes. This maneuver puts pressure on the bleeding point and often stops the flow of blood.

To prevent a resumption of bleeding:

- Don't blow your nose or bend down until several hours after the bleeding episode. Keep your head higher than the level of your heart. Don't pick your nose.
- If re-bleeding occurs, gently blow out to clear your nose of blood clots, and spray both sides of your nose with a decongestant nasal spray containing oxymetazoline (Afrin, others) or phenylephrine (Neo-Synephrine). Pinch your nose again.

To prevent nosebleeds:

- Increase the humidity of the air you breathe in your home. A humidifier or vaporizer can help keep your nasal membranes moist.
- Over-the-counter saline nasal spray or gel may help, especially during winter months.

✚ Medical Help

Seek medical care if:

- You have frequent nosebleeds
- The bleeding lasts for more than 20 minutes
- The bleeding is rapid or the amount of blood loss is great
- Bleeding begins by trickling down the back of your throat
- Other body sites are bruised or bleeding
- The nosebleed follows an accident, a fall or an injury to your head, including trauma that may have broken your nose

Object in ear

A foreign object becoming stuck in the ear is a relatively common problem. Children, in particular, have a penchant for sticking eraser tips, small toys, dried beans or other pieces of food into their ear canals — they may not know any better or they're simply curious about what will happen.

When an object becomes stuck in the ear, it's important for you and your child to stay calm and assess the situation. There may be some pain and temporary hearing loss but, in general, the object can be safely removed with minimal discomfort.

⌂ Home Remedies

If an object becomes lodged in the ear, follow these steps:

- *Don't probe the ear with a tool.* Don't attempt to remove the foreign object by probing with a cotton swab, matchstick or any other tool. To do so is to risk pushing the object farther into the ear and damaging the fragile structures of the middle ear.
- *Remove the object if possible.* If the object is clearly visible, is pliable and can be grasped easily with tweezers, gently remove it.
- *Try using the pull of gravity.* Tilt the head to the affected side. Don't strike the person's head, but shake it gently in the direction of the ground to try to dislodge the object.
- *If the foreign object is an insect, try using oil.* Tilt the person's head so that the ear with the offending insect is turned upward. Try to float the insect out by pouring mineral oil, olive oil or baby oil into the ear. The oil should be warm but not hot. You can ease entry of the oil by straightening the ear canal. Pull the earlobe gently backward and upward. The insect should suffocate and may float out in the oil bath. Don't use oil to remove any object other than an insect. Don't use this method if there's any suspicion of a perforation in the eardrum (pain, bleeding or discharge from the ear).

+ Medical Help

If these methods fail or the person continues to experience pain in the ear, hearing loss or a sensation of something lodged in the ear, seek medical assistance.

Object in eye

Everyone will occasionally get a foreign object in an eye. Often, it's a loose eyelash or a dirt speck blown by the wind. The eye often is able to clear itself by tearing up and blinking.

At other times, the eye doesn't clear itself so easily and you may need assistance. On these occasions, follow the guidelines listed on this page.

You may experience minor discomfort, such as a mild scratchy feeling, in the eyeball after the object has been removed. If you continue to feel discomfort after a day or two, seek medical assistance.

If the object is embedded in the eyeball, don't attempt to remove the object and don't rub the eye. Cover both eyes with a soft pad and seek emergency medical care.

♠ Home Remedies

Clearing your own eye

- If it's a minor issue, such as small particles of dust, blinking several times may remove the particles.
- If blinking doesn't work, try to flush the object out of your eye with clean, lukewarm water or saline solution. Use an eyecup or small clean glass. Position the glass with its rim resting on the bone of your eye socket and pour the fluid in, keeping the eye open.

Clearing someone else's eye

- Wash your hands. Seat the person in a well-lighted area.
- Examine the eye to find the object. Gently pull the lower lid down and ask the person to look up. Then hold the upper lid while the person looks down.
- If the object is floating in the tear film or on the surface of the eye, try flushing it out. If you're able to remove the object, flush the eye with a saline solution or clean, lukewarm water.

Don'ts

- Don't rub the eye, and don't apply patches or ice packs to the eye.
- Don't try to remove an object that's embedded in the eyeball.
- Don't try to remove any object that makes closing the eye difficult.

✚ Medical Help

Seek emergency medical help when:
- You can't remove the object
- The object is embedded in the eyeball
- The person is experiencing abnormal vision
- Pain, vision problems or redness persists

Oral thrush

Oral thrush (candidiasis) is an infection caused by a fungus that accumulates in your mouth. Symptoms may include creamy-white soft patches in your mouth or throat, lesions with a cottage cheese-like appearance, pain, slight bleeding if the lesions are rubbed or scraped, cracking at the corners of your mouth, a cottony feeling in your mouth, or loss of taste.

Oral thrush is most common among babies, young children and older adults. It often occurs when your immune system is weakened by disease or drugs such as prednisone, or when antibiotics disturb the natural balance of microorganisms in your body.

Oral thrush is a minor disorder if you're healthy, but if you have a weakened immune system, symptoms may be more severe and harder to control.

♠ Home Remedies

These suggestions may help during an outbreak of oral thrush:

- *Practice good oral hygiene.* Brush at least twice a day and floss at least once. Replace your toothbrush frequently until the infection clears up. Avoid mouthwash or sprays.
- *Try warm saltwater rinses.* Dissolve 1/2 teaspoon of salt in 1 cup of warm water. Swish the rinse and then spit it out, but don't swallow.
- *Keep baby equipment clean.* If your baby develops thrush, clean pacifiers and bottle nipples with a 50 percent vinegar and water solution. If you use a breast pump, use the vinegar solution to clean detachable parts that come in contact with your milk.
- *Use nursing pads.* If you're breast-feeding and develop a fungal infection, this will help prevent the fungus from spreading to your clothes. Look for pads that don't have a plastic barrier, which can encourage growth of the fungus.

Prevention

The following measures may help prevent fungal infections:

- *Rinse your mouth.* If you have to use a corticosteroid inhaler, be sure to rinse your mouth with water or brush your teeth after taking your medication.
- *Eat yogurt.* Eat fresh-culture yogurt containing *Lactobacillus acidophilus* or *bifidobacterium* or take *acidophilus* capsules when you take antibiotics.
- *Don't ignore vaginal yeast infections.* Treat them immediately.
- *See your dentist regularly — especially if you have diabetes or wear dentures.* Ask your dentist how often you need to schedule a visit. Brush and floss your teeth as often as your dentist recommends. If you wear dentures, be sure to clean them every night.
- *Watch what you eat.* Try limiting the amount of sugar and yeast-containing foods you consume. These foods may encourage fungal growth.

✚ Medical Help

If you or your baby develops painful white lesions inside the mouth, see your doctor or dentist. If thrush develops in older children or adolescents who have no other risk factors, seek medical care. An underlying condition such as diabetes may be the cause.

Osteoporosis

Osteoporosis is a disease that causes your bones to become weak and brittle — so brittle that a minor fall or even mild stress (like bending over or coughing) can fracture a bone. Most of these fractures will occur in the spine, hip or wrist.

Although it's often thought of as a women's disease, osteoporosis affects men as well. And aside from people who have osteoporosis, many others have low bone density that puts them at greater risk of osteoporosis.

To understand osteoporosis, it helps to be aware of the bone remodeling process taking place in your body. Bone continuously changes — new bone is made and old bone is broken down. When you're young, your body builds new bone faster than old bone breaks down.

You generally reach a peak bone mass in your late-20s. After that, bone remodeling changes — you begin to lose slightly more bone than you gain. Your likelihood of developing osteoporosis depends on the bone mass you attained by early adulthood, and how rapidly you lose it later.

In the early stages of bone loss, there is usually no indication of a problem. But once your bones are weakened by osteoporosis, signs and symptoms may include:

- Back pain
- Loss of height
- Stooped posture
- Fracture of the vertebra, wrist, hip or other bone

Risk factors

A diet lacking in calcium, phosphorus and other minerals (along with vitamin D) is a critical factor in the development of osteoporosis. If your bones have too little of these minerals, they become weak and brittle. You'll have a lower peak bone mass and accelerated bone loss later in life.

A number of other factors increase the likelihood that you'll develop osteoporosis. They include:

- Being female
- Getting older
- Having a family history of the disease
- Being of Caucasian or Asian descent
- Having a small body frame

Other risk factors include being inactive, tobacco use, having an eating disorder, excessive alcohol consumption and the use of certain medications such as corticosteroids.

Daily calcium

The Institute of Medicine recommends the following minimum amounts of daily calcium from food and supplements:

- Up to 1 year — 210-270 milligrams (mg)
- Ages 1 to 3 years — 500 mg
- Ages 4 to 8 years — 800 mg
- Ages 9 to 18 years — 1,300 mg
- Ages 19 to 50 years — 1,000 mg
- Age 51 and older — 1,200 mg

The following suggestions may help relieve symptoms and prevent osteoporosis:

Posture

Good posture puts less stress on your spine. When you sit or drive, place a rolled towel in the small of your back. Don't lean over while reading or doing handwork. When lifting, bend at your knees, not your waist, and lift with your legs, keeping your upper back straight.

Calcium

The Institute of Medicine (IOM) provides recommendations for daily amounts of calcium in your diet (see table on page 138).

Dairy products are one, but by no means the only, source of calcium. Almonds, broccoli, spinach, cooked kale, canned salmon with the bones, sardines and soy products, such as tofu and tempeh, also are rich in calcium.

If you find it difficult to get enough calcium, consider taking calcium supplements. The IOM recommends taking no more than 2,500 mg of calcium daily.

Vitamin D

Getting adequate amounts of vitamin D is just as important as calcium. Scientists don't yet know the optimal daily dose of vitamin D, but experts generally recommend that adults get between 400 and 1,000 international units (IUs) daily.

Many people get enough vitamin D from sunlight, but this may not be a good source for everyone. Although vitamin D is present in oily fish, such as tuna and sardines, and in egg yolks, you probably don't eat these on a daily basis. Vitamin D supplements are a good alternative.

Exercise

Exercise will benefit your bones no matter at what age you start, but you'll gain the most benefits if you start exercising regularly when you're young and continue to exercise throughout your life.

Combine strength training with weight-bearing exercises. Strength training will help strengthen your arms and upper spine. Weight-bearing exercises, such as walking, jogging, stair climbing, skipping rope, skiing and impact-producing sports, mainly affect your legs, hips and lower spine.

Don't smoke

Smoking may increase bone loss.

Avoid excessive alcohol

Drinking more than two alcoholic drinks daily may decrease bone formation and reduce your body's ability to absorb calcium.

Because osteoporosis rarely causes signs and symptoms until it's advanced, the National Osteoporosis Foundation recommends bone density testing if you are:

- A woman older than age 65 or a man older than age 70, regardless of risk factors
- A postmenopausal woman with at least one risk factor
- A man between ages 50 and 70 who has at least one risk factor
- Older than age 50 with a history of a broken bone
- A man or woman and take medications, such as prednisone, aromatase inhibitors or anti-seizure drugs
- A postmenopausal woman who has recently stopped taking hormone therapy
- A woman who experienced early menopause

Pink eye

Pink eye, also known as cojunctivitis, is an inflammation or infection of the transparent membrane lining your eyeball. The inflammation causes small blood vessels in the membrane to become more prominent, causing the whites of your eyes to take on a pink or red color.

The condition generally results from a virus or bacteria. Sometimes, it may be due to an allergic reaction. Both viral and bacterial forms are very contagious. Adults and children can develop either type of pink eye, but the bacterial form is more common in children than in adults.

Symptoms of pink eye include redness, itchiness or a gritty feeling in the affected eye, as well as tearing and discharge, blurred vision, and sensitivity to light.

Eyedrops or ointment prescribed by a doctor can treat bacterial pink eye, but there's no treatment for the viral form. Like the common cold, the condition has to run its course. Pink eye generally remains contagious as long as there's tearing and discharge continues to form on the eye.

Viral or bacterial?

You may be able to determine the type of pink eye you have by the discharge.

- *Viral type.* Discharge is usually watery and clear.
- *Bacterial type.* Discharge is often a thick, yellow-green matter.

🏠 Home Remedies

Take these steps:

- *Apply a warm compress.* Soak a clean, lint-free cloth in warm water, squeeze it dry and place it over your gently closed eyelid. Do this several times daily. In case of allergic conjunctivitis, use a cold compress.
- *Control its spread.* To prevent it from spreading to the other eye or to other people, keep your hands away from your eyes and wash your hands frequently. Also change your washcloth and towel daily. Get rid of eye cosmetics, particularly mascara.
- *Don't wear contacts.* If you wear disposable contacts, throw out your current pair. Disinfect nondisposable types thoroughly. Wait until your eyes are no longer red and you don't have any discharge before wearing contacts again.

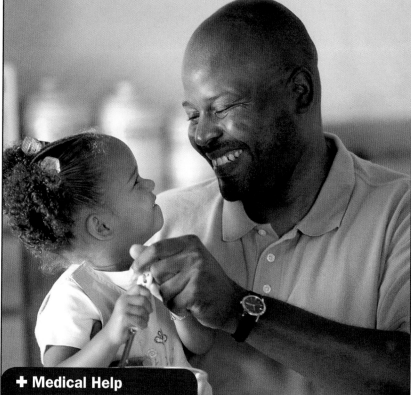

➕ Medical Help

If you think you may have bacterial conjunctivitis, or you have eye pain or your vision is affected, see your doctor. Also see a doctor if your symptoms worsen.

Poison ivy rash

Contact with the poison ivy plant — or its cousins, poison oak and poison sumac — usually causes red, swollen skin, blisters and severe itching. An oily resin triggers the reaction after direct contact between the plant and your skin, but the resin can transfer easily to skin from exposed clothing or pet hair.

Poison ivy rash typically develops within 12 to 48 hours after exposure. Its severity depends on the amount of resin that gets on your skin. Symptoms usually last for a week or two, but may last longer in people who are more sensitive to poison ivy. Some people experience scarring.

♠ Home Remedies

To reduce symptoms that accompany a poison ivy rash:

- *Wash up quickly.* Washing the poison ivy resin off your skin with soap soon after exposure may avert a skin reaction. Be sure to wash under your fingernails. Don't take a bath — this can spread the resin to other parts of your body.
- *Try not to scratch.* Once the rash has broken out, over-the-counter products such as corticosteroid creams, calamine lotion or creams containing menthol can help ease itching.
- *Cool the itch.* Place cool, wet compresses on the rash for 15 to 30 minutes several times a day. Cool-water tub soaks with baking soda (1/2 to 1 cup) or colloidal oatmeal (Aveeno) also may help.
- *Prevent infection.* Cover open blisters with sterile gauze.
- *Try antihistamines at night.* Oral antihistamines may help you sleep better at night.

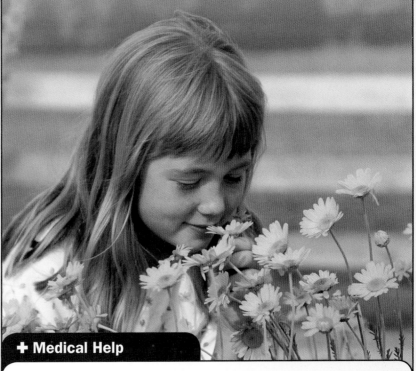

✚ Medical Help

If you have a severe reaction, or your eyes, face or genital area is involved, contact your doctor. Also seek medical help if the blisters begin to ooze pus or you develop a fever greater than 100 F.

Premenstrual syndrome (PMS)

If you routinely experience a wide variety of physical and emotional changes in the days before your period, you may have premenstrual syndrome (PMS). The signs and symptoms tend to recur in a predictable pattern each month, but may be particularly intense in some months and only slightly noticeable in others.

The condition is related to normal hormone cycles and occurs with normal hormone levels. For most women, signs and symptoms disappear as the menstrual period begins, but for some, the physical pain and emotional stress are severe enough to affect their daily routines and activities.

Exactly what causes premenstrual syndrome is unknown, but several factors may contribute to the condition:

Cyclic changes in hormones
Signs and symptoms occur with regular hormonal fluctuations.

Chemical changes in brain
Fluctuations of certain brain chemicals may trigger symptoms.

Depression and stress
These factors may make signs and symptoms more severe.

Poor eating habits
Some symptoms of PMS are linked to low levels of vitamins and minerals. Eating salty foods and drinking alcoholic or caffeinated beverages may also intensify certain symptoms.

PMS Symptoms

Although the list of potential signs and symptoms is long, most women with premenstrual syndrome experience only a few of these problems.

Emotional changes
- Depressed mood and crying spells
- Irritability or anger
- Tension or anxiety
- Mood swings
- Poor concentration
- Lethargy
- Appetite changes and food cravings
- Trouble falling asleep
- Social withdrawal

Physical changes
- Abdominal bloating
- Weight gain from fluid retention
- Swollen hands and feet
- Breast tenderness
- Headache
- Acne flare-ups
- Joint or muscle pain
- Diarrhea or constipation
- Fatigue, nausea and vomiting

🏠 Home Remedies

You can usually manage PMS with a combination of lifestyle changes.

Modify your diet
The following may reduce symptoms:
- Eat smaller, more frequent meals to reduce bloating and the sensation of fullness.
- Limit salt and salty foods to reduce fluid retention.
- Choose foods high in complex carbohydrates, such as fruits, vegetables and whole grains.
- Choose foods rich in calcium, such as fat-free or low-fat dairy products. If you can't tolerate dairy products or aren't getting adequate calcium in your diet, you may consider a daily calcium supplement.
- Avoid caffeine and alcohol.

Exercise regularly
Regular exercise can alleviate many symptoms, such as fatigue. Go for a brisk walk, cycle, swim or do another aerobic activity on most days of the week.

Reduce stress
Stress tends to aggravate the symptoms of PMS.
- Plan ahead for PMS. Don't overbook yourself during the week that you're expecting symptoms to occur.
- Get plenty of sleep.
- Practice various types of relaxation therapy. Progressive muscle relaxation or deep-breathing exercises can help reduce headaches, anxiety or insomnia. Consider yoga, tai chi or meditation.

Take supplements
The following supplements may help improve PMS symptoms:
- *Calcium.* Consuming 1,000 to 1,200 milligrams (mg) of dietary or supplemental calcium daily, such as chewable calcium carbonate (Tums, Rolaids, others), may reduce some symptoms of PMS. Regular use of calcium carbonate also reduces your risk of osteoporosis.
- *Vitamin D.* Research suggests that a high intake of calcium and vitamin D may reduce a woman's risk of PMS.
- *Magnesium.* Taking 400 mg of supplemental magnesium daily may help to reduce fluid retention, breast tenderness and bloating in women with premenstrual syndrome.

Record your symptoms
Keeping a record for a few months may help identify the triggers and timing of your symptoms. You may find that PMS is more tolerable if you see that your symptoms are predictable and short-lived.

➕ Medical Help

If you've had no luck managing premenstrual syndrome with lifestyle changes, and signs and symptoms are seriously affecting your health, mood and daily activities, see your doctor.

Psoriasis

Psoriasis is a disease that causes cells to build up rapidly on the surface of the skin, forming thick silvery scales and itchy, dry red patches. The patches can range from small spots of dandruff-like scaling to major eruptions over large areas of your body. Knees, elbows, trunk and scalp are common locations.

Mild cases of psoriasis may be a nuisance, but more-severe cases can be painful, disfiguring and disabling. Most types of psoriasis go through cycles, flaring for a few weeks or months, and then subsiding or even going into complete remission. Usually, however, the disease returns.

Psoriasis isn't contagious — you can't spread it to other parts of your own body, or to other people, via touch. Factors that may trigger a flare-up include certain types of infections, skin injuries — such as cuts, scrapes or bug bites — stress, cold weather, and smoking.

🏠 Home Remedies

These measures won't cure psoriasis, but they may help improve the appearance and feel of damaged skin:

- *Take daily baths.* Bathing daily helps remove scales and calm inflamed skin. Use lukewarm water and mild soaps that have added oils and fats. Add bath oil, colloidal oatmeal or Epsom salts to the water and soak for at least 15 minutes.
- *Use moisturizer.* Blot your skin after bathing, then immediately apply a heavy, ointment-based moisturizer while your skin is still moist. For very dry skin, oils may be preferable. During cold, dry weather, you may need to apply moisturizer several times a day.
- *Cover the affected areas overnight.* Apply an ointment-based moisturizer to your skin and wrap with plastic wrap overnight. In the morning, remove the covering and wash away scales.
- *Expose your skin to small amounts of sunlight.* Exposing affected skin to short sessions of sunlight three or more times a week can improve lesions. Too much sun can trigger or worsen outbreaks and increase the risk of skin cancer. Be sure to protect healthy skin with sunscreen with a sun protection factor (SPF) of at least 15.
- *Apply medicated cream or ointment.* Apply an over-the-counter cream or ointment containing hydrocortisone or salicylic acid to reduce itching and scaling. If you have scalp psoriasis, try a medicated shampoo that contains coal tar.
- *Avoid psoriasis triggers, if possible.* Find out what may trigger your psoriasis and take steps to avoid it.
- *Avoid drinking alcohol.* Alcohol consumption may decrease the effectiveness of some psoriasis treatments.

✚ Medical Help

If you suspect that you may have psoriasis, see your doctor for a complete examination. Also, talk to your doctor if your psoriasis:

- Progresses beyond the nuisance stage, causing discomfort
- Makes performing routine tasks difficult
- Causes you concern about the appearance of your skin

Raynaud's disease

Raynaud's disease is a condition that causes some areas of your body — such as your fingers, toes, ears and tip of your nose — to feel numb and cool in response to cold temperatures or stress. The small arteries that supply blood to your skin temporarily become narrower, limiting blood circulation to the affected areas.

Women are more likely to have Raynaud's than are men. It's also more common in people living in colder climates.

Raynaud's is more than simply having cold fingers and toes. Symptoms also include:

- A sequence of color changes in your skin in response to the cold or stress
- Numb, prickly feeling or stinging pain as your skin warms or the stress ends

A flare-up may last from less than a minute up to several hours. The affected areas feel cold and numb, usually turning white, then blue, and then red. As circulation improves, the affected areas throb, tingle or swell. Not everyone experiences symptoms in the same sequence.

🏠 Home Remedies

These steps can decrease flare-ups and help you feel better:

- *Don't smoke.* Smoking constricts your blood vessels, causing skin temperature to drop, which may trigger an attack.
- *Exercise.* Regular exercise helps increase blood circulation.
- *Control stress.* Because stress may trigger an attack, learning to avoid stressful situations may help control the disease.
- *Avoid caffeine.* Caffeine products cause your blood vessels to narrow and may increase the signs and symptoms of Raynaud's.
- *Take care of your hands and feet.* If you have Raynaud's, guard your hands and feet from injury. Avoid wearing anything that compresses the blood vessels in your hands or feet, such as tight wristbands, rings or footwear.
- *Try niacin.* Niacin, also known as vitamin B-3, causes blood vessels to dilate, increasing blood flow to skin. Niacin supplements may be useful in treating Raynaud's, although they may have side effects.
- *Don't take certain medications.* Avoid medications or substances that cause blood vessels to narrow, such as phenylephrine, pseudo-ephedrine, amphetamine, ergotamine and ephedra.

During flare-ups

If you're experiencing a flare-up of Raynaud's, your priority is to warm the affected area. To gently warm your fingers and toes:

- Move to a warmer area.
- Place your hands under your armpits.
- Wiggle your fingers and toes.
- Run warm — not hot — water over your fingers and toes.
- Massage your hands and feet.

➕ Medical Help

See your doctor right away if you have a history of severe Raynaud's flare-ups and develop an ulcer or infection in one of your affected fingers or toes.

Restless legs syndrome

Restless legs syndrome (RLS) is a condition in which your legs feel extremely uncomfortable while you're sitting or lying down. People typically describe the unpleasant sensation as crawling, tingling, electric, itchy or aching. When this occurs, you struggle with uncontrollable urges to move around.

The condition can begin at any age and generally worsens as you get older. Women are more likely than men to develop it. RLS can disrupt sleep — leading to daytime drowsiness — and makes traveling very difficult.

Characteristic features of restless legs syndrome include:

- Symptoms start after you've been sitting or lying down for an extended period of time.
- Movement relieves symptoms — at least temporarily.
- Symptoms are typically better during the day and worsen in the evening.
- There's an association with a condition called periodic limb movements of sleep (PLMS), which causes you to involuntarily flex and extend your legs while sleeping.

🏠 Home Remedies

Simple lifestyle changes can play an important role in helping you alleviate symptoms of RLS:

- *Take pain relievers.* Over-the-counter pain relievers such as ibuprofen (Advil, Motrin, others) may relieve mild symptoms.
- *Try baths and massages.* Soaking in a warm bath and massaging your legs can relax your muscles.
- *Apply warm or cool packs.* The use of heat or cold, or alternating use of the two, may lessen the sensations in your limbs.
- *Try relaxation techniques, such as meditation or yoga.*
- *Establish good sleep habits.* Fatigue tends to worsen symptoms of RLS. Create a cool, quiet and comfortable sleeping environment, going to bed at the same time, rising at the same time, and getting enough sleep to feel well rested.
- *Exercise.* Moderate, regular exercise may relieve symptoms of RLS, but overdoing it at the gym may intensify symptoms.
- *Avoid caffeine.* Sometimes cutting back on caffeine-containing products may help relieve symptoms.
- *Cut back on alcohol and tobacco.* These substances may aggravate or trigger symptoms. Test to see whether avoiding them helps.

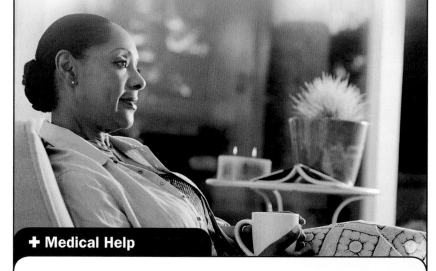

➕ Medical Help

Some people with RLS never seek medical attention because they worry that their symptoms are too difficult to describe or won't be taken seriously. However, if you think you may have RLS or if the above remedies don't improve your symptoms, see your doctor.

Shin splints

The term *shin splints* refers to pain along the shinbone (tibia), the large bone in the front of your lower leg. The pain is caused by inflammation in the bone and the connective tissues that attach muscle to the bone.

Shin splints are associated with athletic activity and typically a result of overuse — training too hard, too fast or for too long. It commonly occurs with runners, basketball players, tennis players and army recruits.

If you develop shin splints, you may notice:
- Tenderness, soreness or pain along the inner part of your lower leg
- Mild swelling

At first, the pain may stop when you stop running or exercising. Eventually, however, the pain may become continuous.

🏠 Home Remedies

In most cases, you can treat shin splints with simple self-care steps:
- *Rest.* Avoid activities that cause pain, swelling or discomfort — but don't give up all activity. While you're healing, try low-impact exercises, such as swimming or bicycling. If pain causes you to limp, consider using crutches until you can walk normally.
- *Ice the affected area.* Apply ice packs for 15 to 20 minutes and four to eight times a day for several days. To protect your skin, wrap the ice packs in a thin towel.
- *Reduce swelling.* Elevate the shin above the level of your heart, especially at night. It may help to compress the area with an elastic bandage or compression sleeve — but loosen the wrap if the pain increases or the area becomes numb.
- *Take an over-the-counter pain reliever.* Try asprin, ibuprofen (Advil, Motrin, others), naproxen (Aleve) or acetaminophen (Tylenol, others) to reduce pain.
- *Wear proper shoes.* Your doctor may recommend a shoe that's especially suited for your foot type, stride and particular sport.
- *Consider arch supports.* Arch supports can help cushion and disperse stress on your shinbones.
- *Resume usual activities gradually.* Returning to usual activities too soon, before you heal, may cause continued pain.

Prevention
- Stretch before running to loosen the muscles in your legs and feet.
- Consider arch supports to prevent shin pain, especially if you have flat arches.
- Cross-train with a sport that places less impact on your shin, such as swimming, walking or biking.
- Consult a trainer to evaluate and adjust your running style.

➕ Medical Help

Seek prompt medical care if:
- Severe pain in your shin follows a fall or accident
- Your shin is hot and inflamed
- Shin pain persists at rest, at night or with walking

Shingles

Shingles (herpes zoster) is a viral infection that causes a painful rash. It's caused by the same virus that causes chickenpox. After you've had chickenpox, the virus lies inactive in nerve tissue near your spinal cord and, years later, may reactivate as shingles.

Pain is usually the first symptom of shingles. For some, the pain can be intense and is sometimes mistaken for a symptom of problems affecting the heart, lungs or kidneys.

A shingles rash usually appears a few days after the pain. It often develops as a band of blisters wrapping around one side of your body from your back to your front. The blisters usually dry up in a few days, forming crusts that fall off over the next few weeks.

While shingles isn't a life-threatening condition, it can be very painful. The blisters contain a contagious virus, so avoid contact with others, especially people with weak immunity, pregnant women and newborns.

♠ Home Remedies

You can relieve some discomfort of shingles with the following:
- Take a cool bath or soak the blisters with cool, wet compresses.
- Apply a lubricating cream or ointment.
- Take over-the-counter pain relievers, such as aspirin, ibuprofen (Motrin, Advil, others), naproxen (Aleve) and acetaminophen (Tylenol, others) to alleviate pain.
- Rubbing over-the-counter creams or ointments on your skin to reduce pain also may be helpful.

Prevention

A shingles vaccine is recommended for all adults age 60 and older, whether or not they've had shingles previously. The vaccine is for prevention, not treatment. Getting the vaccine doesn't guarantee that you won't get shingles, but it will likely reduce the course and severity of the disease. It may also reduce your risk of postherpetic neuralgia, a nerve-related chronic pain condition that can follow shingles.

✚ Medical Help

Contact your doctor if you suspect shingles, especially in the following situations:
- The pain and rash occur near your eyes. If left untreated, this infection can cause permanent eye damage.
- You or someone in your family has a weakened immune system (due to cancer, medications or a chronic medical condition).
- The rash is widespread and painful.

Shoulder pain

Pain can arise from within the shoulder joints and surrounding muscles, ligaments and tendons. The pain usually worsens when you move your arm and shoulder. Pain that doesn't get worse when you move your shoulder is more likely to be "referred pain" caused by a condition or problem in your chest or abdomen.

Treatment of shoulder pain depends on its cause. Bursitis and tendinitis (see pages 35 and 171) are common causes of shoulder pain, as are acute injury and rotator cuff tears. Take note of how the pain began and what makes the pain worse.

Acute shoulder pain
Acute shoulder pain centers on your upper arm, upper back and neck. It may be very painful to put on a coat, extend your arm straight out from your side or reach behind you.

Rotator cuff injury
This type of injury usually results from repetitive overhead motions, such as painting a ceiling, swimming or throwing a baseball, or from trauma, such as falling on your shoulder.

🏠 Home Remedies

To relieve shoulder pain:
- *Rest your shoulder.* Stop doing what caused the pain. Limit heavy lifting or overhead activity for four to seven days until your shoulder starts to feel better.
- *Apply ice and heat.* Use a cold pack, a bag of frozen vegetables or a towel filled with ice cubes for 15 to 20 minutes at a time to help reduce inflammation. Do this every couple of hours. After about two or three days, when the pain and inflammation have improved, hot packs or a heating pad may help relax sore muscles. Limit heat applications to 20 minutes.
- *Use over-the-counter pain medications.* This includes aspirin, ibuprofen (Motrin, Advil, others), naproxen (Aleve) and acetaminophen (Tylenol, others).
- *Do stretching exercises.* After one or two days, do gentle exercises to keep your shoulder muscles limber. If possible, put the shoulder through its full range of motion. Inactivity can cause stiff joints.
- *Take it slow.* Wait until pain is gone before gradually returning to the activity that caused the injury. This may require three to six weeks.
- *Review your technique.* If an activity — such as a racket sport, baseball, golf or weight training — is involved, you may need to alter your technique.

➕ Medical Help

Seek medical care if:
- Your shoulders appear uneven or you can't raise the affected arm
- You have extreme tenderness at your collarbone or shoulder
- You have redness, swelling or fever
- Your shoulder isn't improving after a week of self-care

Call 911 if you have chest pain, difficulty breathing, are sweating, feel faint, or have nausea or vomiting

Sinusitis

Sinusitis occurs when the cavities surrounding your nasal passages (sinuses) become inflamed and swollen. Swelling can close off the passages, making it difficult for the sinuses to drain. Pain may result from the inflammation or from pressure as mucus builds up in the sinus cavities.

Signs and symptoms include pain around your eyes or cheeks, nasal congestion, causing difficulty breathing through your nose, and drainage of a thick, yellow or greenish discharge from the nose or down the back of the throat. There may be aching in your upper jaw and teeth and a reduced sense of taste and smell.

Short-lived (acute) sinusitis is often caused by the common cold. Chronic sinusitis may stem from an infection, allergies, nasal polyps or conditions such as a deviated septum.

The following steps may help relieve symptoms of sinusitis:

- *Apply warm compresses.* Place warm, damp towels around your nose, cheeks and eyes to help ease pain.
- *Drink plenty of fluids.* Fluids help dilute nasal secretions and promote drainage. Avoid beverages that contain caffeine or alcohol, because they can be dehydrating. Alcohol can worsen swelling.
- *Steam your sinuses.* This will ease pain and help mucus to drain. Drape a towel over your head and cautiously inhale steam from a basin of boiling water. Keep the steam directed toward your face. Or take a hot shower, breathing in the warm, moist air.
- *Get plenty of rest.* This will help your body fight infection and speed recovery.
- *Sleep with your head elevated.* This will help your sinuses drain.

Nasal lavage

The rinsing of your nasal passages (lavage) flushes out excess mucus and debris and helps reduce sinus inflammation. Lavage may be performed with a bulb syringe, a specially designed squeeze bottle or a neti pot – a small pot with a long spout, somewhat similar to a teapot. All of these products should be available in pharmacies or medical supply stores.

Fill the squeeze bottle with a mild solution of warm salt water. While standing over a sink, place the tip of the container in one nostril and squeeze, causing the solution to run in that nostril, through your sinuses, and out the other nostril.

With the neti pot, instead of squeezing, pour the solution into a nostril while your head is tipped forward and slightly sideways. As the solution passes through your sinuses, it clears them out.

Beware of decongestant nasal sprays

Decongestant nasal sprays (Afrin, Neo-Synephrine, others) can help open clogged nasal passages, but you should only use them once a day for a short period – up to three days. After a few days of using such a spray, your nasal membranes may become less responsive to the medication and require more spray to alleviate the congestion. When you stop using the spray, your symptoms may become worse — what's known as rebound congestion.

Contact your doctor if your symptoms don't improve within a few days or they worsen, or if you have a history of recurrent or chronic sinusitis. If your sinusitis is the result of a bacterial infection, your doctor may prescribe an oral antibiotic or other medications.

Snoring

Almost half of all adults snore at least occasionally. Snoring occurs when the air you breathe while you're sleeping flows past relaxed tissues in your throat. This causes the tissues to vibrate, creating harsh respiratory sounds.

Depending on its cause, your snoring may be accompanied by restless sleep, gasping or choking at night, morning headache, excessive daytime sleepiness, sore throat, high blood pressure, and irregular heartbeats.

Many factors may affect your airway and lead to snoring:

Mouth anatomy

When you doze off, the muscles in roof of your mouth (palate), tongue and throat relax, which can partially obstruct your airway. Having a low, thick palate or enlarged tonsils or tissues in the back of your throat can narrow the airway further and increase the amount of vibration. Being overweight contributes to narrowing of the airway.

Nasal problems

Chronic nasal congestion or a crooked partition between your nostrils (deviated nasal septum) may be to blame for snoring.

Sleep apnea

Snoring may be associated with obstructive sleep apnea, characterized by loud snoring followed by periods of silence that can last for 10 seconds or more. In this serious condition, your airway is obstructed or becomes so small that the amount of air you breathe is inadequate for your needs. Eventually, a lack of oxygen signals you to wake up and forces your airway open, accompanied by a loud snort or gasping sound. This pattern may be repeated many times during the night.

Alcohol consumption

Snoring can also be brought on by consuming too much alcohol before bedtime. Alcohol relaxes throat muscles and decreases your natural defenses against airway obstruction.

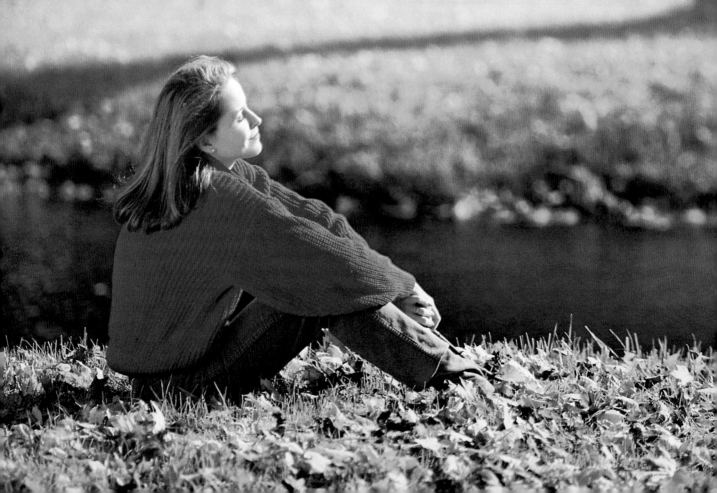

To prevent or ease snoring, try the following suggestions:

Lose weight

Being overweight is a common cause of snoring. Extra bulkiness narrows your airway, and loose tissue in your throat is more likely to vibrate as you breathe.

Sleep on your side

Your tongue is more likely to fall backward into your throat when you sleep on your back, which narrows your airway and partially obstructs airflow. To prevent sleeping on your back, try sewing a tennis ball in the back of your pajama top.

Treat nasal congestion

Allergies or a deviated septum can limit airflow through your nose, forcing you to breathe through your mouth and increasing the likelihood of snoring. Don't use decongestants for more than three days in a row for acute congestion unless directed to do so by your doctor. Correcting a deviated septum may require nasal surgery.

Try nasal strips

Another way to keep nasal passages open and reduce breathing through your mouth is with nasal strips, which can be purchased at most drug stores and pharmacies. Attaching the adhesive strips to your nose before bedtime widens the nasal passages, making it easier to breathe and, possibly, reducing snoring, especially if the vibrations originate in your nose.

Limit or avoid alcohol and sedatives

Avoid alcoholic beverages at least four hours before bedtime. Inform your doctor that you snore before taking sedatives or sleeping pills (hypnotics). These products depress your central nervous system, causing excessive muscle relaxation, including tissues at the base of your throat. Alcohol, sedatives and sleeping pills also blunt your brain's ability to arouse you from sleep. It may take longer for you to start breathing again if you've stopped breathing due to obstructive sleep apnea.

Strengthen your throat muscles

Playing the didgeridoo, a wind instrument that produces a droning sound, may help train your throat muscles and prevent them from narrowing your upper airway. A study from the *British Medical Journal* evaluated use of the instrument by individuals with sleep apnea who complained of snoring. Results show that participants who played the instrument for about 25 minutes a day experienced less daytime sleepiness — a complication of sleep apnea and snoring. However, further study is required.

Keep singing

Singing can also help improve muscle control of your palate and upper throat. A preliminary study found a decrease in snoring among participants who sang prescribed singing exercises for 20 minutes a day for three months. These participants all began snoring as adults, had no nasal problems and were not overweight. More study of this technique is needed.

➕ Medical Help

If your snoring doesn't improve, see your doctor. Inform a pediatrician if your child snores. Children, too, can have obstructive sleep apnea, although most don't. Nose and throat problems, such as enlarged tonsils, and obesity often underlie habitual snoring in children. Treating these conditions can help improve sleep.

Sore throat

The tight, scratchy feeling in your throat may be a familiar sign that a cold or flu (influenza) is on the way. Although uncomfortable, most sore throats aren't harmful and go away on their own in five to seven days. Sometimes, you may look to over-the-counter lozenges or gargles for relief.

Most sore throats are caused by viral or bacterial infections. Viruses and bacteria can enter through your mouth or nose — either because you breathe in particles that are released in the air when someone coughs or sneezes, or because you come into physical contact with an infected person or use shared objects such as utensils and tableware, towels, toys, doorknobs, computer keyboards or telephones.

Sore throats can also be caused by allergies and dry air. When a sore throat involves swollen tonsils, it's sometimes called tonsillitis.

Viral infection

Viruses are typically the source of common colds and the flu, and the sore throat that often accompanies them. Colds usually go away once your system has had time to build up antibodies that destroy the virus — which takes about one week. Antibiotic medications can't help in treating viral infections, so don't look to them for fast, effective relief. Recovery takes time.

Common signs and symptoms of viral infection include:
- Sore or scratchy, dry feeling in the throat
- Hoarseness
- Coughing and sneezing
- Runny nose and postnasal dripping
- Mild fever or no fever

Bacterial infection

Bacterial infections aren't as common as viral infections, but they can be more serious. And the most common bacterial cause of throat infection is strep throat. Often, you develop strep throat within two to seven days of being exposed to someone else with the infection. Children ages 5 to 15 in a classroom setting are the most likely to get it.

Streptococcal bacteria — the cause of strep throat — are highly contagious. They can spread by airborne droplets from a cough or sneeze, or through shared food or drinks. You can also pick up the bacteria from a doorknob or other surface and transfer them to your nose or mouth.

Strep throat, if left untreated, can lead to complications such as kidney inflammation (glomerulonephritis) or rheumatic fever. Strep throat requires medical treatment with antibiotics and pain relievers.

Common signs and symptoms of strep throat are:
- Inflamed, swollen tonsils and lymph nodes
- Pain when swallowing
- Bright red color with white patches in the throat
- Fever, generally more than 101 F, and often accompanied by chills

Until your sore throat has run its course, try these tips:

- *Double your fluid intake.* Fluids such as water, juice, tea and warm soup help keep your mucus thin and easy to clear. Avoid caffeine and alcohol, which can dehydrate you.
- *Gargle with warm salt water.* Mix about 1/2 teaspoon of salt in a full glass of warm water and gargle. This helps soothe your throat and clear it of mucus.
- *Suck on a lozenge or hard candy.* Chewing sugarless gum also helps. These actions stimulate saliva production, which bathes and cleanses your throat.
- *Drink honey mixed with warm tea or warm lemon water.* This is a time-honored method for soothing a sore throat. Due to the risk of infant botulism, a rare form of food poisoning, never give honey to a child younger than age 1.

- *Take pain relievers.* Over-the-counter medications, such as acetaminophen (Tylenol, others), ibuprofen (Advil, Motrin) and aspirin, relieve sore throat pain for four to six hours. Don't give aspirin to children or teenagers.
- *Rest your voice.* If a sore throat affects your voice box (larynx), talking may lead to more irritation and temporary loss of your voice — a condition known as laryngitis. Talking as little as possible may help avoid this.
- *Humidify the air.* Adding moisture to the air prevents the mucous membranes in your sinuses and throat from drying out. This can reduce irritation and promote sleep. Saline nasal sprays also are helpful.
- *Avoid smoke and other air pollutants.* Smoke irritates a sore throat. Stop smoking and avoid environmental smoke, as well as fumes from household products. Keep children away from secondhand smoke.

Prevention

To prevent sore throats, follow some age-old advice:

- Wash your hands frequently or use an alcohol-based hand cleanser, especially during the cold and flu seasons.
- Keep your hands away from your face to avoid getting bacteria and viruses into your mouth or nose.

Seek emergency care if your sore throat is accompanied by any of the following symptoms:

- Drooling
- Difficulty or pain on swallowing or breathing
- Stiff, rigid neck and severe headache
- Temperature higher than 101 F in babies under age 6 months and 103 F in older children or adults
- Rash
- Persistent hoarseness or mouth ulcers lasting two weeks or more

Sprains

Strictly speaking, a sprain occurs whenever you overextend or tear one of your ligaments. Ligaments are the tough, elastic-like bands that connect bone to bone and hold your joints in place. Joint movement that is excessive or beyond normal range — perhaps a violent twist — can tear a ligament partially or completely.

Sprains occur most often in your ankles, knees or the arches of your feet. True sprains are painful and cause rapid swelling. Generally, the greater the pain, the more severe the injury. The severity of a sprain can be:

- *Mild*. A ligament is stretched excessively or tears slightly. The area is tender and somewhat painful, especially with movement. There's not a lot of swelling. You can put weight on the joint.
- *Moderate*. Some fibers are torn but the ligament doesn't rupture completely. The joint is tender, painful and difficult to move. The area may be swollen and discolored from bleeding.
- *Severe*. One or more ligaments tear completely. The area is painful, very swollen and discolored. You're unable to move the joint normally or put any weight on it. The injury may be difficult to distinguish from a fracture or dislocation, both of which require medical care. You may need a cast to hold the joint motionless, or surgery, if the tears cause joint instability.

Preventing sports injuries

To reduce your risk of sprains, strains and other injuries:

- Warm up. Loosen and stretch your muscles at the start of exercise, and gradually increase your level of activity over five to 10 minutes. If you're prone to muscle pain, apply heat before you exercise.
- Cool down. After exercising, ease up gradually with muscle stretches. This may help reduce muscle injury and stiffness.
- Begin gradually. If you're trying out a new sport, increase your level of exertion in stages over several weeks.
- Do cross-training. Combining two or more types of physical activity helps avoid injuries from repetitive stress. You can try multiple activities in the same workout or alternate activites from one day to the next.
- Don't overdo it. Stop an activity immediately if you experience chest pain, irregular heartbeat, dizziness or faintness, pain in an arm or jaw, severe shortness of breath, excessive fatigue, severe joint or muscle pain or joint swelling.

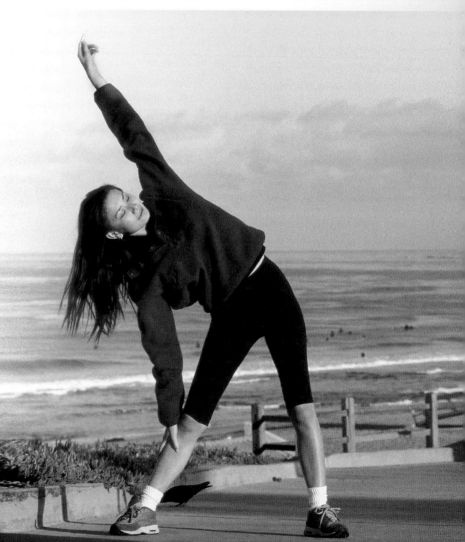

🏠 Home Remedies

To treat a sprain:
- Follow the instructions for R.I.C.E. provided on this page.
- Use over-the-counter pain medications, if needed. Don't exceed the recommended dose unless your doctor advises it.
- After 48 hours, if the swelling is gone, apply gentle heat to the area. Heat can improve blood flow and speed healing.
- Gradually test the injured joint and, if possible, try to use the joint after two days have passed. Mild to moderate sprains usually improve significantly in about one week, although full healing may take up to six weeks.
- Avoid activities that continue to put stress on your injured joint. Repeated minor sprains further weaken the joint.
- Apply cold to sore areas after a workout, even if you're not injured, to prevent inflammation and swelling.

R.I.C.E.

You'll see the term *R.I.C.E.* mentioned frequently in this book. R.I.C.E. is common practice for treating sprained ligaments, muscle strains and joint injuries. The letters stand for Rest, Ice, Compress and Elevate — actions you take in a sequence to promote healing and help prevent further tissue damage.
- **R:** Rest the area to promote tissue healing. Avoid activities that cause more pain, swelling or discomfort.
- **I:** Ice the area immediately, even if you seek medical help. Apply an ice pack or immerse the injury in an icy slush bath for 15 minutes. Repeat every two to three hours during waking hours for the first 2 to 3 days. Cold reduces swelling and inflammation and may also slow bleeding if a muscle or ligament tear has occurred.
- **C:** Compress the area with an elastic bandage until the swelling stops. Don't wrap it tightly or you may hinder circulation. Begin wrapping at the end farthest from your heart. Loosen the wrap if pain increases, if the area becomes numb or if there is swelling below the wrapped area.
- **E:** Elevate the injured area above the level of your heart, especially at night. For example, you can prop up an injured ankle on pillows. Gravity helps reduce swelling by draining away excess blood and fluid.

✚ Medical Help

Seek medical care immediately if:
- You hear a popping sound when the injury occurs and you can't use the joint. If possible, apply cold immediately.
- You have a fever and the area is red and hot.
- You have a severe sprain, as described on page 156. Delayed treatment may cause long-term joint instability or chronic pain.

See your doctor if you're unable to bear weight on the joint after two to three days of self-care or if you don't experience much improvement after about a week.

Stomach flu

What people commonly refer to as stomach flu is also known as viral gastroenteritis. This isn't the same thing as influenza. Real flu (influenza) attacks your respiratory system — your nose, throat and lungs. Viral gastroenteritis is an intestinal infection.

Signs and symptoms

Viral gastroenteritis may appear within one to three days after you're infected. Signs and symptoms range from mild to severe, and usually last just a day or two but occasionally persist as long as 10 days. Signs and symptoms typically include:

- Watery, usually nonbloody diarrhea (bloody diarrhea may indicate a different infection)
- Abdominal cramps and pain
- Nausea, vomiting or both
- Occasional muscle ache or headache
- Low-grade fever

Dehydration — a severe loss of water and essential salts and minerals — is a serious complication of stomach flu. For infants, older adults and people with compromised immune systems, stomach flu can be deadly.

Common causes

The ailment is spread through contact with an infected person or from eating or drinking contaminated food or water. In many cases, transmission follows the fecal-oral route — that is, someone with a virus handles food you eat without washing his or her hands after using the bathroom. Different virus can cause gastroenteritis, including the two most common culprits:

- *Rotavirus.* This type of virus is the most common cause of infectious diarrhea in children. Children usually are infected when they put fingers or objects contaminated with the virus into their mouths. Infected adults usually don't develop signs and symptoms, but can still spread the illness.

  A rotaviral vaccine that's effective in preventing severe symptoms of gastroenteritis is available. Talk to your doctor about whether it's advisable to immunize your child.

- *Noroviruses.* There are several different strains of norovirus, all of which cause similar signs and symptoms. In addition to diarrhea, nausea and vomiting, you may experience muscle ache, headache, fatigue and low-grade fever.

A norovirus infection may sweep through families, communities or large groups traveling, for example, on cruise ships. Most often, you pick up the infection from contaminated food or water, but a person-to-person transmission also is possible.

After exposure to the virus, you're likely to feel sick within 18 to 72 hours. Most people feel better in a day or two, but you're still contagious for at least three days — and up to two weeks — after recovery.

Signs of dehydration

A serious complication of stomach flu is dehydration. Signs and symptoms include:

- Excessive thirst
- Dry mouth
- Deep yellow urine or little or no urine
- Severe weakness, dizziness, lightheadedness or confusion

Keep yourself comfortable and prevent dehydration while you recover with the following steps:

- *Allow your stomach to settle.* No eating and drinking for a few hours after vomiting or diarrhea.
- *Suck on ice chips or take small sips of water.* Try to drink plenty of liquid every day, taking small, frequent sips. Also consider clear sodas, clear broths or noncaffeinated sports drinks.
- *Ease back into eating.* Gradually begin eating bland, easy-to-digest foods such as crackers, toast, gelatin, bananas, rice and chicken. Stop eating if the feeling of nausea returns.

- *Avoid certain products.* These include dairy products, caffeine, alcohol, nicotine, and fatty or highly seasoned foods.
- *Get plenty of rest.*
- *Be cautious with medications.* Use medications such as ibuprofen (Advil, Motrin, others) sparingly, if at all. They can upset your stomach more. Also be cautious with acetaminophen (Tylenol, others), which can cause liver toxicity.

Treating children

If your child has an intestinal infection, your most important goal is to replace lost fluids and salts.

- *Help your child rehydrate.* Let your child's stomach settle for 15 to 20 minutes after any vomiting or diarrhea occurs, then offer small amounts of liquid. It's best to use oral rehydration solutions such as Pedialyte. In children with gastroenteritis, water isn't absorbed well and doesn't adequately replace lost electrolytes. Avoid giving apple juice — it can make diarrhea worse. If you're breast-feeding, let your baby nurse. If bottle-feeding, offer oral rehydration solution or regular formula.
- *Get back to a normal diet slowly.* Gradually introduce bland, easy-to-digest foods, such as rice, crackers, gelatin and bananas.
- *Avoid certain foods.* Dairy products and sugary foods, such as sodas and candy, can make diarrhea worse.
- *Make sure your child gets plenty of rest.*
- *Be cautious with medications.* Giving a child or teenager aspirin may cause Reye's syndrome, a rare but potentially fatal disease. Avoid giving your child over-the-counter anti-diarrheal medications such as Imodium unless advised by your doctor. They can make it harder for your child's body to eliminate the virus.

Continued next page >

If you're an adult, call your doctor if:

- You're not able to keep liquids down for 24 hours
- You've been vomiting for more than two days
- You're vomiting blood or have blood in bowel movements
- You're dehydrated
- You have a fever above 104 F

See your doctor right away if your child:

- Has a fever of 102 F or higher
- Seems lethargic or very irritable
- Is in a lot of discomfort or pain
- Has bloody diarrhea
- Seems dehydrated — watch for signs of dehydration in sick infants and children by comparing how much they drink and urinate with how much is normal for them

If you have an infant, remember that spitting up may be an everyday occurrence for your baby, but vomiting is not. Babies vomit for a variety of reasons, many of which may require medical attention.

Food poisoning culprits

Many bacterial, viral or parasitic agents cause food poisoning, a common cause of stomach flu. This table shows some of the possible contaminants, when you might start to feel symptoms and common ways the organism spreads.

Contaminant	Onset of symptoms	Foods affected and means of transmission
Campylobacter	2 to 5 days	Meat and poultry. Contamination occurs during processing if animal feces comes in contact with the meat. Can also spread via unpasteurized milk and contaminated water.
Clostridium perfringens	8 to 16 hours	Meats, stews and gravies. Commonly spread when serving dishes don't keep food hot enough or the food is chilled too slowly.
Escherichia coli (E. coli) O157:H7	1 to 8 days	Beef contaminated during slaughter. Spread mainly by undercooked ground beef. Other sources include unpasteurized milk and apple cider, alfalfa sprouts, and contaminated water.
Giardia lamblia	1 to 2 weeks	Raw, ready-to-eat produce and contaminated water. Can be spread by an infected food handler.
Hepatitis A	28 days	Raw, ready-to-eat produce and shellfish from contaminated water. Can be spread by an infected food handler.
Listeria	9 to 48 hours	Hot dogs, luncheon meats, unpasteurized milk and cheeses, and unwashed raw produce. Can be spread through contaminated soil and water.
Noroviruses (Norwalk-like viruses)	12 to 48 hours	Raw, ready-to-eat produce and shellfish from contaminated water. Can be spread by an infected food handler.
Rotavirus	1 to 3 days	Raw, ready-to-eat produce. Can be spread by an infected food handler.
Salmonella	1 to 3 days	Raw or contaminated meat, poultry, milk or egg yolks. Survives inadequate cooking. Can be spread by knives, cutting surfaces or an infected food handler.
Shigella	24 to 48 hours	Raw, ready-to-eat produce. Can be spread by an infected food handler.
Staphylococcus aureus	1 to 6 hours	Meats and prepared salads, cream sauces and cream-filled pastries. Can be spread by hand contact, coughing and sneezing.
Vibrio vulnificus	1 to 7 days	Raw oysters and raw or undercooked mussels, clams and whole scallops. Can be spread through contaminated seawater.

Limit your risk of illness from these contaminants by:
- Washing hands well before preparing foods
- Keeping raw meat separate from other foods during food preparation
- Cooking meat to the recommended internal temperature
- Refrigerating food within two hours of cooking (or within one hour if room temperature is above 90 F

Stress and anxiety

Stress is something that just about everyone knows well and experiences often. It's that feeling of pressure, typically a result of too much to do and too little time to do it in. In a busy life, stress is almost unavoidable.

Stress is caused by events that are positive — new job, vacation or marriage — as well as negative — job loss, divorce or death in the family. Stress is not the event itself but rather, your psychological or physical reaction to the event.

Anxiety is a tense feeling that often accompanies stress. It's typically directed toward the future — toward something that may happen soon. Some anxiety can motivate you or help you respond to danger. However, if you have ongoing anxiety that interferes with daily activities and makes it hard to enjoy life, then anxiety can be a problem.

When you experience stress and anxiety, especially if they're severe, your body will respond physically to the threat. Your heart beats faster and breathing quickens. Your blood pressure and blood sugar level rises. Blood flow to your brain and large muscles also increases. After the threat passes, your body slowly relaxes and functions return to normal.

You can usually handle the negative effects of stress when it's occasional, but when stress happens regularly, the effects tend to increase and multiply. Chronic stress is often involved with situations that aren't easily resolved, such as relationship problems, loneliness, financial worries or long workdays.

Signs and symptoms

Stress and anxiety can produce a variety of physical, emotional and behavioral signs and symptoms.

The earliest indications that your body is feeling under stress may include headache, upset stomach, diarrhea, constipation and insomnia. A nervous habit such as nail biting may reappear. You may become irritable with people who are close to you.

Occasionally, this response is so gradual that you, your family and friends don't recognize that there's a problem until your health or relationships change.

Sometimes, the signs and symptoms of stress can lead to illness — perhaps aggravating an existing health problem or possibly triggering a new one, if you're already at risk for that condition.

Controlling stress

Learning strategies to manage stress can help reset your body's response to stressful times. Without these tools, your body may remain on high alert, which, over time, can produce serious health problems. Simple strategies are described on pages 162-163.

Continued next page >

To help control stress and anxiety, follow these suggestions:

- *Learn to relax.* The relaxation therapies described here may help you cope with the physical signs and symptoms. Your goal is to lower your heart rate and blood pressure while also reducing muscle tension.
- *Discuss your concerns.* Talking with a trusted friend helps relieve stress and may provide a more positive perspective on your situation. This may lead to a healthy plan of action.
- *Get plenty of sleep.* A healthy body promotes mental health. Sleep provides more vigor and a refreshed state of mind for tackling major problems.
- *Stay physically active.* Exercise keeps your body healthy and helps burn off excess energy that stress can produce. Aim for at least 30 minutes of daily exercise. Even brief periods of activity can help reduce tension and improve your mood.
- *Eat regular, balanced meals and healthy snacks.*
- *Limit caffeine.* Too much coffee, tea or soda can increase your level of stress.
- *Plan ahead.* Approach daily responsibilities in a practical and organized fashion. Divide big jobs into smaller tasks and take them on, one task at a time, until you reach your goal.
- *Deal with anger.* Anger can and should be expressed, when it's done carefully. First, count to 10 and compose yourself. Then, respond to strong emotions.
- *Be realistic.* Set goals you can achieve. Concentrate on what's important. Setting unrealistically high goals invites failure.
- *Get away.* A change of pace or change of scene may help you develop a whole new outlook.
- *Avoid self-medication.* At times people rely on medication or alcohol for stress relief. Such substances tend to only mask the underlying problem.
- *Make time to enjoy life.* Going for walks or to the movies, golfing with friends or getting together for a game of cards helps relieve inner pressures.
- *Nurture your inner spirituality.* Nature, art, music, meditation and prayer, as well as religious services, can help build inner strength and perspective.
- *Develop a support network.* Family members, friends and co-workers whom you can turn to for support may be helpful when coping with stress.

Relaxation techniques are an important part of stress management. Relaxation isn't just about finding quiet time or enjoying a hobby. It's a process that helps you repair the toll that stress takes on your mind and body. Relaxation techniques usually involve refocusing your attention on something calming and increasing awareness of your body.

Relaxation therapy
Relaxation therapy includes many techniques, ranging from paced respiration and deep breathing to meditation and progressive muscle relaxation. Most involve the repetition of a single word, phrase or muscular activity, which allows you to "empty" your mind of external thoughts and stressors.

Contact a doctor or mental health professional if stress feels overwhelming or you're unable to function well, physically or emotionally.

Massage

A number of studies indicate that massage can help control the signs and symptoms of stress and anxiety by relaxing your muscles and calming your mind.

Yoga

Several studies indicate that regularly practicing yoga may help reduce daily stress and anxiety. Kundalini yoga, a type of yoga that's been studied specifically for anxiety disorder, combines poses and breathing techniques with chanting and meditation.

Aromatherapy

Aromatherapy is the science of using oils from various plants to treat illness and promote health. The oils are often vaporized and inhaled or used in massage. It's believed that compounds in the oils activate certain brain chemicals that have a relaxing effect.

Art and music therapy

You can use drawing, painting, clay and sculpture to express your inner thoughts and emotions when talking about them is difficult. The creation and interpretation of art is thought to be therapeutic. Listening or playing music — even during medical procedures — has also been shown to have relaxing and calming effects.

Stuffy nose

A stuffy nose develops when delicate tissue in the nose becomes swollen, often because of blood vessels that are inflamed. The sinus passageways narrow, preventing the easy drainage of mucus and resulting in a "stuffy" feeling. Nasal congestion is just an annoyance for most older children and adults, but it can be serious for infants, who may have a hard time breathing and breast-feeding as a result. The causes of a stuffy nose may include:

- Common cold
- Obstructions such as nasal polyps, tumors and enlarged adenoids
- Deformities of the nose and nasal chambers. Deformities such as a deviated septum may result from an injury that occurred years earlier.
- Allergies. Inhaled substances, such as pollen, mold or house dust, can trigger an inflammatory response.
- Vasomotor rhinitis. Specific triggers such as smoke, air conditioning or vigorous exercise may also cause nasal inflammation.

🏠 Home Remedies

To treat a stuffy nose:
- Regularly and gently blow your nose if mucus or debris is present.
- Breath steam to loosen the mucus and clear your sinuses, or take a warm shower or sit in the bathroom with the shower running.
- Drink plenty of liquids.
- Nonprescription oral decongestants (liquid or pills) may be helpful, but limit nonprescription decongestant nasal sprays or nose drops to no more than three days of use. Taken longer than that, they can make the problem worse.
- Try saline nasal drops or spray or nasal lavage (see page 151). These are safe to use as long as needed.

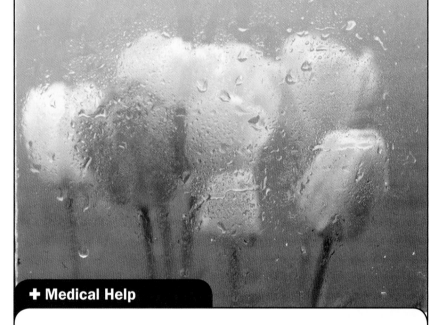

➕ Medical Help

See your doctor if:
- Your symptoms last more than 10 days.
- You have a high fever, particularly if it lasts more than three days.
- Your nasal discharge is green in color, and accompanied by sinus pain or fever.
- You have asthma or emphysema, or you're taking immune-suppressing medications.
- You have blood in your nasal discharge or a persistent clear discharge after a head injury.

Sunburn

You know sunburn when it happens: red, painful skin that feels hot to the touch. Sunburn usually appears within a few hours after sun exposure and may take from several days to several weeks to fade. Severe sunburn may include swelling and small fluid-filled blisters. It can also cause headache, fever and fatigue.

Within a few days, your body starts to heal itself by "peeling" the top layer of damaged skin. After peeling, your skin may temporarily have an irregular color and pattern.

Prevention is the best medicine

To protect yourself from sunburn:

- Try to avoid being outdoors from 10 a.m. to 4 p.m. when the sun's ultraviolet radiation is at its peak.
- Cover exposed areas, wear a broad-brimmed hat and use a sunscreen with a sun protection factor (SPF) of at least 15.
- Protect your eyes. Choose sunglasses that block 99 to 100 percent of ultraviolet rays. For more protection, choose wraparound sunglasses or those that fit close to your face.

♠ Home Remedies

Once sunburn occurs, you can't do much to limit skin damage. However, the following tips may reduce your pain and discomfort:

- *Take anti-inflammatory medication.* Take aspirin, ibuprofen (Advil, Motrin, others) or naproxen (Aleve) until redness and soreness subside. Aspirin isn't recommended for children or teenagers.
- *Apply cold compresses.* Apply a towel dampened with cool tap water to the affected skin. Or take a cool bath or shower.
- *Apply moisturizers.* A moisturizing cream, aloe vera lotion or low dose (0.5 percent to 1 percent) hydrocortisone cream may decrease pain and swelling, and speed up healing.
- *If blisters form, don't break them.* Blisters form a protective layer to damaged skin. Breaking them slows the healing process and increases the risk of infection. If needed, lightly cover blisters with gauze. If blisters break on their own, apply an antibacterial cream.
- *Drink plenty of fluids.* Exposure to sun and heat causes fluid loss through your skin. Be sure to replenish those fluids to prevent dehydration — when your body doesn't have enough water and other fluids to carry out normal functions.
- *Treat peeling skin gently.* Peeling is simply your body's way of getting rid of the top layer of damaged skin. While your skin is peeling, continue to use moisturizing cream.
- *Beware of topical '-caine' products.* Some of these products, such as benzocaine, claim to relieve sunburn pain. But some dermatologists warn against using such products because they can irritate the skin or cause an allergic reaction.

✚ Medical Help

See your doctor if the sunburn:

- Is blistering and covers a large portion of your body
- Is accompanied by a high fever, extreme pain, confusion or nausea
- Doesn't respond to at-home care within a few days

Also, seek medical care if you notice signs or symptoms of an infection:

- Increasing pain, tenderness or swelling
- Yellow drainage (pus) from an open blister
- Red streaks, leading away from the open blister, which may extend in a line upward along the arm or leg

Sweating and body odor

Sweating is your body's normal response to a buildup of body heat. You sweat when you exercise or exert yourself, when you're in a warm environment, or when you're anxious or under stress. This type of sweating is both natural and healthy.

Sweating varies widely from person to person. Many women perspire more heavily during menopause. Drinking hot beverages, or beverages containing alcohol or caffeine, can trigger a light sweat for some individuals. Some people simply inherit a tendency to sweat heavily, especially on the soles of their feet and palms of their hands.

For most people, sweating, or perspiration, is a nuisance that feels uncomfortable and dampens clothing. Body odor is probably more troublesome. Although your sweat is practically odorless, it may take on an unpleasant or offensive odor when it comes into contact with bacteria on your skin.

Odor is more likely to develop at locations, such as your armpits and feet, that are more protected (for example, in shoes and socks) and tend to stay damp and warm. Sweating and body odor may also be influenced by your mood, your diet, some drugs and medical conditions, and even your hormone levels.

Because it's almost impossible to define what's a normal amount of sweating for everybody, try to learn what's normal for you. That may help you pinpoint any unusual changes.

A "cold sweat" is usually your body's response to serious illness, anxiety or severe pain. A cold sweat should receive immediate medical attention if there are signs of lightheadedness or chest and stomach pains.

Antiperspirants and deodorants

If you're concerned about sweating and body odor, the solution may be a simple one. Antiperspirants and deodorants can provide similar results but they work in different ways:

- Antiperspirants contain aluminium-based compounds that temporarily block the sweat pore, thereby reducing the amount of perspiration that reaches your skin.
- Deodorants are usually alcohol-based and turn your skin acidic, making it less attractive to bacteria. Deodorants don't reduce perspiration but often contain fragrances to mask the odor.

The question of whether to choose an antiperspirant or deodorant depends on how much you sweat and how comfortable you are with that amount of sweat.

The following suggestions may help you reduce sweating and body odor:

- *Bathe daily.* Regular bathing helps keep the amount of bacteria on your skin in check.
- *Dry your feet thoroughly.* Microorganisms thrive in the damp spaces between your toes. Use over-the-counter foot powders to help absorb sweat.
- *Wear shoes made of natural materials.* Shoes made of materials such as leather or fabric help prevent sweaty feet by allowing your feet to breathe.
- *Rotate your shoes.* Shoes won't completely dry overnight, so try not to wear the same pair two days in a row if you have trouble with sweaty feet.
- *Wear the right socks.* Cotton and wool socks absorb moisture and help keep your feet dry. If you're active, moisture-wicking athletic socks are a good choice.
- *Change your socks often.* Change socks once or twice a day, drying your feet thoroughly each time. Women may prefer pantyhose with cotton soles.
- *Air your feet.* Go barefoot when you can, or at least slip out of your shoes now and then.
- *Choose natural-fiber clothing.* Wear fabrics such as cotton, wool and silk, which allow your skin to breathe. For exercise, you may prefer high-tech fabrics that can wick moisture away from your skin.
- *Apply antiperspirants nightly.* At bedtime, apply antiperspirants to sweaty hands or feet. Try perfume-free antiperspirants.
- *Try relaxation techniques.* Techniques such as yoga, meditation or biofeedback can help you control the stress that triggers perspiration.
- *Change your diet.* If certain foods or beverages cause you to sweat more than usual or your perspiration to smell, consider eliminating them from your diet.

➕ Medical Help

Consult your doctor if you experience any of the following:
- You suddenly begin to sweat much more or less than usual.
- Sweating disrupts your daily routine.
- You experience night sweats for no apparent reason.
- You notice a change in body odor.

Excessive sweating associated with shortness of breath requires immediate medical attention. This could be a sign of a heart attack.

Swimmer's ear

Swimmer's ear, or otitis externa, is an infection of the ear canal. Your ear canal has features that helps keep it clean and prevent infection, especially the substance you may know as earwax, or cerumen. Persistent moisture in the ear — for example, from frequent swimming — may result in a loss of earwax and breakdown of your defense against ear infection.

Swimmer's ear is most often caused by bacteria that are common in the environment. Infections caused by fungi or viruses are less common. Similar inflammation or infection may occur from scraping your ear canal while cleaning your ear or from hair sprays or hair dyes.

The signs and symptoms are generally mild at the onset, but may get worse if the infection isn't treated or it spreads. Signs and symptoms include:
- Redness in the ear canal
- Mild discomfort
- Drainage of clear fluid

These signs and symptoms may develop into ear pain, swelling, drainage of pus, and decreased or muffled hearing.

♠ Home Remedies

If the discomfort is mild and there's no drainage from your ear, you can do the following:
- Place a warm (not hot) heating pad over your ear.
- Take aspirin or other over-the-counter pain medications (be sure to follow the label instructions).

Prevention

Follow these tips to prevent swimmer's ear:
- Keep your ears dry. Dry only your outer ear slowly and gently with a soft towel or cloth. Tip your head to the side to help water drain from your ear canal. Don't clean inside the ear canal unless you're instructed to do so by your doctor.
- Avoid getting water in your ear canal when bathing. Use a cotton ball coated with petroleum jelly to keep water out of your ears during showers and baths.
- Protect your ears. Avoid substances that may irritate your ears, such as hair sprays or hair dyes.
- Try a homemade preventive treatment. A mixture of 1 part white vinegar and 1 part rubbing alcohol may help prevent the growth of bacteria and fungi that can cause swimmer's ear. Apply before and after swimming. Pour 1 teaspoon of the solution into each ear and let it drain back out. Similar over-the-counter solutions may be available at your drugstore.

✚ Medical Help

See a doctor if you're experiencing any signs or symptoms of swimmer's ear, even if they are mild. Seek immediate medical care if you experience severe pain, significant drainage, fever or swelling.

Swimmer's itch

Swimmer's itch is a rash caused by certain parasites that normally live on waterfowl and freshwater snails. On warm, sunny days — especially in calm freshwater lakes or ponds — these parasites can be released into the water.

During your swim, the parasites might burrow into your skin, where they cause an itchy rash. Fortunately, humans aren't suitable hosts for the parasites, which soon die.

Swimmer's itch is generally characterized by:

- Itching that may begin within an hour or two, or as long as two days, after swimming
- A red, raised rash

Swimmer's itch usually affects only exposed skin — skin not covered by swimsuits, wet suits or waders. Although uncomfortable, swimmer's itch is usually short-lived and typically clears on its own within a few days.

🏠 Home Remedies

As much as you're tempted, don't scratch the affected areas. To relieve itching, try these remedies:

- Cover affected areas with a clean, wet washcloth.
- Soak in a bath sprinkled with Epsom salts, baking soda or oatmeal.
- Stir water into baking soda until it makes a paste and then apply it to the affected areas.

Prevention

There's no evidence that applying sunscreen, lotions or creams helps prevent swimmer's itch. To reduce the risk of itch:

- *Choose swimming spots carefully.* Avoid swimming in areas where swimmer's itch is a known problem or signs warn of possible contamination. Also avoid swimming or wading in marshy areas where snails are commonly found.
- *Avoid the shoreline, if possible.* If you're a strong swimmer, head to deeper water for your swim because you may be more likely to develop the itch if you spend a lot of time in shallow water.
- *Rinse after swimming.* Rinse exposed skin with fresh water immediately after the swim, then vigorously dry your skin with a towel. Launder your swimsuits often. You might even alternate between different swimsuits.
- *Take care of your pool.* If you have a pool, keep it well maintained and chlorinated.

➕ Medical Help

Talk to your doctor if you have a rash after swimming that lasts more than one week. If you notice pus at the rash site, consult your doctor.

Teething

Teething occurs when a baby's teeth first begin to push through the gums. Although the timing varies widely, most babies begin teething by about age 6 months. The two bottom front teeth (lower central incisors) are usually the first to appear, followed by the two top front teeth (upper central incisors).

Classic signs and symptoms of teething include:
- Drooling, which may begin about two months before the first tooth appears
- Irritability or crankiness
- Swollen gums
- Chewing on solid objects

Many parents suspect that teething causes fever and diarrhea, but researchers say this isn't true. Teething may cause signs and symptoms in the mouth and gums, but it doesn't cause problems elsewhere in the body.

🏠 Home Remedies

If your teething baby seems uncomfortable, consider these simple tips:
- *Rub your baby's gums.* Use a clean finger, moistened gauze pad or damp washcloth to massage your baby's gums. The pressure can ease your baby's discomfort.
- *Offer a teething ring.* Try one made of firm rubber. The liquid-filled variety may break under the pressure of your baby's chewing. If a bottle seems to do the trick, fill it with water. Prolonged contact with sugar from formula, milk or juice may cause tooth decay.
- *Keep it cool.* A cold washcloth or chilled teething ring can be soothing. Don't give your baby a frozen teething ring, however. Contact with extreme cold may hurt, doing your baby more harm than good. If your baby eats solid foods, offer items such as applesauce or yogurt.
- *Dry the drool.* Excessive drooling is part of the teething process. To prevent skin irritation, keep a clean cloth handy to dry your baby's chin. Have your baby sleep on an absorbent sheet.
- *Try an over-the-counter product.* If your baby is especially cranky, acetaminophen (Tylenol, others) or ibuprofen (Advil, Motrin, others) may help. Don't give your baby products that contain aspirin, however, and be cautious about teething medications that can be rubbed directly on a baby's gums. The medication may be washed away by your baby's saliva before it has any chance of doing good — and too much of the medication may numb your baby's throat, which may interfere with his or her normal gag reflex.

➕ Medical Help

Teething can usually be handled at home. Contact the doctor if your baby develops a fever, seems particularly uncomfortable, or has other signs or symptoms of illness. The problem may be something other than teething.

Tendinitis

Tendinitis is an inflammation or irritation of a tendon — one of the thick fibrous cords that attach muscles to bones. It can occur in any tendon, but is most common around your shoulders, elbows, wrists and heels. Common names for various tendinitis problems are tennis elbow, golfer's elbow, pitcher's shoulder, swimmer's shoulder and jumper's knee.

Signs and symptoms occur just outside the joint, at the point where a tendon attaches to a bone. They typically include:
- Pain, described as a dull ache
- Tenderness
- Mild swelling

Although tendinitis can be caused by injury from a sudden, single action, the condition is much more likely to stem from the repetition of a particular movement over time. Most people develop tendinitis because their jobs or their hobbies involve repetitive motions that aggravate the tendons needed to perform the tasks.

Tendinitis is also common in people whose daily activities involve awkward positions, frequent overhead reaching, vibration and forceful exertion.

🏠 Home Remedies

Although rest is a key part of treating tendinitis, prolonged inactivity can cause stiffness in your joints. After a few days of completely resting the injured area, gently move it through its full range of motion to maintain joint flexibility.
- Follow the instructions for R.I.C.E. (see page 157).
- Gently move the joint through its full range four times a day. Otherwise rest it. A sling, elastic bandage or splint may help.
- Take an anti-inflammatory medication such as aspirin, ibuprofen (Advil, Motrin, others), naproxen (Aleve) or products containing acetaminophen (Tylenol, others) to reduce discomfort.

Prevention
To prevent tendinitis:
- Ease up. Avoid activities that place excessive stress on your tendons, especially for prolonged periods. If you notice pain, stop and rest.
- Mix it up. If one activity causes a persistent pain, try something else. Incorporate cross-training into your exercise program.
- Improve your technique. If your technique in an activity is flawed, you could be setting yourself up for tendon problems.
- Stretch first. Before you exercise, take time to stretch in order to maximize the range of motion in your joints.

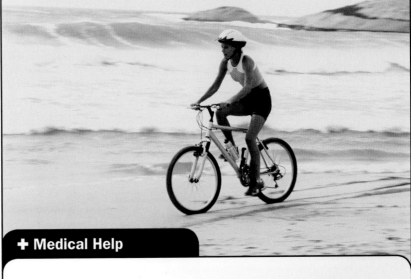

➕ Medical Help

See your doctor if you have a fever, the area is inflamed or your symptoms don't improve within two weeks.

Thumb pain

Pain at the base of your thumb may be the first sign of osteoarthritis in your hands, or you may be experiencing thumb arthritis or tendinitis of the thumb.

With any of these conditions, you may notice pain when you grip, grasp, pinch or apply force with your thumb. You may also experience swelling, and decreased strength and range of motion. It becomes difficult to perform simple tasks, such as writing, opening jars, turning the key in your door or car ignition, or trying to hold small objects.

With osteoarthritis of the hands, the pain may be limited to one joint or extend to many. It's more common in women than in men. Arthritis pain can be the result of a previous injury, repetitive activity or heredity. A common cause of thumb tendinitis is overuse of the wrist.

🏠 Home Remedies

To help relieve thumb pain:

- *Take it easy.* Modify behaviors and avoid activities that cause pain.
- *Rest your thumb.* Use a splint to stabilize the wrist and thumb. Remove the splint at least four times a day to move and stretch the joints to maintain flexibility.
- *Use over-the-counter pain medications if the pain is severe.*
- *Apply heat or cold.* Alternate between heat and cold to help relieve swelling and pain and to soothe your joints. Heat can help ease pain, decrease joint stiffness and relax tense muscles. Experiment with hot packs or electric heating pads on their lowest settings, soaking your hands and wrists in warm water, or simply taking a warm shower or bath. Cold can be effective for reducing pain during flare-ups or after you've had too much physical activity. Applying ice packs or soaking your hands in cool or cold water has a numbing effect that dulls hand and wrist pain.
- *Exercise your thumb daily.* While your hands are warm, move your thumb in wide circles. Bend it to touch each of the other fingers on your hand.
- *Modify household equipment.* Consider purchasing adaptive equipment, such as jar openers, key turners and large zipper pulls. Enlarge the grasp on garden tools, kitchen utensils and writing devices — or buy items with large handles. Replace traditional door handles, which you must grasp with your thumb, with levers.

➕ Medical Help

If you have persistent swelling, stiffness or pain at the base of your thumb, you're unable to fully extend your thumb, or your thumb "catches" in a bent position, seek medical advice. Seek medical care immediately if the pain limits activities or is too severe to tolerate most days.

Tick bites

Spring and summer months are usually the time to worry about tick bites. Although the bites are often harmless, ticks can pass on organisms that may cause serious illnesses. Fortunately, antibiotic treatment is usually successful, particularly when treatment is started early.

Two of the most common tick-related diseases are Lyme disease and Rocky Mountain spotted fever. Although both illnesses can mimic other conditions, each may be identified by a telltale rash. Other tick-borne diseases include ehrlichiosis and anaplasmosis.

Lyme disease

Several days to weeks after a bite, a red, circular-shaped rash, often with a central clearing, may develop around the bite. Other indications may include:

- Flu-like signs and symptoms
- Pain that shifts from one joint to another
- Muscle aches

Rocky Mountain spotted fever

During the first week, a rash of red spots or blotches may appear on your wrists and ankles and eventually spread up the arms and legs to the chest. Other signs and symptoms include:

- High fever and chills
- Severe headache
- Abdominal pain
- Fatigue and loss of appetite

🏠 Home Remedies

To reduce your risk of getting a tick bite or becoming ill from the bite:

- When walking in wooded or grassy areas, wear shoes, long pants tucked into socks and light-colored, long-sleeved shirts. Avoid low bushes and long grass.
- Tick-proof your yard by clearing brush and leaves. Keep woodpiles in sunny areas.
- Check yourself and your pets often for ticks after being in wooded or grassy areas. Shower immediately after leaving these areas because ticks often remain on your skin for hours before biting.
- Insect repellents often repel ticks. Use products containing DEET or permethrin. Be sure to follow label precautions.

If you're bitten by a tick

- Remove the tick promptly and carefully. Use tweezers to grasp the tick near its head or mouth and pull gently and steadily to remove the whole tick without crushing it.
- If possible, seal the tick in a jar. Your doctor may want to see the tick if you develop signs and symptoms of illness after a tick bite.
- Use soap and water to wash your hands. Also wash the area around the tick bite after handling the tick.

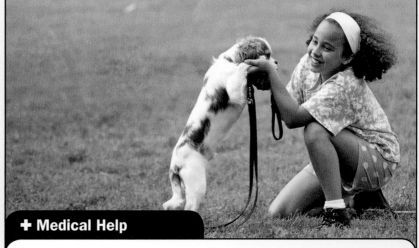

➕ Medical Help

Call your doctor if you can't completely remove the tick or you don't feel well. Also see your doctor if the tick was attached to your body for 36 hours or more, or you develop a rash, fever, stiff neck, muscle aches, joint pain and inflammation or flu-like symptoms.

Toenail fungal infections

Fungi are microscopic organisms that can invade your skin through tiny cuts or small separations between the nail and nail bed. Fungal infections occur more in toenails than in fingernails because toenails are often confined in a dark, warm moist environment inside your shoes — conditions perfect for the growth and spread of fungi.

This stubborn, but harmless, problem often begins as a tiny white or yellow spot on your toenail. Depending on the type of fungus, your nails may discolor, thicken, distort in shape, or turn brittle, crumbly or ragged. The nail surface becomes dull, with no luster or shine.

Toenail fungal infections are more common among older adults. Other risk factors include perspiring heavily, working in a humid or moist environment, wearing footwear that inhibits good ventilation, having diabetes and having a damaged nail.

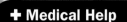

♠ Home Remedies

To help prevent nail fungal infections, try the following:
- Avoid toenails that are too long or too short. Trim nails straight across and file down thickened areas.
- Keep your toenails dry and clean. Dry your feet thoroughly, including between the toes, after bathing.
- Change your socks often, especially if your feet sweat excessively. Take your shoes off occasionally during the day and after exercise. Synthetic socks that wick away moisture may keep your feet drier than do cotton or wool socks.
- Use antifungal spray or powder on your feet and inside your shoes.
- Don't trim or pick at the skin around your nails.
- Avoid walking barefoot in damp public places such as swimming pools, showers and locker rooms.

Two home remedies that may be worth trying are:
- *Vinegar.* There's no evidence that a vinegar soak can cure nail fungus but some studies suggest that it may inhibit the growth of certain bacteria. Soak your feet for 15 to 20 minutes in a mixture of 1 part vinegar to 2 parts warm water. If your skin becomes irritated, try soaking only two to three times a week, or increase the proportion of water in the mixture.
- *Vicks VapoRub.* As with vinegar, there's no scientific proof that this product works on nail fungus, but anecdotal reports claim it does. You apply the product to infected nails but there's no consensus on how often.

✚ Medical Help

If self-care measures aren't effective and the condition of your nails bothers you or causes problems, see your doctor or podiatrist.

Toothache

Tooth decay is the primary cause of toothaches. Bacteria that live in your mouth thrive on the sugars and starches in your food. These bacteria form a sticky plaque that clings to the surface of your teeth.

Decay-producing acid forms in plaque and attacks the hard outer coating (enamel) of your teeth. The erosion caused by plaque forms tiny openings (cavities) in tooth surfaces. The first sign of decay may be a sensation of pain when you eat something sweet, very cold or very hot. A toothache often indicates that your dentist needs to check your teeth.

Tooth decay can occur more rapidly in people who have dry mouth, people who consume a lot of soft drinks or sports drinks or suck on hard candies or cough drops, people who eat a lot of high-sugar foods, and people who abuse methamphetamine.

♠ Home Remedies

Until you're able to visit your dentist, try these self-care tips to help relieve toothache:

- Take an over-the-counter (OTC) pain reliever.
- Apply an OTC antiseptic containing benzocaine directly to the irritated tooth and gum. Direct application of oil of cloves (eugenol) also may help. Don't place aspirin or another painkiller directly against your gums, as it may burn your gum tissue.
- Thoroughly clean all parts of your mouth, including your teeth — don't avoid the painful areas.
- Use warm water to brush your teeth.
- Use toothpaste designed for sensitive teeth.
- Avoid foods or beverages that are hot, cold or sweet enough to trigger pain.

Prevention

Taking good care of your teeth is the best way to avoid tooth decay and cavities.

- Brush your teeth at least twice a day — ideally after every meal — using fluoride-containing toothpaste.
- Use floss or an interdental cleaner to remover food particles wedged between your teeth.
- If you can't brush after eating, try to rinse your mouth with mouthwash or water.
- Drink water that has fluoride added to it. The fluoride added to regular tap water has helped decrease tooth decay significantly. But today, many people drink bottled water that doesn't contain fluoride.

✚ Medical Help

Contact your dentist if you have signs of infection, such as swelling, pain when you bite, red gums or a foul-tasting discharge. If fever accompanies the pain, seek emergency care.

Traveler's diarrhea

Nothing can ruin a vacation or business trip faster than loose stools and abdominal cramps. Traveler's diarrhea usually isn't serious but it can be very disruptive and unpleasant.

A trip to a foreign country by no means guarantees gastrointestinal discomfort. But if you visit a place where the climate, social conditions or sanitary practices are different from yours at home, you have an increased risk of getting traveler's diarrhea.

It's possible that the condition stems from the stress of travel or a change in your regular diet. But almost always an infectious agent is to blame, including viruses, bacteria or parasites. You often get traveler's diarrhea from food or water contaminated by feces.

The sickness strikes abruptly, usually lasts three to seven days and is rarely life-threatening. You generally don't require medical treatment other than replacing lost fluids, which can be made up with canned fruit juices, weak tea, clear soup and carbonated beverages.

♠ Home Remedies

Traveler's diarrhea tends to resolve itself but these medications may help relieve symptoms:

- *Anti-motility agents.* These agents, including loperamide (Imodium) and medications containing diphenoxylate (Lomotil), provide prompt but temporary relief by slowing the transit time of food through your digestive tract and allowing more time for absorption.
- *Bismuth subsalicylate (Pepto Bismol).* This over-the-counter medication can decrease the frequency of your stools and shorten the duration of your illness. However, it isn't recommended for children, pregnant women or people who are allergic to aspirin.

Prevention

To reduce your risk of traveler's diarrhea:

- Avoid tap water or spring water. Drink only bottled water. Sodas, beer or wine served in their original containers are acceptable.
- Avoid ice cubes in your beverage. They may have been made with contaminated water.
- Use bottled water or boiled water to brush your teeth. Keep your mouth closed while showering.
- Don't eat any food from street vendors.
- Avoid salads, buffet foods, undercooked meats, raw vegetables, grapes, berries, fruits that have been peeled or cut, and unpasteurized milk and dairy products.
- Eat vegetables and fruits that you can peel yourself, such as bananas or oranges.
- Eat yogurt or take probiotic supplements. Probiotics contain beneficial, or "good," bacteria that helps maintain a proper microorganic balance in your intestinal tract.

✚ Medical Help

If you have severe dehydration, persistent vomiting, bloody stools or a high fever, or if your symptoms last for more than a few days, seek medical help. Be especially cautious with children, because traveler's diarrhea can cause severe dehydration in a short time.

Ulcer

Peptic ulcers are open sores that develop on the inner lining of your esophagus, stomach or upper small intestine. It wasn't too long ago that lifestyle factors, such as a love of spicy foods or a stressful job, were thought to be at the root of most ulcers. Doctors now know that bacterial infection — not stress or diet — is a primary cause of ulcers.

Burning pain is the most common symptom of an ulcer, and the pain is aggravated whenever stomach acid comes in direct contact with the ulcerated area. The pain typically may:

- Be felt anywhere from your navel up to your breastbone
- Last from a few minutes to several hours
- Be worse when your stomach is empty
- Flare at night
- Be relieved temporarily by eating certain foods or taking acid-reducing medication
- Disappear and then return for a few days or weeks

♠ Home Remedies

To prevent ulcers or help existing ulcers heal, try the following:

- *Don't smoke.* Smoking may interfere with the protective function of your stomach lining, making it more susceptible to the development of an ulcer. Smoking also increases stomach acid.
- *Limit or avoid alcohol.* Excessive use of alcohol irritates and erodes the lining in your stomach and intestines, which can cause inflammation and bleeding.
- *Avoid nonsteroidal anti-inflammatory drugs (NSAIDs).* These products can irritate your stomach lining. If you use pain relievers regularly, use acetaminophen (Tylenol, others).
- *Control acid reflux.* If you have an esophageal ulcer — usually associated with acid reflux — you can take steps to help manage the reflux. These include avoiding spicy or fatty foods, avoiding lying down after meals, reducing your weight and raising the head of your bed.
- *Pay attention to your diet.* While an ulcer is healing, it's advisable to watch what you eat and to control stress. Acidic or spicy foods may increase stomach acid, increasing ulcer pain. The same is true for stress. If stress is severe, it may delay the healing of an ulcer.

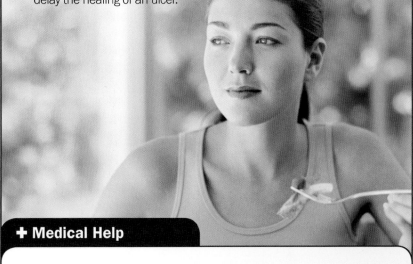

✚ Medical Help

An ulcer isn't something that you should treat on your own, without a doctor's help. Over-the-counter antacids and acid blockers may relieve the gnawing pain, but the relief is short-lived. If you have signs or symptoms of an ulcer, see your doctor for treatment.

Vaginal yeast infection

A vaginal yeast infection is a type of vaginitis — inflammation of the vagina — typically caused when the balance of microorganisms that are normally present in your vagina becomes altered. These changes may result in an overgrowth of yeast, which can lead to a yeast infection. The signs and symptoms of infection can range from mild to severe, including:

- Itching and irritation in the vagina and at the entrance to the vagina (vulva)
- Burning sensation, especially during intercourse or while urinating
- Red, swollen vulva
- Vaginal pain and soreness
- Thick, white, odor-free vaginal discharge with a cottage cheese appearance

You're more susceptible to a yeast infection if you are pregnant or have diabetes, or if you're taking antibiotics, cortisone or birth control pills.

♠ Home Remedies

Treatment options include one-day, three-day and seven-day courses of medications for yeast infections. The active ingredient in these creams or suppositories is clotrimazole (Gyne-Lotrimin), miconazole (Monistat) or tioconazole (Vagistat). Some of these products also come with an external cream that is applied to the labia and vulva to soothe itching. Follow package directions and complete the entire course of treatment, even if you're feeling better right away.

To ease discomfort until an antifungal medication takes full effect, apply a cold compress, such as a damp washcloth, to the labial area. You may also take probiotic supplements or suppositories. Probiotics contain beneficial bacteria, such as *Lactobacillus acidophilus*, which may help restore the balance of microorganisms in your vagina. One study found that suppositories containing L. acidophilus improved symptoms of vaginal yeast infections, while other studies of oral preparations of L. acidophilus found little benefit. Eating yogurt that contains active lactobacillus cultures is a healthy habit that may, in addition, help reduce recurrent vaginal yeast infections.

Prevention

To help prevent vaginal yeast infections, try the following:

- Don't douche. The vagina doesn't require cleansing other than normal bathing. Repetitive douching disrupts the balance of organisms that normally live in the vagina. And douching won't clear up an infection of the vagina.
- Avoid potential irritants, such as scented tampons or pads.
- Wear cotton underwear and pantyhose with a cotton crotch. Don't wear underwear to bed. Yeast thrives in moist environments.
- Change out of wet swimsuits and damp clothing as soon as possible.

✚ Medical Help

Make an appointment to see your doctor if:

- This is the first time you've experienced a yeast infection
- You're not sure whether you have a yeast infection
- Your symptoms don't go away after self-treating with antifungal creams and suppositories
- You develop other symptoms

Varicose veins

Varicose veins are gnarled, enlarged veins that you can see just under the surface of your skin. They may be blue or dark purple in color. Any vein may become varicose, but the veins most commonly affected are those in your legs and feet.

For many people, varicose veins don't cause any pain and are primarily a cosmetic concern. But for some people, they cause aching pain and discomfort. Sometimes varicose veins signal a higher risk of other circulatory problems.

If painful signs and symptoms do occur, they may include:
- Achy feeling in your legs
- Burning, throbbing, muscle cramping and swelling in your lower legs
- Worsened pain after sitting or standing for a long time
- Itching around one or more of your veins
- Skin ulcers near your ankle, which may signal a vascular disease that requires medical attention.

♠ Home Remedies

These steps may decrease the discomfort of varicose veins, and help prevent or slow their development, as well. They include:
- *Exercise.* Get your legs moving. Walking is a great way to encourage blood circulation in your legs.
- *Watch your weight, and your diet.* Shedding excess pounds takes pressure off your veins. Follow a low-salt, high-fiber diet to prevent the swelling that may result from water retention and constipation.
- *Watch what you wear.* Avoid high heels. Low-heeled shoes work calf muscles more, which is better for your veins. Don't wear tight clothes around your waist, legs or groin. Tight panty-leg girdles, for instance, can cut off blood flow.
- *Elevate your legs.* To improve circulation in your legs, take short breaks daily to elevate your legs above the level of your heart. For example, lie down with your legs resting on three or four pillows.
- *Avoid long periods of sitting or standing.* Make a point of changing your position frequently to encourage blood flow. Try to move around at least every 30 minutes.
- *Don't sit with your legs crossed.* Some doctors believe this position can increase circulation problems.
- *Wear compression socks when traveling or standing for long periods of time.*

✛ Medical Help

If you're concerned about how your veins look and feel and self-care measures haven't helped, consult your doctor. See your doctor if you develop skin ulcers or if the veins become sore or reddened and one leg is more swollen than the other.

Warts

Common warts are caused by a virus that triggers a rapid growth of cells on the outer layer of your skin. The warts look like small, grainy bumps that are rough to the touch. They may be painful and unsightly, but they're usually harmless and often disappear on their own without treatment. Common warts aren't cancerous.

There are more than 200 types of warts. Common warts usually occur on your hands and fingers. Other types of warts include:

- Plantar warts, which occur on the soles of your feet
- Genital warts, which develop in your genital area
- Flat warts, which often appear on your face, hands and legs

Like other infectious diseases, wart viruses pass from person to person. It can take a wart as long as two to six months to develop after your skin has been exposed to the virus.

♠ Home Remedies

Unless you have an impaired immune system or diabetes, try these home remedies to remove warts:

Salicylic acid
Wart-removal products are available at drugstores, either as a topical solution or patch. For common warts, look for products containing 17 percent salicylic acid (Compound W, Occlusal-HP), which peels off the infected skin. These products require daily use, often for a few weeks. For best results, soak your wart in warm water for 10 to 20 minutes before applying the product. File away any dead skin with a nail file or pumice stone between treatments. Just be careful — the acid in these products can irritate or damage healthy skin around the wart. If you're pregnant, talk with your doctor before using an acid solution.

Duct tape
One study employed a "duct tape therapy" that involved covering warts with duct tape for six days, then soaking the warts in warm water and rubbing them with an emery board or pumice stone. The process was repeated for as long as two months. Researchers hypothesized that this unconventional therapy worked by irritating the wart and triggering the body's immune system to attack the virus. More recent research has disputed these findings and found that duct tape wasn't effective for treating warts. Still, the low cost and convenience of this treatment may make it worth trying, regardless.

✚ Medical Help

Most warts disappear on their own or with self care. Prompt treatment by a doctor, however, may decrease the chance that the warts will spread. Also visit your doctor if your warts are a cosmetic nuisance, bothersome, painful or rapidly multiplying.

Watery eyes

Tears lubricate your eyes and help wash away particles of dust and grit. Watery eyes occur when an excess production of tears overwhelms your eyelids or when the fluid drains too slowly through your tear ducts.

One of the most common causes of watery eyes is an age-related change affecting your eyelids. As you get older, the muscles in your eyelids tend to relax, which may prevent the inner lid from lying flat against the eye's surface. The result is a pooling of tears in the corners of your eyes. The tears remain and may become stagnant, irritating your eyes.

Another common age-related cause of tearing is when a tear duct becomes blocked, preventing the drainage of fluid from the eye. Other causes include dryness and irritation from the environment. Watery eyes commonly accompany infections such as pink eye. They can also result from allergies, including an allergic reaction to preservatives in eyedrops or contact lens solutions.

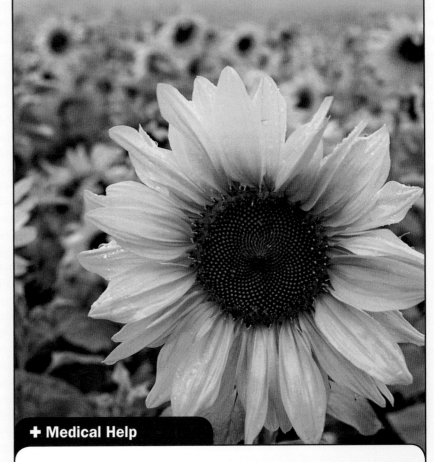

♠ Home Remedies

To help treat and prevent watery eyes:
- Apply a warm compress over closed eyelids two to four times a day for 10 minutes.
- Don't rub your eyes.
- Replace mascara and other types of eye makeup at least every three months. These products can become contaminated with bacteria transferred by the applicator.
- Follow proper directions for the wearing, cleaning and disinfecting of contact lenses.

+ Medical Help

Seek medical care if the condition continues despite self-care efforts and interferes with your daily activities, or if you develop eye pain or new onset of impaired vision.

Wrinkles

Wrinkles are a natural part of aging. As you grow older, your skin gets thinner, drier, less elastic and less able to protect itself from damage. As a result, wrinkles, lines and creases form on your skin.

Some people don't seem to age as quickly as others do. Although genetics is the most important factor in determining skin texture, another major contributor to wrinkles is spending too much time in the sun. Smoking also can cause premature aging of your skin.

Cosmetic products that promise youthful skin are often expensive and usually fail to deliver any significant improvements. When wrinkles become bothersome, people often turn to medications, resurfacing techniques, fillers, injectables and surgery to help smooth and invigorate their skin.

🏠 Home Remedies

These measures may help slow the process of aging skin:

- *Protect your skin from the sun.* Shield your skin — and help prevent future wrinkles — by limiting the amount of time you spend in the sun. Always wear protective clothing and hats outdoors. Also, use sunscreen when outdoors, even in winter.
- *Choose products with built-in sunscreen.* When selecting skin-care products, choose those with a built-in sun protection factor (SPF) of at least 15. Also, be sure to select products that block both types of ultraviolet (UVA and UVB) rays.
- *Use moisturizers.* Dryness turns plump skin cells into shriveled ones, creating fine lines and wrinkles long before you're due. Though moisturizers can't prevent wrinkles, they may temporarily mask tiny lines and creases. Also avoid harsh soaps and hot water when bathing.
- *Don't smoke.* Even if you've smoked for years or smoked heavily when you were younger, you can still improve your skin tone and texture and prevent future wrinkles by quitting smoking.

Beware of nonprescription wrinkle creams

The effectiveness of anti-wrinkle creams depends in part on the active ingredient or ingredients they contain. Retinol, alpha hydroxy acid, kinetin, coenzyme Q10, copper peptides and antioxidants may result in slight to modest improvements in wrinkles. However, wrinkle creams containing these ingredients that are sold over-the-counter contain lower concentrations of these active ingredients than do prescription creams. Therefore, the results — if any — are limited and usually short-lived.

➕ Medical Help

If you're concerned about the appearance of your skin, see your dermatologist. He or she can help you create a personalized skin-care plan by assessing your skin type and evaluating your skin's condition. A dermatologist can also recommend medical wrinkle treatments.

Wrist and hand pain

Think of all the things you do each day using your wrists, hands and fingers. You may not even be aware of the many nerves, blood vessels, muscles and small bones that work together as you perform a task as simple as turning a key in the door — until the movement becomes painful.

Pain may be caused by sudden injuries such as sprains or fractures. But long-term medical problems also may cause wrist and hand pain, such as arthritis, carpal tunnel syndrome and the wear and tear from overuse or repetitive movements.

The amount of pain may vary, depending on what's causing it. For example, pain from osteoarthritis is often described as similar to a dull toothache, while tendinitis usually causes a sharp, stabbing pain. The location of pain also may provide clues as to what is causing signs and symptoms.

Ganglion cysts

Ganglion cysts are fluid-filled lumps that usually appear along tendons and joints of your wrists and hands. Ganglions are sometimes painful and, if bothersome, may require treatment. Seek medical care immediately if a lump becomes painful and inflamed or if a cyst breaks through the skin and begins to drain.

🏠 Home Remedies

To relieve wrist and hand pain:
- Follow the instructions for R.I.C.E. (see page 157).
- Use over-the-counter pain medications, if needed.

Prevention

To prevent wrist and hand problems:
- Build bone strength with a diet that includes adequate amounts of calcium and vitamin D to prevent fractures.
- Use tools with large handles so you don't have to grip them as hard.
- Remove rings from your fingers before doing manual labor. If you injure your hand, remove rings before your fingers become swollen.
- Take frequent breaks to rest muscles you're using regularly, and try to vary activities so you're not always using the same muscles.
- Do flexibility and strengthening exercises.
- Try out special ergonomic devices that can make you more comfortable, improve posture and protect your wrists and hands.

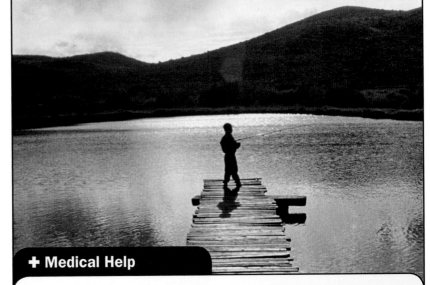

➕ Medical Help

Minor sprains and strains usually respond to rest, ice and over-the-counter pain medications. But if pain and swelling last longer than a few days or becomes worse, see your doctor. Seek medical care immediately if:
- You suspect a fracture
- A fall or accident has caused rapid swelling and moving the area is painful
- The area is hot and inflamed and you have a fever

Emergency care

Emergencies don't happen every day, but when they do there is usually little time to react and help may not be immediately at hand. With preparation, you can respond effectively when a person appears injured, seriously ill or in distress. Perhaps this preparation may never be needed but on the chance it is, your quick action could some day save a life.

Take a certified first-aid training course to learn life-saving skills, such as cardiopulmonary resuscitation (CPR) and the Heimlich maneuver, and to recognize signs of heart attack, shock and traumatic injury. Check with your local Red Cross, county emergency services, public safety office or the American Heart Association for information on first aid and related courses that are offered in your community.

In this section, we discuss some of the basic steps you may take in case of an emergency until medical help arrives.

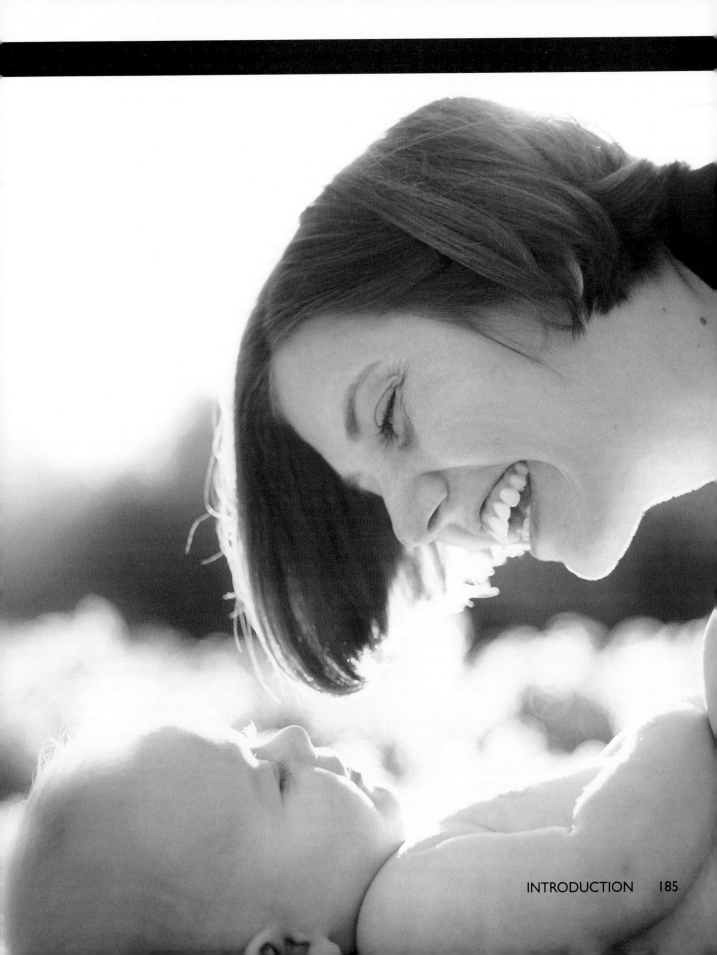

Allergic reaction (anaphylaxis)

Anaphylaxis is a severe, potentially life-threatening allergic reaction. It can occur rapidly after you're exposed to something that you're allergic to, such as peanuts or venom from a bee sting.

Your immune system produces chemicals that help protect you from many foreign substances, including bacteria and viruses. Infrequently, your system over-reacts. During anaphylaxis, it releases a flood of chemicals that puts your entire body into shock. Your blood pressure drops suddenly and your airways constrict, preventing normal breathing.

Anaphylaxis requires an immediate trip to the emergency room and an injection of epinephrine to reduce your body's allergic response. If your condition isn't treated quickly, it can lead to unconsciousness or death.

Signs and symptoms

An anaphylactic reaction is most likely to occur soon after exposure to the allergy trigger, or allergen. Even if, in the past, you only experienced a mild reaction to the allergen, you still may be at risk of a severe reaction when you're exposed to it now.

Signs and symptoms usually occur within seconds or minutes of exposure. In rare cases, the reaction occurs more than half an hour after exposure. Anaphylactic signs and symptoms include:

- Skin reactions, such as hives, swollen eyes, itching and skin that is flushed, pale or cool and clammy
- Constricted airways and swollen lips, tongue or throat, which can cause wheezing and trouble breathing
- Weak and rapid pulse
- Nausea, vomiting or diarrhea
- Dizziness or fainting

Triggers

A number of allergens can trigger anaphylaxis, depending on how sensitive you are to different substances. Common anaphylactic triggers include:

- Foods such as peanuts, tree nuts (walnuts, pecans), fish, shellfish, milk and eggs
- Insect stings from bees, yellow jackets, wasps, hornets and fire ants
- Certain medications, especially penicillin

What to do

If someone is having a severe allergic reaction and showing signs of shock, quick action is essential. Even if you're not positive of the cause, take the following steps immediately:

- Call 911 or emergency medical help.
- Check the person's pulse and breathing and, if necessary, use cardiopulmonary resuscitation (CPR) or other first aid.
- If the person has medications to treat an allergy attack, such as an epinephrine auto-injector or antihistamine tablets, give them immediately.

Using an auto-injector

Many people at risk of anaphylaxis carry a device called an auto-injector. This device is a spring-loaded syringe that can inject a single dose of medication when pressed against the thigh. The device is generally very easy to use and instructions are often printed on the side.

If you require an auto-injector, make sure that you, as well as the people closest to you, know how to administer the drug. If family or friends are with you in an anaphylactic emergency, they could save your life. Medical personnel responding to a call for help also may give you an injection of epinephrine or another medication to treat your symptoms.

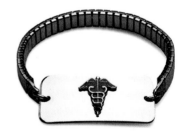

If you have a drug allergy, carry allergy identification at all times. Drug-alert necklaces and bracelets are available at drugstores.

Burns

The most serious burns — third-degree burns — are an emergency involving all layers of skin and causing permanent tissue damage (see page 33). The burned areas may be charred black or appear dry and white. If smoke inhalation accompanies the burn, breathing may be difficult. You may have carbon monoxide poisoning or other toxic effects.

For severe burns

Call 911 or emergency medical help. Until an emergency unit arrives, follow these steps:

1. *Don't try to remove burned clothing.* However, do make sure the victim is not in contact with smoldering materials or exposed to smoke or heat.
2. *Don't immerse large burns in cold water or ice.* Doing so could cause a drop in body temperature and reduce blood pressure and circulation, putting the body in shock.
3. *Elevate the body part or parts that are burned.* Raise them above heart level, if possible.
4. *Gently cover the burned area.* Use a cool, moist, sterile bandage, cloth or towel.

For electrical burns

An electrical burn may appear minor or not show on a person's skin, but the damage can extend deep into underlying tissues below the surface. If a strong electrical current passes through the body, internal damage, such as a heart rhythm disturbance or cardiac arrest, can occur.

Sometimes the jolt associated with an electrical burn can throw a person to the ground or against a wall, resulting in fractures or other injuries.

Call 911 or a medical emergency number if the person who has been burned is in pain, is confused, or is experiencing any changes in breathing, pulse or consciousness.

While waiting for medical help, follow these steps:

1. *Don't touch.* The person may still be in contact with the electrical source. Touching the person may pass the current through you.
2. *Turn off the power source, if possible.* If you're unable to do so, try to move the source away from both you and the injured person using a dry, nonconducting object made of cardboard, plastic or wood. Don't attempt this if the voltage is over 600 volts, such as a downed power line.
3. *Check for breathing and pulse.* If absent, begin cardiopulmonary resuscitation (CPR) on the individual immediately.

For chemical burns

Make sure the cause of the burn has been removed. Flush chemicals off the skin's surface with cool running water for at least 10 minutes. If the burning chemical is a powder-like substance such as lime, brush it off your skin before flushing.

Remove clothing and jewelry that has been contaminated by the chemical. Then, wrap the area with a dry, sterile dressing (if possible) or clean cloth.

Seek emergency assistance if:
- The person shows signs of shock, such as fainting, pale complexion or breathing in a notably shallow manner
- The chemical burn has penetrated through the upper skin layer, and the burned area exceeds 3 inches in diameter
- The chemical burn occurred on an eye, face, hand, foot, groin or buttock, or over a major joint

If you're unsure whether a chemical substance is toxic, provide the chemical container or a complete description of the substance to medical personnel.

Bleeding

Bleeding may occur externally through cuts and tears in the skin or internally from ruptured blood vessels, sometimes exiting through natural openings of the body such as the mouth. Most injuries don't cause life-threatening bleeding, but in situations where substantial blood is lost, shock, unconsciousness and death may result.

To stop severe bleeding, follow these steps:

1. Lay a bleeding person down and, if possible, cover his or her body with a blanket or jacket to prevent the loss of heat.

2. If possible, position the person's head slightly lower than his or her trunk or elevate the legs. This position reduces the risk of fainting by increasing blood flow to the brain. If possible, elevate the site that's bleeding.

3. While wearing gloves, remove any obvious dirt or debris from the wound. Don't remove objects that are embedded in the skin. Don't probe into the wound or attempt to clean or rinse it out. Your primary concern is to stop the bleeding.

4. Apply direct pressure on the wound, using a sterile bandage, clean cloth, article of clothing or, if nothing else, your hands.

5. Hold continuous pressure on the wound for at least 20 minutes without checking to see if the bleeding has stopped. Then, maintain pressure by binding the wound with a bandage or clean cloth and adhesive tape. Don't apply a tourniquet except as a last resort.

6. Don't remove the gauze or bandage. If bleeding continues and begins to seep through the material you're holding on the wound, add more absorbent layers of material on top of it.

7. If direct pressure on the wound doesn't stop the bleeding, you can apply pressure to the main artery that delivers blood to the area of the wound. Squeeze the artery against nearby bone while keeping your fingers flat. With the other hand, continue to apply pressure on the wound.

8. Immobilize the body part that's injured — in other words, try to keep it in a stabile position — once the bleeding has been stopped. Leave the bandages in place and call 911 or your local emergency number. Transport the injured person to an emergency room as soon as possible if there is severe bleeding or signs of shock.

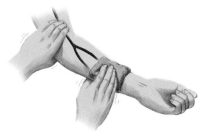

To stop bleeding, apply pressure directly to the wound using a sterile bandage, gauze or clean cloth.

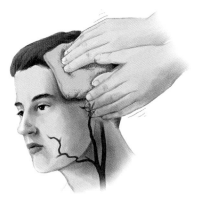

If bleeding continues despite pressure applied directly to the wound, maintain pressure and also apply pressure to the nearest major artery between the injury and the heart.

Cardiopulmonary resuscitation

Cardiopulmonary resuscitation (CPR) can save lives in a range of emergencies, such as a heart attack or near drowning, in which someone's breathing or heartbeat has stopped.

Ideally, CPR involves two separate elements: chest compressions combined with mouth-to-mouth rescue breathing. But what you are able to perform in an emergency situation depends on your knowledge and comfort level. If you're untrained or unsure of your skills, you may do "hands-only" CPR (chest compressions) and not mouth-to-mouth rescue breathing.

The bottom line is: It's far better to do something than to do nothing at all — the difference could save a person's life.

Before you begin

When assessing an emergency situation, determine if the person is conscious or unconscious.
1. If the person is unresponsive and appears to be unconscious, tap or shake the shoulder and ask loudly, "Are you OK?"
2. If there's no response, and another person is able to help you, one of you should call 911 or a local emergency number while the other begins CPR.

3. If you're alone but have immediate access to a telephone, call the emergency number before starting CPR.
4. Begin CPR or hook up an automatic external defibrillator (AED), if a device is immediately available. Voice prompts from the device will guide you step-by-step on its use. If advised to do so by the voice prompts, deliver one shock, then begin CPR.
5. For children, perform CPR first, then call 911. If you're alone with an infant or a child age 1 to 8 years, perform two minutes of CPR before calling for help or using an AED.

Continued next page >

How AEDs work

An automatic external defibrillator (AED) is a device that senses your heart's rhythm during cardiac arrest and, in some cases, delivers an electric shock to get your heart beating again.

A short instructional video typically accompanies the AED that explains how to use and maintain the device. Watch the video after your purchase, and periodically review how to use it later on.

In an emergency, the AED will essentially make decisions for you. Voice instructions guide you through the defibrillation process, explaining how to check for breathing and pulse, and how to position electrode pads on the person's chest.

Once the pads are in place, the AED automatically measures the heart rhythms. If a shock is needed, the device will instruct you on delivering it. The AED will also guide you through CPR. The process can be repeated as needed until emergency responders take over.

CPR

When performing cardiopulmonary resuscitation (CPR), your actions should be performed in a specific sequence that's best described as the ABC method — which stands for Airway, Breathing and Circulation.

A: Open the airway

1. Put the person on his or her back on a firm surface. Kneel next to the neck and shoulders.
2. Put your palm on the person's forehead and gently tilt the head back. With your other hand, lift the chin forward to open the airway.
3. Take five to 10 seconds to check for normal breathing. Look for chest motion, listen for breath sounds, and feel for breath on your cheek and ear. (Gasping is not normal breathing.)
4. If breathing isn't normal and you're trained in CPR, perform mouth-to-mouth breathing. If you're not trained in emergency procedures or uncertain about your ability to perform them, proceed directly to the chest compressions (see page 191.)

B: Breathe for the person

Rescue breathing can be mouth-to-mouth or mouth-to-nose if the mouth is seriously injured or can't be opened.

1. With the airway open (head tilted, chin lifted) pinch the nostrils shut and cover the person's mouth with yours, making a seal.

2. Prepare to give two breaths. Give the first breath. If the chest rises, give the second breath. If the chest doesn't rise, repeat the head-tilt, chin-lift maneuver, then give the second breath.
3. If there's no breathing, coughing or movement, begin chest compressions described in "C" to restore air and blood circulation.

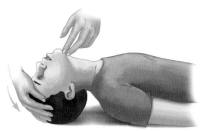

Put your palm on the forehead and gently tilt the head back. With your other hand, gently lift the chin forward to open the airway.

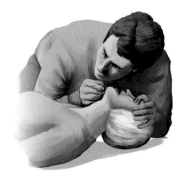

Take five to 10 seconds to check for normal breathing. Look for chest motion, listen for breath sounds, and feel for breath on your cheek and ear.

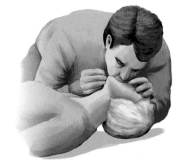

With the airway open, pinch the nostrils shut and cover the person's mouth with yours. Give the breath.

CPR

C: Restore circulation

If an automatic external defibrillator (AED) is immediately available, turn it on and follow the voice prompts (see page 189). Otherwise, you may start chest compressions:

1. Place the heel of one hand over the center of the individual's chest, between the nipples. Place your other hand on top of the first hand. Keep your elbows straight and your shoulders directly above your hands.

2. Use your upper body weight (not just your arms) to push straight down on (compress) the chest about one to two inches. Push hard at a rate of about 100 compressions a minute — faster than one compression a second.

3. After 30 compressions, tilt the head back and lift the chin up to open the airway. Give two rescue breaths. That's one cycle (remember the expression "30, then 2"). If you're not trained in CPR, you can skip the rescue breathing and do only chest compressions.

4. Continue doing cycles of 30 compressions and two rescue breaths. If the individual has not begun moving after five cycles (about two minutes) and an AED becomes available, apply it and follow the prompts. Administer one shock, then resume CPR — starting with chest compressions — for another five cycles before administering a second shock.

5. Continue CPR until there are signs of movement or until emergency medical responders can take over.

CPR for children

For children 1 to 8 years old, use one or two hands (depending on the child's size) and breathe more gently. If you're alone, do five cycles (two minutes) of CPR before calling 911.

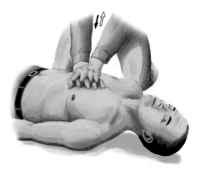

Coordinate chest compressions with rescue breathing.

Hands-only CPR saves lives

The American Heart Association (AHA) states that bystanders can effectively use hands-only CPR — chest compressions without rescue breaths — on people over the age of 8 in emergency situations if the bystanders have witnessed the event. Hands-only CPR involves:

1. Calling 911 or a local medical emergency number.

2. Giving chest compressions, pushing hard and fast in the center of the chest and avoiding interruptions. The compressions continue until emergency medical responders arrive and say to stop. Bystanders should also try to perform traditional CPR (with rescue breaths) if they don't witness the event.

CPR

CPR for infants

The procedure for giving cardio-pulmonary resuscitation (CPR) to an infant (under 12 months old) is similar to the one used for adults. Loudly call out the infant's name and stroke or gently tap the shoulder. Do not shake the child. If there's no response, have someone call 911 while you:

- Place the infant on his or her back on a firm, flat surface, such as a table or the floor.
- Gently tilt the head back and lift the chin to open the airway.
- In no more than 10 seconds, check for signs of breathing: Look for chest motion, listen for breath sounds, and feel for breath on your cheek and ear.
- If you see blockage in the mouth, remove it with a sweep of your finger. Be careful not to push the object deeper into the airway. If you still detect no breathing, start CPR.
- Cover the mouth and nose with your mouth.
- Prepare to give two gentle breaths. Use the strength of your cheeks to deliver puffs of air instead of deep breaths from your lungs.
- After the first breath, watch to see if the chest rises. If it does, give a second breath. If it doesn't, repeat the head-tilt, chin-lift maneuver and give the second breath.
- Begin chest compressions to

restore circulation. Place two fingertips of one hand in the center of the infant's chest, just below the nipple line.
- Gently push down one-third to one-half the depth of the chest. Allow the chest to come back up. Count aloud as you push in fairly rapid rhythm (a rate of about 100 compressions a minute).
- After 30 compressions, give two rescue breaths. This will complete a cycle. If someone else can help you provide CPR, one person does 15 chest compressions and the other person delivers the two rescue breaths.
- Perform CPR for five cycles before making an emergency call for help, unless someone else can make the call while you attend to the infant.
- Continue CPR until you see signs of life or until emergency responders arrive.

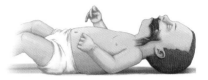

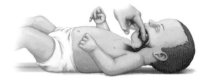

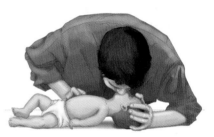

Before giving CPR to an infant, tilt the child's head back to open the airway. If you see an object in the infant's mouth, remove it with a sweep of your finger. Alternate compression of the infant's chest with gentle breaths from your mouth.

Choking

Choking occurs when an object becomes lodged in your throat or windpipe, stopping the flow of air to your lungs. The blockage, in turn, cuts off the circulation of oxygen-rich blood to your brain and other vital organs. If the blockage isn't cleared rapidly, the condition can prove fatal.

A common cause of blockage is food — often from eating too fast or while laughing, talking or doing some form of physical activity.

The universal sign of choking is hands clutched to the throat. If a person in distress doesn't give this indication, look for other signs:

- Inability to talk
- Difficulty breathing or noisy breathing
- Inability to cough forcefully
- Skin, lips and nails turning blue or dusky
- Loss of consciousness

Five-and-five approach

For situations in which a person is choking, the Red Cross recommends that you take a "five-and-five" approach:

1. Give five blows to the back between the shoulder blades using the heel of your hand.
2. Deliver five abdominal thrusts These thrusts are known as the Heimlich maneuver.
3. Continue to alternate between five back blows and five abdominal thrusts until the blockage is dislodged.

If you're alone, do the five-and-five approach before calling 911 or a local emergency number. If another person is present, have that person call for help while you give first aid.

If the person becomes unconscious during the procedure, perform CPR with chest compressions (see pages 189-192).

The Heimlich maneuver

The Heimlich maneuver is perhaps the best known technique for clearing an obstructed airway. It should be used on someone only if there's a complete or near-complete blockage of the airway. To perform the maneuver:

1. Stand behind the person. Wrap your arms around the person's waist. Tip the person forward slightly.
2. Make a fist with one hand. Place it slightly above the person's navel.
3. Grasp the fist with your other hand. Press hard into the abdomen with a quick, upward thrust, as if trying to lift the person up.
4. Continue the five-and-five cycle until the blockage is dislodged.

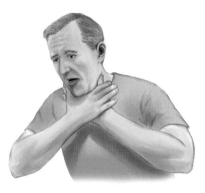

Typically, a person who is choking is unable to communicate except by hand motions.

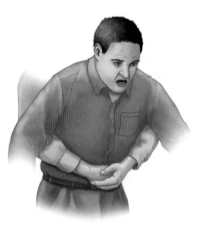

The Heimlich maneuver should be performed if the person can't speak, cough or effectively exchange air.

Choking

When a child is choking

If the child is older than 1 year, use abdominal thrusts only (see page 193). If the child is under 1 year, sit down and hold the child facedown on your forearm, which should be resting on your thigh. The infant's head is slightly lower than the chest.

Gently but firmly thump between the shoulder blades with the heel of your hand five times. The combination of gravity and force should release the object that's blocking the airway.

If the blockage isn't released, hold the infant on your forearm, face up with the head lower than the trunk. Place two fingers on the breastbone and give five quick chest compressions.

Repeat the back blows and chest thrusts if breathing doesn't resume. Call for emergency help. If you open the airway but there's no breathing, begin cardiopulmonary resuscitation (CPR) for infants (see page 192).

When a person is unconscious

1. Lower the person on his or her back to the floor, if he or she isn't already lying down.
2. Try to clear the airway. If there is visible blockage in the throat, reach a finger into the mouth and sweep out the cause of the blockage. Be careful not to push the object deeper into the airway.

3. Begin CPR if the object remains lodged and the person doesn't respond to the above measures. Chest compressions used in CPR could help to dislodge the object. Remember to recheck the mouth periodically.

When you're alone

If you're alone and choking, you're not able to deliver back blows to yourself. However, you can perform abdominal thrusts to dislodge the blockage.
1. Make a fist and place it above your navel, with the thumb side toward your abdomen.
2. Grasp your fist with the other hand and bend over a hard surface — a chair or counter top will do.
3. Shove your fist inward and upward. Continue to do so until the object dislodges.

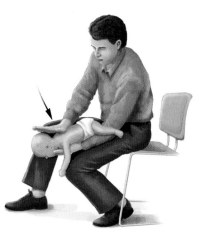

A gentle slap on the back can help clear the airway of a choking infant.

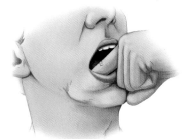

A finger sweep is the simplest way to clear an obstruction from the throat.

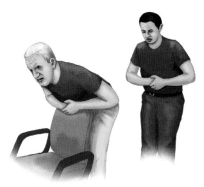

If help is unavailable, you can perform the Heimlich maneuver on yourself.

Fracture

A bone fracture usually occurs as a result of a fall, blow or other traumatic event. If you suspect a fracture, protect the injury from further damage. Don't try to re-align the injured bone. Instead, try to immobilize it in a stabile position — including any joint above and below the injury. A firm pillow or other firm item may help you.

A fracture requires medical attention. If a broken bone is the result of major trauma, call 911 or your local emergency number.

Signs and symptoms

Signs and symptoms of a fracture may include:

- Swelling or bruising over a bone
- Limb deformity
- Sharp pain that intensifies when the affected area is moved or pressure is put on it
- Loss of function in injured area
- Broken bone that has poked through the skin

If bleeding occurs with the broken bone, apply pressure to stop the bleeding. If possible, elevate the wound to lessen blood flow. Maintain pressure on the wound for at least 15 minutes. If bleeding continues, reapply pressure until it stops.

If you've been trained in the procedure and professional help isn't available, you may use a simple splint to immobilize a fractured area. A sling may help immobilize a fractured arm. An open fracture can get infected, so cover the wound with sterile gauze before applying a splint.

If the person appears faint or pale, or is breathing in a shallow, rapid fashion, treat the person for shock (see page 200). Lay the person down, elevate the legs and cover him or her with a blanket to keep warm. Lay the person on the uninjured side if vomiting occurs.

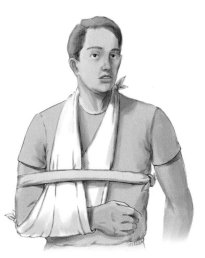

A simple sling can effectively immobilize an injured elbow.

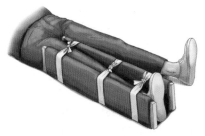

A splint can be made of wood, metal or any rigid material. Pad the splint with gauze or cloth, then fasten the splint to the limb with gauze or strips of cloth, tape or other material.

Heart attack

Some heart attacks occur suddenly, but most start slowly, with mild pain or discomfort. The symptoms may come and go, over minutes or over hours.

If you suspect you're having a heart attack, call for emergency help immediately. Most people wait several hours before seeking assistance — either because they don't recognize the signs and symptoms or because they deny something could be wrong.

Each year, more than a million Americans have a heart attack — and many die because of delayed treatment. Among those who survive, most permanent damage to the heart happens in the first few hours after onset.

Minutes matter

A heart attack occurs when an artery that supplies oxygen to your heart muscle becomes blocked. Arterial blockage is often caused by a buildup of fatty deposits called plaques. Without oxygen, heart cells are destroyed, causing pain or pressure. With each passing minute, more of the heart muscle is deprived of oxygen and deteriorates or dies.

Signs and symptoms

About half the people who have heart attacks experience warning signs hours, days or even weeks in advance. Not all of the signs and symptoms listed here will occur,

but the more of them you have, the more likely it's a heart attack.
- Pain, pressure, tightness, squeezing or burning in the chest lasting more than a few minutes (the sensation may come and go, triggered by exertion and relieved by rest)
- Pain in one or both arms, neck or jaw, or between the shoulder blades (with or without chest pain)*
- Shortness of breath (with or without chest pain)*†
- Stomach pain or discomfort*
- Nausea or vomiting*
- Rapid, fluttering or pounding heartbeats
- Lightheadedness or dizziness
- Sweating
- Unusual fatigue for no apparent reason
- Anxiety or sense of doom

Signs and symptoms of heart attack vary widely and may differ between sexes. Some people, especially those with diabetes, have "silent" heart attacks — mild symptoms or none at all.

Get help fast

Don't wait if you suspect a heart attack. Immediately call 911 or a local emergency number. Paramedics can treat you on the way to the hospital. If you can't access an emergency number, have someone drive you to the nearest hospital. Driving yourself can put others at risk.

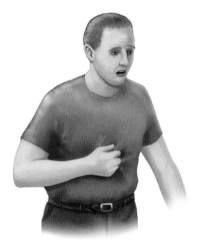

The symptoms of a heart attack vary, but you may experience pain, pressure or a squeezing sensation in your chest along with sweating and shortness of breath.

* These symptoms are slightly more common in women than in men. Most women have some form of chest discomfort with a heart attack, but it might not be the main symptom.
† Shortness of breath without chest pain is a more common symptom of heart attack in people over age 65 and in people with diabetes.

Heart attack

While waiting for help

- Chew aspirin, if recommended — either one regular-strength (325 mg) tablet or four baby (81 mg each) tablets. This may help reduce the damage to your heart by making your blood less likely to clot. Chew even if you're on daily aspirin therapy because chewing (vs swallowing) speeds absorption. Don't follow this step if you're allergic to aspirin, or you have bleeding problems, or your doctor previously told you not to take aspirin.
- Take nitroglycerin, if prescribed. Using this medication according to instructions can temporarily open your blood vessels and improve blood flow to your heart. Never take anyone else's nitroglycerin medication.

When providing assistance

If you're helping someone while waiting for paramedics to arrive:

- Have the person chew aspirin (see bullet point above).
- If the person becomes unconscious, begin cardiopulmonary resuscitation, or CPR (see pages 189-192). If you're not fully trained in the procedure, you can do "hands-only" CPR. Most 911 dispatchers can instruct you in CPR until help arrives.
- In the initial minutes, a heart attack can trigger ventricular fibrillation, a condition in which the heart quivers uselessly. Without immediate attention, ventricular fibrillation leads to sudden death. The timely use of an automatic external defibrillator (AED) — which helps shock the heart back into a normal rhythm — can provide emergency assistance before the person having a heart attack reaches a hospital. For more on AEDs see page 189.

Prevention

A healthy lifestyle can help you prevent a heart attack by controlling risk factors that contribute to the narrowing of the arteries that supply blood to your heart. Aspects of a healthy lifestyle include:

- Not smoking and avoiding secondhand smoke
- Staying physically active
- Eating a heart-healthy diet
- Maintaining a healthy weight
- Managing stress
- Getting regular medical checkups
- Controlling blood pressure and cholesterol

You may also be advised to take a daily aspirin.

Poisoning

Any substance swallowed, inhaled, injected or absorbed by the body that interferes with the body's normal function can be, by definition, a poison.

Pesticides and household cleaning supplies are well-known poisons, but there are many other less familiar substances that may poison you. In fact, almost any nonfood substance is poisonous if taken in large enough doses.

Signs and symptoms

Poisoning can be a serious medical emergency. Look for these warning signs if you suspect poisoning:

- Unconsciousness
- Burns or redness around the mouth and lips
- Breath that smells like chemicals or gasoline
- Vomiting, difficulty breathing, drowsiness or confusion
- Uncontrollable restlessness or agitation or having seizures
- Burns, stains and odors on the person, on clothing, or on the furniture, rugs or other objects in the surrounding area
- Empty medication bottles or scattered pills

What you can do

If someone is unconscious and you think that he or she has ingested poison, call immediately for emergency medical help.

If the person is awake and alert, take the following steps:

- If the person has been exposed to poisonous fumes, such as carbon monoxide, get him or her into fresh air immediately. Avoid breathing in the fumes yourself.
- Call the poison control center at 800-222-1222. In some communities, a local number may be listed with other emergency numbers in the front of the telephone book.
- When you call for emergency assistance, have the following information ready, if possible:
  - The poisoned person's condition, age and weight
  - The ingredients listed on the product container, if available
  - The approximate time that the poisoning took place
  - Your name, phone number and location
- Follow the directions provided by the poison control center for treatment.
- Don't allow the person to eat or drink anything unless instructed to do so. Don't administer ipecac syrup to induce vomiting.
- Monitor vital signs and changes in the poisoned person. If breathing stops, begin cardiopulmonary resuscitation, or CPR (see pages 189-192). Watch for symptoms of shock (see page 201).
- If poison has spilled on the person's clothing, skin or eyes, remove the clothing, using gloves. Rinse the skin in a shower or flush the eyes with water (see page 136).
- Take the poison container or packaging with you to the hospital, if available.

Caution with kids

Children under age 5 are often exposed to poisons because they're curious and they're unaware of the danger. If infants and toddlers live in or visit your home:

- Keep potential poisons in cabinets located out of reach, or with safety locks.
- Keep the poison control phone number handy: 800-222-1222.

Seizure

A seizure occurs when sudden, abnormal brain cell activity affects the way your brain coordinates information. A seizure can produce temporary confusion, uncontrollable jerking movements, and complete loss of consciousness. Some seizures are more severe than others. However, all seizures should be treated as medical emergencies.

Seizures caused by epilepsy are perhaps the best known kind, but several other disorders can produce them, including head injury, heart rhythm problem and sudden withdrawal from medications. In rare cases, a seizure may be the first sign of a brain tumor.

People with diabetes may experience insulin shock, which may produce a form of seizure that is treated differently than other seizures.

What you can do
When you're with a person who is having a seizure:
1. Keep the person from injuring himself or herself. If vomiting occurs, turn the person's head so that the vomit is expelled and isn't breathed in. Clear the area around the person of furniture or other objects to reduce his or her risk of injury during uncontrolled body movements. Although the person may briefly stop breathing, breathing almost invariably returns without need for cardiopulmonary resuscitation (CPR).
2. After the seizure is over, position the person on his or her side to allow for normal breathing and for vomit, blood and other fluids to drain from the mouth. Blood may be present if he or she bit the tongue or cheek. The person may be confused for awhile. Monitor changes until there's a complete return of mental function.
3. Seek emergency assistance during a seizure if necessary. Call for immediate help if:
   - The person has never had a seizure before
   - The episode lasts more than a few minutes
   - The seizure reoccurs
4. Treat any bumps, bruises or cuts that may have occurred during the seizure, particularly if there was a fall.

Insulin shock
A person with diabetes may experience a seizure if his or her blood sugar drops too low. This form of seizure is called insulin shock or insulin reaction.

If you're with someone experiencing insulin shock, give the person some kind of carbohydrate or sugar, if possible. Fruit juices, candy or sugar-containing soft drinks are effective.

If the person is unable to swallow, try putting a teaspoon of syrup in his or her cheek every few minutes. If the person is unconscious, you may need to administer a glucagon injection under the skin using a special injector. If recovery isn't prompt, seek immediate medical attention.

Seizure in a child
Sometimes, a high fever in an infant or child can cause what's known as a febrile seizure. If this situation occurs, stay calm and follow these steps:
- Place your child on his or her side, at a location where there's no chance of falling
- Stay close to watch and comfort your child
- Remove any hard or sharp objects near your child
- Loosen any tight or restrictive clothing
- Don't restrain your child or interfere with your child's movements
- Don't attempt to put anything in your child's mouth

A first-time seizure should be evaluated by your doctor as soon as possible, even if it lasts only a few seconds. If the seizure lasts longer than 5 minutes or is accompanied by vomiting, stiff neck, breathing difficulty or extreme sleepiness, seek emergency medical attention.

Shock

Shock may result from trauma, heatstroke, allergic reaction, severe infection, poisoning, dehydration or other causes. When you're in shock, there's a reduction of blood flow throughout your body — a change that lowers your blood pressure and reduces the supply of oxygen to organs and other vital tissues. Shock can come on suddenly or it can have a delayed onset. The condition can be life threatening.

Signs and symptoms

Various signs and symptoms may appear when a person is in shock:

- Change in skin color and feel. The skin may look pale or gray, and feel cool and clammy.
- The pulse may be weak and rapid as blood pressure drops. Breathing may be slow and shallow, or rapid and deep (hyperventilation).
- The eyes lack luster and seem to stare. Sometimes the pupils are dilated.
- The person may become unconscious. If not, the person may feel faint, dizzy or weak, or become confused, or extremely anxious or agitated.

What you can do

If you suspect that a person is going into shock, even if there were no warning signs immediately after an injury, call 911 or a local emergency number for medical help. There may be a delayed reaction. While waiting for emergency responders to arrive:

1. Lay the person down on his or her back with a cushion or other prop elevating the feet higher than the head. If raising the legs will cause pain or further injury, keep the body flat. Keep movement to a minimum.

2. Keep the person warm and comfortable. Loosen tight collars, belts and clothing that constricts. Cover the person with a blanket. If the ground or floor is cold, place a blanket underneath. If it's hot, place the person in the shade or a cool area, if possible. Even if the person complains of thirst, give nothing by their mouth.

3. Watch for warning signs of shock. Check for breathing and a pulse. If the signs are absent, begin cardiopulmonary resuscitation, or CPR (see pages 189-192).

4. If the person vomits or bleeds from the mouth, turn the person on his or her side to prevent choking.

5. Start treatment for bleeding or injuries, such as broken bones, if you can. Immobilize a fracture or take other first-aid steps.

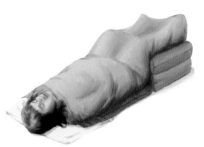

With the onset of shock, keep the person warm, and elevate legs and feet above the level of the heart in order to maximize the flow of blood to the head.

Stroke

In the United States, stroke is the third-leading cause of death and the No. 1 cause of adult disability. Only heart disease and cancer cause more deaths each year.

A stroke is a "brain attack" — it happens when blood supply to a part of your brain is interrupted or severely reduced. Within a few minutes of being deprived of oxygen and nutrients, brain cells in that area begin dying.

A stroke is a medical emergency, and prompt treatment is crucial. Almost 2 million brain cells die each minute during a typical stroke. As the American Heart Association notes, "Time lost is brain lost."

Signs and symptoms

To help you recognize a stroke, many major health organizations urge you to remember the five signs and symptoms with this slogan: "Give me five: Walk, talk, reach, see, feel."

- *Walk.* Is balance suddenly a problem?
- *Talk.* Is speech suddenly slurred or the face droopy?
- *Reach.* Has one side of the body suddenly become weak or numb?
- *See.* Is vision suddenly all or partially lost?
- *Feel.* Is a headache sudden and severe?

Signs and symptoms may last only minutes, or they may persist for hours. Warning signs should be taken very seriously.

What you can do

If you suspect that you're experiencing warning signs of stroke, call 911 or a local emergency number immediately.

If you're calling for another person, monitor him or her closely while waiting for the emergency responders. If needed, be ready to take these actions:

- If breathing stops, begin cardiopulmonary resuscitation, or CPR (see pages 189-192). Minor breathing difficulty may be relieved simply by resting the person's head and shoulders on a pillow.
- If vomiting occurs, turn the person's head to the side so that the vomit can drain out of the mouth instead of being breathed into the lungs. Don't allow the person to eat or drink anything.
- If paralysis occurs, protect the paralyzed limbs from injury that might occur when the person moves about or is transported.

What's a TIA?

A transient ischemic attack (TIA), has the similar signs and symptoms of a stroke but usually lasts only a few minutes and causes no permanent damage. Often called a ministroke, a TIA can serve as a warning — each TIA attack increases your risk of stroke.

If you think you've had a TIA, call your doctor immediately.

After a TIA, your risk of a stroke increases immediately and may be as high as 10 to 20 percent over the next three months. The doctor may identify potentially treatable conditions that may help you prevent a future stroke — for example, high blood pressure, high cholesterol or diabetes. The doctor also may prescribe medication to prevent blood clots or a procedure to remove the build-up of plaques in your arteries.

Index

MAYO CLINIC *BOOK OF ALTERNATIVE MEDICINE*

Medical Editor Brent Bauer, M.D.
Senior Director, Content Nicole Spelhaug
Senior Product Manager, Books and Newsletters Christopher Frye
Managing Editor Karen Wallevand
Contributing Editors Richard Dietman, Kevin Kaufman
Executive Editor, Design Development Daniel Brevick
Art Directors Stewart Jay Koski, Paul Krause
Photographers Scott Dulla, Joseph Kane, Richard Madsen, Matthew C. Meyer
Editorial Research Librarians Anthony Cook, Amanda Golden
Proofreaders Miranda Attlesey, Donna Hanson
Indexer Steve Rath
Administrative Assistants Beverly Steele, Terri Zanto Strausbauch

MAYO CLINIC *BOOK OF HOME REMEDIES*

Medical Editors Philip Hagen, M.D., Martha Millman, M.D.
Senior Director, Content Nicole Spelhaug
Senior Product Manager, Books and Newsletters Christopher Frye
Managing Editor Kevin Kaufman
Contributing Editor Karen Wallevand
Art Directors Stewart Jay Koski, Rick Resnick
Editorial Research Librarians Anthony Cook, Amanda Golden
Proofreaders Miranda Attlesey, Donna Hanson
Indexer Steve Rath
Administrative Assistants Beverly Steele, Terri Zanto Strausbauch

TIME HOME ENTERTAINMENT

Publisher Jim Childs
Vice President, Business Development & Strategy Steven Sandonato
Executive Director, Marketing Services Carol Pittard
Director, Retail & Special Sales Tom Mifsud
Executive Publishing Director Joy Butts,
Editorial Director Stephen Koepp
Editorial Operations Director Michael Q. Bullerdick
Director, Bookazine Development & Marketing Laura Adam
Finance Director Glenn Buonocore
Associate Publishing Director Megan Pearlman
Assistant General Counsel Helen Wan
Assistant Director Special Sales Ilene Schreider,
Senior Book Production Manager Susan Chodakiewicz
Design & Prepress Manager Anne-Michelle Gallero
Brand Manager, Product Marketing Nina Fleishman
Associate Prepress Manager Alex Voznesenskiy
Special thanks to Christine Austin, Jeremy Biloon, Rose Cirrincione, Lauren Hall Clark, Jacqueline Fitzgerald, Christine Font, Jenna Goldberg, Hillary Hirsch, Suzanne Janso, David Kahn, Mona Li, Amy Mangus, Robert Marasco, Kimberly Marshall, Amy Migliaccio, Nina Mistry, Dave Rozzelle, Ricardo Santiago, Adriana Tierno, Vanessa Wu

Published by Time Home Entertainment Inc.
Time Home Entertainment Inc.
135 W. 50th St.
New York, NY 10020

ISBN 10: 0848741226
ISBN 13: 9780848741228

Book of Alternative Medicine
First edition: January 2007
Second edition: April 2010

Book of Home Remedies
First edition: October 2010

1 2 3 4 5 6 7 8 9 10

We welcome your comments and suggestions on Mayo Clinic Book of Alternative Medicine & Home Remedies. Please write to us at Time Home Entertainment Inc. Books, Attention: Book Editors, P.O. Box 11016, Des Moines, IA 50336-1016. If you would like to order more copies of this book or any of our hardcover Collector's Edition books, please call 800-327-6388 (Monday through Friday, 7 a.m. to 8 p.m., or Saturday, 7 a.m. to 6 p.m. Central time).

For bulk sales to employers, member groups and health-related companies, contact Mayo Clinic Health Management Resources, 200 First St. SW, Rochester, MN 55905, or send an email to SpecialSalesMayoBooks@Mayo.edu.

Mayo Clinic Book of Alternative Medicine & Home Remedies is intended to supplement the advice of your personal physician, whom you should consult regarding individual medical conditions. MAYO, MAYO CLINIC and the Mayo triple-shield logo are marks of Mayo Foundation for Medical Education and Research.

We do not endorse any company or product.

Photo credits: Stock photography from Artville, BananaStock, Brand X Pictures, Comstock, Corbis, Creatas, Digital Stock Art, Digital Vision, EyeWire, Food Shapes, Image Ideas, Image Source, PhotoAlto, Photodisc, Pixtal, Rubberball and Stockbyte. The individuals pictured are models, and the photos are used for illustrative purposes only. There is no correlation between the individuals portrayed and the conditions or subjects being discussed.

Jacket design by Anne-Michelle Gallero

In this book we discuss a variety of products and practices. Our intent is for this information to serve as discussion points between the reader and his or her doctor. Because we say a therapy may be beneficial or we give it a "green light" does not mean we are endorsing any specific product.